T0226841

Disorders of the Platelets

Editor

A. KONETI RAO

HEMATOLOGY/ONCOLOGY CLINICS OF NORTH AMERICA

www.hemonc.theclinics.com

Consulting Editors
GEORGE P. CANELLOS
H. FRANKLIN BUNN

June 2013 • Volume 27 • Number 3

ELSEVIER

1600 John F. Kennedy Boulevard • Suite 1800 • Philadelphia, Pennsylvania, 19103-2899

http://www.theclinics.com

HEMATOLOGY/ONCOLOGY CLINICS OF NORTH AMERICA Volume 27, Number 3
June 2013 ISSN 0889-8588, ISBN 13: 978-1-4557-7102-8

Editor: Patrick Manley
Developmental Editor: Donald Mumford

Hematology/Oncology Clinics (ISSN 0889-8588) is published bimonthly by Elsevier Inc., 360 Park Avenue South, New York, NY 10010-1710. Months of issue are February, April, June, August, October, and December. Business and Editorial Offices: 1600 John F. Kennedy Blvd., Ste. 1800, Philadelphia, PA 19103—2899. Customer Service Office: 3251 Riverport Lane, Maryland Heights, MO 63043. Periodicals postage paid at New York, NY and at additional mailing offices. Subscription prices are $367.00 per year (domestic individuals), $599.00 per year (domestic institutions), $179.00 per year (domestic students/residents), $417.00 per year (Canadian individuals), $732.00 per year (Canadian institutions) $496.00 per year (international individuals), $732.00 per year (international institutions), and $241.00 per year (international and Canadian students/residents). International air speed delivery is included in all *Clinics* subscription prices. All prices are subject to change without notice. **POSTMASTER:** Send address changes to *Hematology/Oncology Clinics of North America*, Elsevier Health Sciences Division, Subscription Customer Service, 3251 Riverport Lane, Maryland Heights, MO 63043. Customer Service (orders, claims, online, change of address): Elsevier Health Sciences Division, Subscription Customer Service, 3251 Riverport Lane, Maryland Heights, MO 63043. Tel: 1-800-654-2452 (U.S. and Canada); 314-447-8871 (outside U.S. and Canada). Fax: 314-447-8029. E-mail: journalscustomerservice-usa@elsevier.com (for print support); journalsonlinesupport-usa@elsevier.com (for online support).

Reprints. For copies of 100 or more, of articles in this publication, please contact the Commercial Reprints Department, Elsevier Inc., 360 Park Avenue South, New York, New York 10010-1710; Tel.: 212-633-3813, Fax: 212-462-1935, E-mail: reprints@elsevier.com.

Hematology/Oncology Clinics of North America is covered in *MEDLINE/PubMed (Index Medicus)*, *EMBASE/Excerpta Medica*, and *BIOSIS*.

Printed and bound by CPI Group (UK) Ltd, Croydon, CR0 4YY

Transferred to digital print 2012

Contributors

CONSULTING EDITORS

GEORGE P. CANELLOS, MD
William Rosenberg Professor of Medicine, Department of Medical Oncology, Dana-Farber Cancer Institute, Boston, Massachusetts

H. FRANKLIN BUNN, MD
Professor of Medicine, Harvard Medical School, Division of Hematology, Brigham and Women's Hospital, Boston, Massachusetts

EDITOR

A. KONETI RAO, MD, FACP
Sol Sherry Professor of Medicine, Professor of Thrombosis Research and Pharmacology, Chief, Hematology Section, Department of Medicine, Co-Director, Sol Sherry Thrombosis Research Center, Temple University School of Medicine, Philadelphia, Pennsylvania

AUTHORS

VAHID AFSHAR-KHARGHAN, MD
Section of Benign Hematology, M.D. Anderson Cancer Center, Houston, Texas

GOWTHAMI M. AREPALLY, MD
Associate Professor of Medicine, Division of Hematology, Department of Medicine, Duke University Medical Center, Durham, North Carolina

WADIE F. BAHOU, MD
Professor of Medicine/Hematology, Director, Stony Brook Stem Cell Facility Center; Department of Medicine, Health Sciences Center, Stony Brook University, Stony Brook, New York

LAWRENCE F. BRASS, MD, PhD
Professor of Medicine and Pharmacology, Perelman School of Medicine, University of Pennsylvania, Philadelphia, Pennsylvania

BENG H. CHONG, PhD, MBBS, FRACP, FRCPA, FRCP (Glasgow)
Director, Department of Haematology, St George Hospital; Professor of Medicine (Conjoint), Department of Medicine, St George Clinical School, University of New South Wales, Kogarah, New South Wales, Australia

REYHAN DIZ-KÜCÜKKAYA, MD
Istanbul Bilim University Medical Faculty, Division of Hematology, Department of Internal Medicine, Hematology and Oncology Clinic, Avrupa Florence Nightingale Hospital, Sishane, Istanbul, Turkey

PAUL HARRISON, BSc, PhD, FRCPath
School of Immunity and Infection, University of Birmingham Medical School, Birmingham, United Kingdom

WALTER H.A. KAHR, MD, PhD
Division of Haematology/Oncology, Department of Paediatrics and Department of Biochemistry; Program in Cell Biology, Research Institute, The Hospital for Sick Children, University of Toronto, Toronto, Ontario, Canada

LEVON KHACHIGIAN, PhD
Director, Centre for Vascular Research, University of New South Wales, Kensington, Sydney, New South Wales, Australia

GAURAV KISTANGARI, MD
Staff, Department of Hospital Medicine, Cleveland Clinic, Cleveland, Ohio

RITEN KUMAR, MD, MSc
Division of Haematology/Oncology, Department of Paediatrics, The Hospital for Sick Children, University of Toronto, Toronto, Ontario, Canada

GRACE M. LEE, MD
Hematology/Oncology Fellow, Division of Hematology, Department of Medicine, Duke University Medical Center, Durham, North Carolina

JOSÉ A. LÓPEZ, MD
Chief Scientific Officer, Puget Sound Blood Cancer; Division of Hematology, University of Washington Medical Center; Department of Biochemistry, University of Washington, Seattle, Washington

MARIE LORDKIPANIDZÉ, BPharm, PhD
Centre for Cardiovascular Sciences, Institute of Biomedical Research, College of Medical and Dental Sciences, University of Birmingham, Edgbaston, Birmingham, United Kingdom

KEITH R. McCRAE, MD
Professor of Molecular Medicine, Department of Cellular and Molecular Medicine, Taussig Cancer Institute, Cleveland Clinic, Cleveland, Ohio

JOSE PERDOMO, PhD
Department of Medicine, St George Clinical School, University of New South Wales, Kogarah; Center for Vascular Research, University of New South Wales, Kensington, Sydney, New South Wales, Australia

A. KONETI RAO, MD, FACP
Sol Sherry Professor of Medicine, Professor of Thrombosis Research and Pharmacology, Chief, Hematology Section, Department of Medicine, Co-Director, Sol Sherry Thrombosis Research Center, Temple University School of Medicine, Philadelphia, Pennsylvania

TIMOTHY J. STALKER, PhD
Research Assistant Professor, Department of Medicine, Perelman School of Medicine, University of Pennsylvania, Philadelphia, Pennsylvania

PERUMAL THIAGARAJAN, MD
Departments of Pathology and Medicine, Michael E. DeBakey Veterans Affairs Medical Center, Baylor College of Medicine, Houston, Texas

MAURIZIO TOMAIUOLO, PhD
Postdoctoral Fellow, Department of Medicine, Perelman School of Medicine, University of Pennsylvania, Philadelphia, Pennsylvania

HAN-MOU TSAI, MD
iMAH Hematology Associates, New Hyde Park, New York

PHILIP YOUNG-ILL CHOI, MBBS
Department of Medicine, St George Clinical School, University of New South Wales, Kogarah; Center for Vascular Research, University of New South Wales, Kensington, Sydney, New South Wales, Australia

Contents

> Once released into the circulation by megakaryocytes, circulating platelets can undergo rapid activation at sites of vascular injury and resist unwarranted activation, which can lead to heart attacks and strokes. Historically, the signaling mechanisms underlying the regulation of platelet activation have been approached as a collection of individual pathways unique to agonist. This review takes a different approach, casting platelet activation as the product of a signaling network, in which activating and restraining mechanisms interact in a flexible network that regulates platelet adhesiveness, cohesion between platelets, granule secretion, and the formation of a stable hemostatic thrombus.

> Platelet function tests have been traditionally used to aid in the diagnosis and management of patients with bleeding problems. Given the role of platelets in atherothrombosis, several dedicated platelet function instruments are now available that are simple to use and can be used as point-of-care assays. These can provide rapid assessment of platelet function within whole blood without the requirement of sample processing. Some tests can be used to monitor antiplatelet therapy and assess risk of bleeding and thrombosis, although current guidelines advise against this. This article discusses the potential utility of tests/instruments that are available.

> Technological advances in protein and genetic analysis have altered the means by which platelet disorders can be characterized and studied in health and disease. When integrated into a single analytical framework, these collective technologies are referred to as systems biology, a unified approach that links platelet function with genomic/proteomic studies to provide insight into the role of platelets in broad human disorders such as cardiovascular and cerebrovascular disease. This article reviews the historical progression of these applied technologies to analyze platelet function, and demonstrates how these approaches can be systematically developed to provide new insights into platelet biomarker discovery.

of HIT. Once HIT is recognized, an alternative anticoagulant should be initiated to prevent further complications.

Since the last review in 2007 of thrombotic thrombocytopenic purpura (TTP) and microangiopathic hemolytic anemia in the *Clinics*, further understanding of the nature of TTP and atypical hemolytic uremic syndrome (aHUS) has led to increasing use of rituximab in the treatment of TTP and the approval in 2011 of eculizumab for the treatment of aHUS. With this new armamentarium, distinction of aHUS from TTP has become more critical than ever. This article updates the new knowledge, highlights the difference between aHUS and TTP, and presents a scheme for their diagnosis and management.

Inherited disorders of platelet function are characterized by highly variable mucocutaneous bleeding manifestations. The platelet dysfunction arises by diverse mechanisms, including abnormalities in platelet membrane glycoproteins, granules and their contents, platelet signaling and secretion mechanisms: thromboxane production pathways and in platelet procoagulant activities. Platelet aggregation and secretion studies using platelet-rich plasma currently form the primary basis for the diagnosis of an inherited platelet dysfunction. In most such patients, the molecular and genetic mechanisms are unknown. Management of these patients needs to be individualized; therapeutic options include platelet transfusions, 1-desamino-8D-arginine vasopressin (DDAVP), recombinant factor VIIa, and antifibrinolytic agents.

Platelet membrane glycoproteins play a key role in hemostasis and thrombosis. Although disorders of platelet membrane glycoproteins are rare, their effects on the lives of those affected are very important. Severe deficiencies manifest themselves early during childhood with mucocutaneous bleeding. Mild deficiencies may not be diagnosed until adulthood or until the hemostatic system is stressed by surgery or trauma. The diagnosis of these disorders requires detailed laboratory investigation. Management of bleeding in patients with inherited platelet disorders requires both preventive measures and the treatment of individual bleeding episodes according to severity. The study of platelet membrane disorders also has yielded important insights into the functions of affected proteins, information that has produced some of the most successful antithrombotic drugs currently in use.

Platelet transfusion therapy has become an integral part of the treatment
of patients with hematological and solid tumor malignancy receiving chemotherapy. Since its introduction almost 60 years ago, several advances
and refinements have been introduced in the collection, storage, and administration to improve the safety and efficacy of platelet transfusion. This
review summarizes the current practice and clinical approach to patients
with thrombocytopenia. Existing evidence-based guidelines for appropriate platelet transfusion is reviewed.

HEMATOLOGY/ONCOLOGY CLINICS OF NORTH AMERICA

FORTHCOMING ISSUES

August 2013
Breast Cancer
Harold J. Burstein, MD, *Editor*

October 2013
Sarcoma
Andrew Wagner, MD, *Editor*

December 2013
Prostate Cancer
Christopher Sweeney, MD, *Editor*

RECENT ISSUES

April 2013
Chronic Lymphocytic Leukemia
Jennifer R. Brown, MD, *Editor*

February 2013
Neutropenia
Christoph Klein, MD, *Editor*

December 2012
Rare Cancers
Guy Eslick, MD, *Editor*

DOWNLOAD
Free App!

Review Articles
THE CLINICS

NOW AVAILABLE FOR YOUR iPhone and iPad

Preface

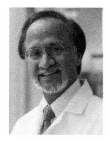

A. Koneti Rao, MD
Editor

In 1990, I had the opportunity to serve as a guest editor along with Dr Robert Colman of an issue of the *Hematology/Oncology Clinics of North America* on "Platelets in Health and Disease." It is in this continuum that I am delighted to organize the present issue focusing on platelets and its disorders. Reflecting back over the last 2 decades, there have been tremendous advances in our understanding of platelet function and pathology—new proteins and pathways have been defined, novel methods to assess platelet function has developed, and important breakthroughs have occurred into the mechanisms and management of well-recognized platelets disorders. A small part these exciting advances in the platelet field is captured in this issue.

Platelets, the youngest members of the hematologic cell community, have gone from being "dust" on a peripheral smear to major players in hemostasis, thrombosis, inflammation, and atherosclerosis—all in a span of little over a century. The rapid increase in our understanding of the basic biology of the megakaryocyte and platelets has been stupendous and gallops forward with ever-increasing new roles of platelets in diverse clinically relevant processes. This now encompasses cancer metastasis and the elimination of bacteria from the blood, in addition to atherosclerosis and inflammation. Platelets have gone from cells once considered incapable of protein synthesis to those that possess the spliceosome and are capable of activation-driven synthesis of biologically important proteins as well as creating progeny under certain conditions—all remarkable for anucleate fragments. This has led to a better understanding of disease-causing alterations in platelet number and function.

This issue of the *Hematology/Oncology Clinics of North America* begins with a review of the normal and complex mechanisms of platelet activation and inhibition. It lays foundation for the subsequent articles that delve into the intricacies of the role of platelets in disease. The next 2 articles focus on the approaches to evaluate platelet function and biology. The first article provides an overview of the various approaches available from a clinical perspective and their role. The second article expands into the application of state-of-the-art genomics and proteomics—to understand basic biology of platelets and the aberrations in platelet disorders.

Hematol Oncol Clin N Am 27 (2013) xiii–xiv
http://dx.doi.org/10.1016/j.hoc.2013.04.001
0889-8588/13/$ – see front matter © 2013 Published by Elsevier Inc.

hemonc.theclinics.com

A series of 5 articles focus on the current understanding of clinical aspects, molecular basis, pathogenesis, and management of patients with thrombocytopenia of diverse origin. One review brings us up to date on the advances in our understanding of congenital thrombocytopenias, an area that has yielded major insights recently. The second article presents the current concepts of immune thrombocytopenias, both primary and secondary. Another review addresses the important topic of drug-induced thrombocytopenias; this is followed by a review on heparin-induced thrombocytopenia, an entity that continues to remain a paradox and is associated with substantial morbidity. Thrombotic thrombocytopenic purpura with all its ramifications is the subject of a separate review that also incorporates the newer insights into the burgeoning role of complement abnormalities in the hemolytic uremic syndrome.

Some of the seminal concepts in platelet physiology have had their roots in specific inherited disorders of platelet function. The last 2 decades have seen important advances in understanding the molecular basis of some of them. Two reviews tackle this area. One article provides an overview of the inherited disorders of platelet function and describes those with defects in platelet granules, secretion, and signal transduction. The second article provides a complementary review of disorders that arise from abnormalities in membrane glycoproteins. From a therapeutic perspective, platelet transfusion therapy remains the bedrock of management of platelet bleeding disorders. In the concluding article of this volume, the current concepts in the important area of platelet transfusion therapy are described.

Overall, the reviews in this issue are presented with the clinician in mind, and this is reflected in the contributions from each of the authors. I am thankful to them for this, and for bringing out the remarkable intricacies of these anucleate fragments of the multinucleated megakaryocyte. I thank also the editors at Elsevier for pulling all of this together.

A. Koneti Rao, MD
Hematology Section, Department of Medicine
Sol Sherry Thrombosis Research Center
Temple University School of Medicine
Philadelphia, PA 19140, USA

E-mail address:
koneti@temple.edu

Harnessing the Platelet Signaling Network to Produce an Optimal Hemostatic Response

Lawrence F. Brass, MD, PhD[a],*, Maurizio Tomaiuolo, PhD[b],
Timothy J. Stalker, PhD[c]

KEYWORDS

- Platelets • Hemostasis • Vascular injury • Signal transduction • Networks
- G protein–coupled receptors • G proteins • Integrins

KEY POINTS

- Circulating platelets possess the ability to undergo rapid activation at sites of vascular injury and resist unwarranted activation, which can lead to heart attacks and strokes.
- The signaling mechanisms underlying the regulation of platelet activation have been approached as a collection of individual pathways unique to agonist.
- This review takes a different approach, casting platelet activation as the product of a signaling network, in which activating and restraining mechanisms interact in a flexible network that regulates platelet adhesiveness, cohesion between platelets, granule secretion, and the formation of a stable hemostatic thrombus.

INTRODUCTION: THE CONTRIBUTION OF PLATELETS TO THE HEMOSTATIC RESPONSE

Platelets have evolved to be the primary cellular component of the hemostatic response to injury, replacing the nucleated thrombocytes found in most nonmammalian species. After maturing from megakaryocyte-derived proplatelets, platelets circulate in an essentially quiescent state for 10 days in humans, and about half of that in mice. During that time, the quiescent state is maintained by extrinsic regulators such as nitrogen monoxide (NO) and prostacyclin (PGI_2) by the presence of healthy endothelium, which separates platelets from activators within the vessel wall; and, perhaps most critically, by the absence of physiologic platelet activators such as

Disclosure: The authors have no conflicts of interest to disclose.
[a] Department of Medicine, University of Pennsylvania Perelman School of Medicine, 915 BRB-II, 421 Curie Boulevard, Philadelphia, PA 19104, USA; [b] Department of Medicine, University of Pennsylvania Perelman School of Medicine, 922 BRB-II, 421 Curie Boulevard, Philadelphia, PA 19104, USA; [c] Department of Medicine, University of Pennsylvania Perelman School of Medicine, 910 BRB-II, 421 Curie Boulevard, Philadelphia, PA 19104, USA
* Corresponding author.
E-mail address: brass@mail.med.upenn.edu

Hematol Oncol Clin N Am 27 (2013) 381–409
http://dx.doi.org/10.1016/j.hoc.2013.02.002
0889-8588/13/$ – see front matter © 2013 Elsevier Inc. All rights reserved.

collagen, thrombin, and adenosine diphosphate (ADP). Hemostatic thrombi form when the vessel wall has been breached. Pathologic thrombi form in response to vessel wall disease in the arterial system, stasis and inflammation in the venous system, and the inappropriate presence of platelet activators anywhere in the vascular system. Even in a healthy vascular system, differences in local conditions within arteries and veins affect platelet activation. Because pressures and flow rates are higher, hemostasis in the arterial system requires activated platelets to form the initial obstacle to blood loss, accelerate the production of thrombin, and provide a stable base and protected environment in which fibrin can accumulate. However, platelet activation is not limited to the arterial system; it occurs in the venous system and in capillaries as well and contributes to the hemostatic response in those locations. Patients with marked thrombocytopenia develop petechiae because of small leaks in the microcirculation that are otherwise prevented by platelets.

The primary goal of the hemostatic response is to limit blood loss when penetrating injuries occur. Many of the attributes of platelets that allow them to sense and respond rapidly to vascular injury are the same attributes that contribute to heart attacks and strokes when misdirected. The hemostatic response is sometimes modeled as occurring in 3 overlapping phases: initiation, extension, and stabilization. Initiation occurs when moving platelets become tethered to von Willebrand factor (VWF)/collagen complexes within the injured vessel wall and remain in place long enough to become activated by collagen. Extension occurs when additional platelets adhere to the initial monolayer, extending it in the lateral and luminal directions. Locally generated thrombin plus ADP and thromboxane A_2 (TXA$_2$) released by platelets play an important role in this step, activating platelets via G protein–coupled receptors (GPCRs). Subsequent intracellular signaling activates the integrin $\alpha_{IIb}\beta_3$ on the platelet surface. Activated platelets stick to each other via bridges formed by the binding of fibrinogen, fibrin or VWF to activated $\alpha_{IIb}\beta_3$. Stabilization refers to the events that help to consolidate the platelet plug and prevent premature disaggregation, in part by amplifying signaling within the platelet. The net result of these 3 phases is a hemostatic plug comprising activated platelets and cross-linked fibrin, a structure stable enough to withstand the forces generated by flowing blood in the arterial circulation.

This model for thinking about the hemostatic response can be helpful, because it emphasizes the initial role of collagen and VWF in anchoring platelets to a site of injury and the subsequent roles of thrombin, ADP, and TxA$_2$. Platelets require some form of initial tethering to remain in place long enough to become fully activated. Moving platelets are pushed to the periphery of the blood stream by the flow properties of blood and the presence of red cells at the center of the blood stream. In the first seconds after injury, plasma VWF joins VWF already present in the vascular wall in becoming anchored to collagen. Flow forces working on the anchored VWF expose cryptic binding sites for platelet glycoprotein (GP) Ibα, allowing platelets to become tethered without requiring prior activation. In the absence of functional VWF, platelets can still be activated by collagen, thrombin, ADP, and TxA$_2$, but in vivo, they are unable to remain at the site of injury long enough for the initial layers of the hemostatic thrombus to form. Hence, VWF deficiency or dysfunction results in a bleeding disorder, as do disorders affecting secretion. As platelet activation progresses, additional VWF is released locally from platelet storage granules.[1]

However, although useful in some respects, a limitation of thinking about platelet activation as successive waves of initiation, extension, and stabilization is that it does not completely describe what has been observed at sites of injury. Recent studies of platelet activation after penetrating injuries in the microcirculation show that platelet activation is not uniform throughout the hemostatic mass.[2–8] Instead of a homogeneous mass, there is a core of fully activated, stably adherent platelets overlaid by a shell of less-activated, mostly unstable platelets (**Fig. 1**). As the response to injury continues, the shell persists even as the stable core expands, suggesting that not all of the platelets associated with the hemostatic response become fully activated. Rather than a homogeneous mass in which all platelets are activated to the same extent and fibrin is dispersed throughout the mass, the hemostatic thrombus retains regional heterogeneity and a hierarchical structure. Fibrin is found primarily in the parts of the thrombus core that are closest to the site of injury. At present, observations such as these are still largely limited to flow chambers and the cremasteric and mesenteric microcirculations in rodent models, but they raise several questions. Do the same events occur when penetrating injuries occur in larger vessels? What normally limits the growth of the hemostatic response and prevents inappropriate vascular occlusion? What goes wrong in pathologic settings such as dyslipidemia or plaque rupture? How is the hemostatic response regulated to produce an optimal outcome?

THE PLATELET SIGNALING NETWORK: THE FOREST AND THE TREES

The molecular mechanisms that underlie the hemostatic response have been the subject of intense scrutiny for many years, reflecting the relevance of this process to clinical medicine and the lives of humans. To the extent that space allows, the remainder of this article summarizes what has been learned. However, before diving into the trees, it is worth considering the forest. Largely for experimental reasons, it has generally been more practical to tease apart platelet activation 1 molecule at a time. Studies with genetically modified mice have helped this process considerably, even although mouse platelets turn out to be different from human platelets in several critical ways. The results make it possible to draw models such as the one in **Fig. 2**, which

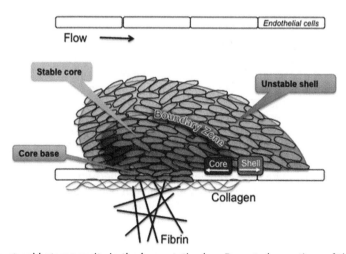

Fig. 1. Structural heterogeneity in the hemostatic plug. Recent observations of the platelet response to acute vascular injury in vivo show that there are distinct regions within the hemostatic thrombus where platelets are either more or less activated and where fibrin tends to accumulate. A stable core of closely packed, fully activated platelets is overlaid by an outer shell of less-stable, less-activated platelets, with a boundary zone in between. Fibrin is found within the thrombus core and in a fibrin network formed from fibrinogen that escapes before hemostasis can be achieved.

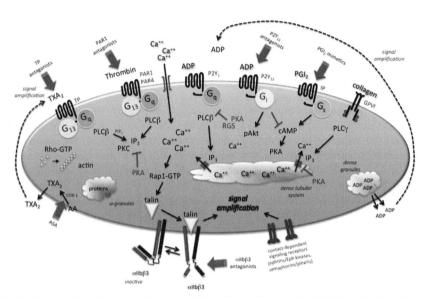

Fig. 2. An overview of some of the major signaling pathways of platelet activation. Targets for antiplatelet agents that are in clinical use or in clinical trials are indicated in blue. Inhibitors are in red. AA, arachidonic acid; IP3, inositol-1,4,5-trisphosphate; PAR, protease-activated receptor; PGI2, prostaglandin I2; PKA, protein kinase A; PKC, protein kinase C; PLC, phospholipase C; RGS, regulator of G protein signaling; TXA2, thromboxane A2.

summarizes key steps in platelet activation. Knowledge of platelet signaling pathways has aided the development of several antiplatelet agents that have entered clinical practice or are in clinical trials.

However, **Fig. 2** has important limitations. One limitation is that it has little to say about the events that lead to granule secretion in activated platelets. Resting platelets store and activated platelets secrete numerous molecules that support platelet activation and the hemostatic response. Some of these molecules also help to drive events such as wound healing and angiogenesis. Patients lacking storage granules have a clinical bleeding disorder. The presence of both proangiogenic and antiangiogenic factors within platelet storage granules has fueled recent debates about differential selectivity in either the storage or the release of these molecules in vivo.[9–12]

A second limitation of models such as the one shown in **Fig. 2** is that it falls short in answering questions that are critical for understanding platelet activation. Why does platelet activation require such complexity? Why are there so many platelet agonists and so many signaling pathways? If they are merely redundant, why does it seem that genetic or pharmacologic ablation of so many individual molecules has a meaningful effect on platelet function? An answer to some of these questions may come from thinking about signaling networks rather than signaling pathways.

One way of illustrating such networks is shown in **Fig. 3**. In a network-centric view of platelet activation, instead of responding to a single agonist via a single signaling pathway, platelets accumulating at a site of injury respond to the mixture of inputs (agonists) to which they are exposed. This mixture varies over both time and space, creating agonist concentration gradients. Positive and negative feedback in the form of soluble molecules (some released by platelets, others by damaged cells) plus contact-dependent interactions between adjacent platelets play an important

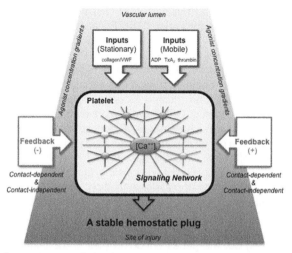

Fig. 3. A network-centric view of platelet activation. Signaling in platelets is represented as a balanced network, in which the effects of multiple inputs (mainly agonists) are modulated by positive and negative feedback. Signaling pathways communicate with each other and share nodal points in the network. The extent of activation of any given platelet varies according to the combination and concentration of the agonists to which the platelet is exposed and the sum of the feedback to which it is subjected. Gradients of agonist concentration are expected to be highest at the vessel wall near the site of injury (*bottom*) and lowest in the thrombus shell (*top*). Referring to the model in **Fig. 1**, platelets in the core of the thrombus are most subject to thrombin, collagen, and contact-dependent feedback, whereas those in the shell are affected primarily by soluble mediators such as ADP and TxA$_2$.

role in modulating platelet reactivity. Information flow within the platelet sums the effects of these inputs and nodal points in the signaling network provide links between them. This view of platelet activation can be tied to the structure shown in **Fig. 1** by considering, first, how declining gradients of different platelet agonists originating near the point of injury differentially affect the platelet activation state as the distance from the point of injury grows and, second, how the closer proximity of platelets in the thrombus core facilitates the binding of cell surface ligands to receptors on the surface of adjacent platelets.

NORMAL PLATELET ACTIVATORS IN VIVO

Once vascular injury has occurred, platelets are principally activated by locally exposed collagen, locally generated thrombin, platelet-derived TXA$_2$, and ADP that has either been released from damaged cells or secreted from platelet dense granules. The flow pattern of circulating red cells facilitates platelet adhesion to collagen by pushing platelets closer to the vessel wall, allowing GPIbα on the platelet surface to be snared by the A1 domain of VWF bound to collagen. Human platelets express 15,000 to 25,000 copies of GPIbα in a multiprotein complex with GPIbβ, GPIX, and GPV. Mutations in GPIbα that prevent its expression on the platelet surface or impair its receptor function produce an inherited recessive bleeding disorder (Bernard-Soulier syndrome) because platelet adhesion to the vessel wall is impaired. Macrothrombocytopenia arises in this disorder in part from a failure to form the normal linkages between GPIbα complex and filamin in the platelet membrane cytoskeleton.[13]

Once platelets are captured at the damaged vessel wall, the primary drivers for platelet activation are collagen, thrombin, ADP, TXA$_2$, and, to a more limited extent, epinephrine (see **Fig. 2**). With the exception of collagen, each of these agonists signals through 1 or more members of the GPCR superfamily. Properties that are common to this class of receptors make them well suited for their tasks in platelets. Most bind their ligands with high affinity and, because they act as exchange factors, each occupied receptor can theoretically activate multiple G proteins, amplifying the initial signal. Binding studies show that agonist GPCRs are expressed on the platelet surface in low numbers, ranging from a few hundred (ADP and epinephrine) to a few thousand (thrombin) per cell.[14–20] The duration of GPCR signaling is subject to receptor internalization, receptor desensitization, and the accelerated inactivation of G proteins by members of the RGS (regulator of G protein signaling) family. This multiplicity of mechanisms allows for tight regulation of platelet activation.

Human platelets express at least 10 heterotrimeric G proteins, including at least 1 G$_s$, 4 G$_i$ (G$_{i1}$, G$_{i2}$, G$_{i3}$ and G$_z$), 3 G$_q$ family members (G$_q$, G$_{11}$ and G$_{16}$), and 2 G$_{12}$ family members (G$_{12}$ and G$_{13}$). Much has been learned about the critical role of these G proteins by knocking out the genes encoding their α subunits in mice.[21] Less is known about the G$_{\beta\gamma}$ isoforms that are expressed in platelets and the selectivity (if any) of their individual contributions to platelet activation.

Most of the time agonist-initiated platelet activation begins with the activation of a phospholipase C (PLC) isoform, which by hydrolyzing membrane phosphatidylinositol-4,5-bisphosphate (PIP$_2$) produces the second messenger (inositol-1,4,5-trisphosphate [IP$_3$]) needed to increase the cytosolic Ca^{2+} concentration. This situation leads to integrin activation via an intracellular pathway that includes a Ca^{2+}-dependent exchange factor (CalDAG-GEF), a switch (predominantly Rap1b), an adaptor (RIAM), and proteins that interact directly with the integrin cytosolic domains (kindlin and talin).[22] Which isoform of PLC is activated depends on the agonist. Collagen activates PLCγ2 using a mechanism that depends on scaffold molecules and protein tyrosine kinases. Thrombin, ADP, and TXA$_2$ activate PLCβ using G$_q$ as an intermediary. The α subunit of G$_q$ binds directly to the phospholipase, activating it.

It is the binding of bivalent fibrinogen to $\alpha_{IIb}\beta_3$ that enables platelets to stick to one another, forming an aggregate. Other proteins that can substitute for fibrinogen include fibrin, VWF, and fibronectin. Average expression levels of $\alpha_{IIb}\beta_3$ range from approximately 50,000 per cell on resting platelets to 80,000 on activated platelets. Mutations in $\alpha_{IIb}\beta_3$ that prevent its expression or suppress its function produce a bleeding disorder (Glanzmann thrombasthenia) because platelets are unable to form stable aggregates. Antiplatelet agents such as eptifibatide (Integrilin), tirofiban (Aggrastat), and abciximab (ReoPro) take advantage of this situation by blocking $\alpha_{IIb}\beta_3$.

Platelet Activation by Collagen

Under static conditions, collagen can activate platelets without the assistance of cofactors, but under arterial flow conditions, VWF plays an essential role. Collagen polymers are better platelet agonists than collagen monomers.[23,24] Platelets can adhere to monomeric collagen but require the more complex structure found in fibrillar collagen for optimal activation.[25] Four collagen receptors have been identified on human and mouse platelets. Two bind directly to collagen (integrin $\alpha_2\beta_1$ and GPVI); the other 2 ($\alpha_{IIb}\beta_3$ and GPIbα) bind to collagen via VWF (**Fig. 4**). Of these receptors, GPVI is the most potent signaling receptor.[26] The structure of the GPVI extracellular domain places it in the immunoglobulin superfamily. Its ability to generate signals rests on its constitutive association with the immunoreceptor tyrosine-based activation domain (ITAM)-containing Fc receptor γ-chain (FcRγ). Platelets from mice that lack either

GPVI or FcRγ have impaired responses to collagen, as do platelets in which GPVI has been depleted or blocked.[27–30] Loss of FcRγ impairs collagen responses in part because of loss of a necessary signaling element and in part because of its role in helping GPVI reach the platelet surface. $\alpha_2\beta_1$ supports adhesion to collagen and acting as a source of further signaling after engagement.[31,32] Human platelets with reduced expression of $\alpha_2\beta_1$ have impaired collagen responses,[33,34] as do mouse platelets that lack β_1 integrins when the ability of these platelets to bind to collagen is tested at high shear.[30,35]

Signaling through GPVI can be studied in isolation with the snake venom protein, convulxin, or with synthetic collagen-related peptides, both of which bind to GPVI, but not to other collagen receptors. Each of these entities causes clustering of GPVI, leading to the phosphorylation of FcRγ by Src family tyrosine kinases constitutively associated with a proline-rich domain in GPVI.[36] Phosphorylation creates an ITAM motif recognized by the tandem SH2 domains of the tyrosine kinase Syk. Association of Syk with the GPVI/FcRγ-chain complex activates Syk, produces signaling complexes based on the scaffold proteins LAT and SLP-76, and leads to the activation of PLCγ2. Loss of Syk impairs collagen responses.[29] PLCγ2 hydrolyzes PIP$_2$ to form IP$_3$ and diacylglycerol (DAG). IP$_3$ opens Ca^{2+} channels in the platelet dense tubular system, increasing the cytosolic Ca^{2+} concentration through passive efflux. Depletion of the Ca^{2+} stores within the dense tubular system triggers Ca^{2+} influx across the platelet plasma membrane. The changes in the cytosolic Ca^{2+} concentration that occur when platelets adhere to collagen under flow can be visualized in real time.[37,38] Diacylglycerol activates the more common protein kinase C (PKC) isoforms that are expressed in platelets, allowing the serine/threonine phosphorylation events that are needed for platelet activation.

Collectively, collagen receptors support the capture of fast-moving platelets at sites of injury, cause activation of the captured platelets, and stimulate the cytoskeletal reorganization that allows the previously discoid platelets to flatten out and adhere more closely to the exposed vessel wall. As noted earlier, VWF supports this process. It increases the density of potential binding sites for collagen per platelet, because the number of copies of GPIbα and $\alpha_{IIb}\beta_3$ greatly exceeds the number of copies of GPVI and $\alpha_2\beta_1$. Because VWF is highly multimeric, it also increases the number of binding sites per collagen molecule. This situation increases the likelihood that platelets encounter an available binding site and, once bound, are able to increase the number of contacts with collagen by bringing additional receptors into play. GPVI and GPIbα are able to bind collagen and VWF without prior platelet activation, but once activation begins, $\alpha_2\beta_1$ and $\alpha_{IIb}\beta_3$ are able to bind their respective ligands as well. Some of the integrin-activating signaling occurs downstream of GPVI, but there is evidence that the GPIb-IX-V complex can signal as well, as can $\alpha_2\beta_1$ and $\alpha_{IIb}\beta_3$ once they are engaged.

Platelet Activation by Thrombin

Thrombin is able to activate platelets at concentrations as low as 0.1 nM. Although other platelet agonists can also cause phosphoinositide hydrolysis, none seems to be as efficiently coupled to PLC as thrombin. Within seconds of the addition of thrombin, the cytosolic Ca^{2+} concentration increases 10-fold, triggering downstream Ca^{2+}-dependent events, including the activation of phospholipase A$_2$ and integrin activation via the Rap1b-mediated pathway. All of these responses, but not shape change, are abolished in platelets from mice lacking $G_{q\alpha}$.[39] Thrombin also activates Rho in platelets, leading to rearrangement of the actin cytoskeleton and shape change, responses that are greatly reduced or absent in mouse platelets that lack

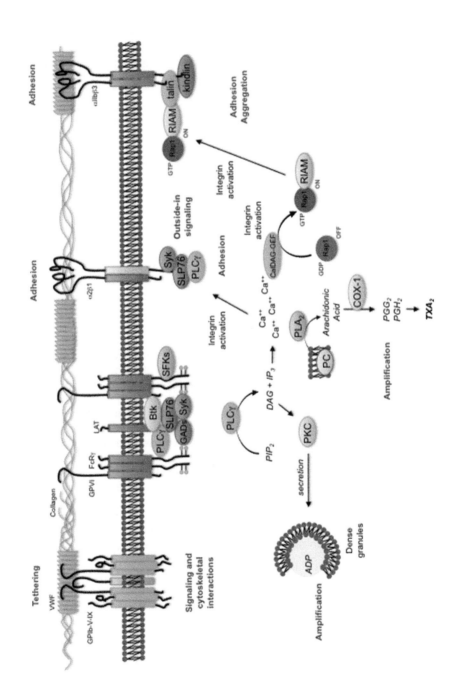

$G_{13\alpha}$.[40] Thrombin is able to inhibit adenylyl cyclase activity in human platelets, either directly (via a G_i family member) or indirectly (via released ADP).[41,42]

Platelet responses to thrombin are mediated by members of the protease-activated receptor (PAR) family of GPCRs. There are 4 members of this family, 3 of which (PAR1, PAR3, and PAR4) can be activated by thrombin. PAR1 and PAR4 are expressed on human platelets; mouse platelets express PAR3 and PAR4. Receptor activation occurs when thrombin cleaves the extended N terminus of each of these receptors, exposing a new N terminus that serves as a tethered ligand.[43] Synthetic peptides based on the sequence of the tethered ligand domain of PAR1 and PAR4 are able to activate the receptors, mimicking at least some of the actions of thrombin. PAR3 was originally identified after gene ablation studies showed that platelets from mice lacking PAR1 were still fully responsive to thrombin.[44] Approximately half of PAR1$^{-/-}$ mice die in utero, but this seems to be caused by loss of receptor expression in the vasculature, rather than in platelets.[45] Whereas human PAR3 has been shown to signal in response to thrombin, PAR3 on mouse platelets primarily serves to facilitate PAR4 cleavage.[46] Activation of PAR4 requires higher concentrations of thrombin than are required for activation of PAR1, apparently because it lacks the hirudinlike sequences that can interact with the anion-binding exosite of thrombin and facilitate receptor cleavage.[46–49] Kinetic studies in human platelets suggest that thrombin signals first through PAR1 and subsequently through PAR4.[50,51]

Considerable evidence shows that PAR family members are sufficient to activate platelets. Peptide agonists for either PAR1 or PAR4 cause platelet aggregation and secretion.[43,48] Conversely, simultaneous inhibition of human PAR1 and PAR4 abolishes responses to thrombin,[52] as does deletion of the gene encoding PAR4 in mice.[53] However, there are differences between mice and humans: optimal thrombin responses in human platelets require both PAR1 and PAR4, whereas those in mouse platelets are mediated by PAR3-facilitated cleavage of PAR4. PAR1 and PAR4 are coupled to at least G_q and G_{13}. There is conflicting evidence about whether G_i-dependent signaling in thrombin-activated platelets is entirely mediated by secreted ADP or occurs in part by a direct interaction between PARs and G_{i2}.[54–56] However, given the ability of PAR1 to directly couple to G_{i2} in cells other than platelets, it is likely that both occur. This hypothesis is consistent with a recent observation that expression of an RGS-resistant variant of $G_{i2\alpha}$ enhances thrombin responses in mouse platelets, even when the contribution of secreted ADP is blocked.[57] On the other hand, a requirement for PAR family members does not preclude the involvement of other participants in platelet responses to thrombin. GPIbα has a high affinity thrombin binding site within residues 268 to 287.[58,59] Deletion or blockade of this site reduces platelet responses to thrombin, particularly at low thrombin concentrations,[60–64] and impairs PAR1 cleavage on human platelets.[63] PAR1 antagonists have been developed and are undergoing clinical trials.[65] The early results show that blocking PAR1 may have

---

Fig. 4. Platelet activation by collagen. Platelets use several different molecular complexes to support platelet activation by collagen. These complexes include (1) VWF-mediated binding of collagen to the GPIb-IX-V complex and integrin $\alpha_{IIb}\beta_3$ and (2) a direct interaction between collagen and both the integrin $\alpha_2\beta_1$ and the GPVI/FcRγ-chain complex. Clustering of GPVI results in the phosphorylation of tyrosine residues in the FcRγ cytoplasmic domain, followed by the activation of the tyrosine kinase, Syk. One consequence of Syk activation is the activation of PLCγ_2, leading to phosphoinositide hydrolysis, secretion of ADP, and the production of TXA$_2$. COX-1, cyclooxygenase 1; DAG, diacylglycerol; PG, prostaglandin; PI3K, phosphatidylinositol 3-kinase; PKC, protein kinase C; PLA$_2$, phospholipase A$_2$.

some clinical usefulness, but can also increase bleeding risk in patients receiving other antiplatelet agents.[66–68]

Platelet Activation by ADP

ADP is stored in platelet dense granules and released on platelet activation. It is also released from damaged cells at sites of vascular injury, serving as a stimulus for activating tethered platelets and stabilizing the hemostatic plug. Aggregation studies show that all of the other platelet agonists are dependent to some extent on released ADP to elicit maximal platelet aggregation, although this dependence varies with the agonist and is dose related. Drugs that block platelet ADP $P2Y_{12}$ receptors have proved to be effective antiplatelet agents despite the fact that ADP, when added alone, is a less potent platelet agonist than thrombin.

When added to platelets in vitro, ADP causes an increase in cytosolic Ca^{2+}, TXA_2 formation, protein phosphorylation, shape change, aggregation, and secretion. It also inhibits cyclic adenosine monophosphate (cAMP) formation. These responses are half-maximal at approximately 1 μM ADP. However, even at high concentrations, ADP is a comparatively weak activator of PLC. Instead, its usefulness as a platelet agonist rests more on its ability to activate other pathways.[69,70] Human and mouse platelets express 2 distinct receptors for ADP, denoted $P2Y_1$ and $P2Y_{12}$. Both receptors are members of the purinergic class of GPCRs.[17–19,71,72] $P2Y_1$ receptors couple to G_q. $P2Y_{12}$ receptors couple to G_i family members. Optimal activation of platelets by ADP alone requires activation of both receptors, but the potentiation by ADP of platelet responses to other agonists seems to be mainly caused by $P2Y_{12}$. Knockouts of $P2Y_1$ and $P2Y_{12}$ in mice produce effects consistent with those predicted by pharmacologic studies on human platelets.[17,54] A third purinergic receptor on platelets, $P2X_1$, is an adenosine trisphosphate (ATP)-gated Ca^{2+} channel.[73–76] Platelet dense granules contain ATP as well as ADP, and studies suggest that there are conditions in which $P2X_1$ activity is essential for platelet activation.[77–79] $P2X_1$ is also functional on megakaryocytes.[80]

When $P2Y_1$ is blocked or deleted, ADP is still able to inhibit cAMP formation, but its ability to cause an increase in cytosolic Ca^{2+}, shape change, and aggregation is greatly impaired, as it is in platelets from mice that lack $G_{q\alpha}$.[39] $P2Y_1{}^{-/-}$ mice have a minimal increase in bleeding time and show some resistance to thromboembolic mortality after injection of ADP, but no predisposition to spontaneous hemorrhage. Primary responses to platelet agonists other than ADP are unaffected and when combined with serotonin, which is a weak stimulus for PLC in platelets, ADP can still cause aggregation of $P2Y_1{}^{-/-}$ platelets. Taken together, these results show that platelet $P2Y_1$ receptors are coupled to $G_{q\alpha}$ and responsible for activation of PLC. $P2Y_1$ receptors can also activate Rac and the Rac effector, p21-activated kinase (PAK),[81] but do not seem to be coupled to G_i family members.

$P2Y_{12}$ was independently identified by 2 groups.[19,72] As had been predicted by inhibitor studies and by the phenotype of a patient lacking functional $P2Y_{12}$,[82] platelets from $P2Y_{12}{}^{-/-}$ mice do not aggregate normally in response to ADP.[83] $P2Y_{12}{}^{-/-}$ platelets retain $P2Y_1$-associated responses, including shape change and PLC activation, but lack the ability to inhibit cAMP formation in response to ADP. The G_i family member associated with $P2Y_{12}$ seems to be primarily G_{i2}, because platelets from $G_{i2\alpha}{}^{-/-}$ mice have an impaired response to ADP,[84,85] whereas those lacking $G_{i3\alpha}$ or $G_{z\alpha}$ do not.[85,86] Conversely, expression of a $G_{i2\alpha}$ variant that is resistant to the inhibitory effects of RGS proteins produces a gain of function in mouse platelets stimulated with ADP.[57] Absence of $P2Y_{12}$ produces a hemorrhagic phenotype in humans, albeit a mild one.[19,82,87] Deletion of either $P2Y_1$ or $P2Y_{12}$ in mice prolongs the bleeding time and impairs platelet responses not only to ADP but also to thrombin and TXA_2, particularly at low concentrations.[83,88,89] Because the receptors for thrombin and TXA_2 can cause robust activation of PLC, the contribution of ADP when thrombin or TXA_2 are present seems to be largely because of its ability to activate G_{i2}.[90] Downstream effectors for $G_{i2\alpha}$ include Src family members[91] as well as PI3 kinase and Rap1b.

Platelet Activation by TXA_2

TXA_2 is produced from arachidonate in platelets by the aspirin-sensitive cyclooxygenase 1 (COX-1) pathway. When added to platelets in vitro, stable TXA_2 analogues such as U46619 cause shape change, aggregation, secretion, phosphoinositide hydrolysis, protein phosphorylation, and an increase in cytosolic Ca^{2+} and have little, if any, direct effect on cAMP formation. Similar responses are seen when platelets are incubated with exogenous arachidonate.[92] TXA_2 can diffuse across the plasma membrane and activate nearby platelets.[93] Like secreted ADP, release of TXA_2 amplifies the initial stimulus for platelet activation and helps to recruit additional platelets.[94] This process is effective locally, but is limited by the brief ($\sim$30 second) half-life of TXA_2 in solution, helping to confine the spread of platelet activation to the original area of injury.

Only 1 gene encodes TXA_2 receptors, but 2 splice variants are produced that differ in their cytoplasmic tails. Human platelets express both.[95] Loss of $G_{q\alpha}$ abolishes U46619-induced IP_3 formation, but does not prevent shape change,[39] which can be blocked by knocking out $G_{13\alpha}$.[40] Although in cells other than platelets, TXA_2 receptors have been shown to couple to G_i family members,[96] in platelets the inhibitory effects of U46619 on cAMP formation seem to be largely mediated by secreted ADP. These observations have previously been interpreted to mean that platelet TXA_2 receptors are coupled to G_q and $G_{12/13}$, but not to G_i family members. However, the enhanced response observed in mouse platelets carrying an RGS protein-resistant $G_{i2\alpha}$ variant suggests that this is still an open issue.[57]

The biological relevance of TXA_2 to normal platelet function is supported by genetic and pharmacologic evidence. $TP^{-/-}$ mice have a prolonged bleeding time. Their platelets are unable to aggregate in response to TXA_2 agonists and show delayed aggregation with collagen, presumably reflecting the role of TXA_2 in platelet responses to collagen.[97] A group of Japanese patients with impaired platelet responses to TXA_2 analogues have proved to be either homozygous or heterozygous for an R60L mutation in the first cytoplasmic loop of TP.[98] However, the most compelling case for the contribution of TXA_2 signaling in human platelets comes from the successful use of aspirin as an antiplatelet agent. When added to platelets in vitro, aspirin abolishes TXA_2 generation. Aspirin also blocks platelet activation by arachidonate and impairs responses to thrombin and ADP. The defect in thrombin responses appears as a shift in the dose/response curve, indicating that TXA_2 generation is supportive of platelet activation by thrombin, but not essential.

Platelet Activation by Epinephrine

Compared with thrombin, epinephrine is a weak activator of human platelets when added on its own. Nonetheless, there are reports of human families in which a mild bleeding disorder is associated with impaired epinephrine-induced aggregation and reduced numbers of catecholamine receptors.[99,100] Epinephrine responses in platelets are mediated by α_{2A}-adrenergic receptors.[20,101,102] In both mice and humans, epinephrine is able to potentiate the effects of other agonists so that the combination is a stronger stimulus for platelet aggregation than either agonist alone. Potentiation is often attributed to the ability of epinephrine to inhibit cAMP formation, but as is discussed later, there are clearly other effects as well. In contrast to other platelet agonists, epinephrine has no detectable direct effect on PLC and does not cause shape change, although it can trigger phosphoinositide hydrolysis indirectly by stimulating TXA_2 formation.[103] Taken together, these results suggest that platelet α_{2A}-adrenergic receptors are coupled to G_i, but not G_q or G_{12} family members. Human and mouse platelets express 4 members of the G_i family: G_{i1}, G_{i2}, G_{i3}, and G_z.[104] Of these members, $G_{z\alpha}$ has the slowest rate of intrinsic guanosine triphosphate (GTP) hydrolysis and is the only one that is not a substrate for pertussis toxin. Knockout studies show that epinephrine responses in platelets are abolished when $G_{z\alpha}$ is deleted. Loss of $G_{i2\alpha}$ or $G_{i3\alpha}$ has no effect.[85,86] G_z also seems to be responsible for the ability of epinephrine to activate Rap1b.[85,105] Therefore, it seems that in mouse platelets, α_{2A}-adrenergic receptors couple to G_z, but not G_{i2} or G_{i3}.

CRITICAL EVENTS

Thus far, this review has focused on platelet activation mechanisms from the perspective of individual agonists, many of which trigger a common set of pathways. In this section, some of those pathways are considered.

Phosphoinositide Hydrolysis

With the exception of epinephrine, platelet activation begins with the activation of PLC which, by hydrolyzing membrane phosphatidylinositol-4,5-bisphosphate (PIP_2), produces IP_3 and (DAG), the second messengers needed to increase the cytosolic Ca^{2+} concentration and activate some of the PKC isoforms found in platelets. As already noted, how PLC is activated varies with the agonist. Collagen activates $PLC\gamma_2$ using adaptor molecules and tyrosine kinases. Thrombin, ADP, and TXA_2 activate PLCβ isoforms using $G_{q\alpha}$ and (less efficiently if at all) $G_{\beta\gamma}$ derived from G_i. Regardless of which PLC isoform is activated, the subsequent increase in the Ca^{2+} concentration triggers downstream events, including integrin activation and TXA_2 formation. Thrombin provides a robust stimulus for phosphoinositide hydrolysis and causes the largest and fastest increase in cytosolic Ca^{2+}. Collagen and ADP are more dependent on the synthesis and release of TXA_2 to achieve a maximal response.

Cytosolic Ca^{2+} and Integrin Activation

Resting platelets maintain their cytosolic free Ca^{2+} concentration at approximately 0.1 μM by (1) limiting Ca^{2+} influx and (2) pumping Ca^{2+} out of the cytosol across the plasma membrane or into the dense tubular system (smooth endoplasmic reticulum). This action consumes ATP. In activated platelets, $[Ca^{2+}]_i$ can spike 10-fold to greater than 1 μM with potent agonists like thrombin. Measurements made of large populations of platelets suggest that this increase occurs rapidly and uniformly in response to potent agonists such as thrombin and less potently with agonists such as ADP and collagen. However, observations made with single platelets suggest that the Ca^{2+} response is heterogeneous, occurring to a different extent in different platelets, with some showing spiking behavior rather than a sustained increase and some not responding at all.[106–108] The molecular basis of this heterogeneity is not fully understood, although simulation studies suggest that platelet size is a factor.[108]

The increase in cytosolic Ca^{2+} that occurs during platelet activation derives from 2 sources. The first part is caused by the IP_3-mediated release of Ca^{2+} from the platelet dense tubular system. The second part occurs when depletion of the dense tubular system Ca^{2+} pool triggers store operated Ca^{2+} entry through a conformational change in STIM1, a protein in the dense tubular system membrane, binding of STIM1 to Orai1 in the plasma membrane, allowing an influx of plasma Ca^{2+}.[109] These events can be separated by chelating extracellular Ca^{2+}, thereby precluding Ca^{2+} influx. The increase in $[Ca^{2+}]_i$ activates the GTP-binding protein, Rap1b, via the Ca^{2+}-dependent guanine nucleotide exchange factor (GEF), CalDAG-GEF.[110] Activated Rap1b has been shown to bind to RIAM, bringing it to the plasma membrane, where it can bind talin. This situation allows talin to bind to the cytoplasmic domain of $\alpha_{IIb}\beta_3$, triggering integrin activation and exposing a binding site for fibrinogen.[22]

TXA₂ Production

The initial events of platelet activation lead to the activation of phospholipase A_2, which cleaves phosphatidylcholine and other membrane phospholipids, liberating arachidonate from the C2 position of the glycerol backbone. Arachidonate can be transformed into many bioactive compounds, but in platelets, TXA_2 is the key product. TXA_2 synthesis begins with COX-1, which forms prostaglandin (PG) G_2 and PGH_2 from arachidonate in a 2-step process (see **Fig. 4**). The PGH_2 is then metabolized to TXA_2 by thromboxane synthetase.[111] Evidence suggests that phospholipase A_2 activation in platelets can occur in more than 1 way. It can clearly happen in response to an increase in cytosolic Ca^{2+}, because the addition of a Ca^{2+} ionophore is sufficient to cause phospholipase A_2 activation.[112] There is also evidence that mitogen-activated protein kinase pathway signaling activates phospholipase A_2, although not necessarily by direct phosphorylation of phospholipase A_2.[113,114] TXA_2 formation is promoted by platelet aggregation and may, therefore, also occur as a consequence of integrin signaling, although this has not been tested directly.[115] TXA_2 can diffuse out of the platelet, activating nearby receptors in an autocrine or paracrine fashion before it is hydrolyzed to inactive TXB_2. Even although TXA_2 is a potent platelet activator, its half-life in aqueous solution is short (about 30 seconds), which has implications for both its duration of action and its impact downstream from a growing thrombus. This situation may be especially relevant for the model of the hemostatic response shown in **Fig. 1**, which postulates that declining gradients of soluble platelet agonists originating in the thrombus core contribute to the heterogeneity in platelet activation that we and others have observed within the hemostatic mass.

Shape Change and Rearrangement of the Actin Cytoskeleton

Activated platelets lose their characteristic discoid shape, either assuming a globular shape with filopodial extensions if they are activated in suspension or flattening out and developing lamellopodia if they are activated on a suitable surface. Shape change reflects loss of the circumferential microtubule ring and rearrangement of the actin cytoskeleton of the platelet, a process mediated by monomeric G proteins in the Rho and Rac families. When platelets in suspension are activated by soluble agonists, shape change precedes platelet aggregation. The soluble agonists (thrombin, ADP, and TXA_2) that trigger shape change typically act through receptors that are coupled to members of the G_q and G_{12} families. Epinephrine is unable to cause shape change, because its receptors are coupled solely to G_z.

At least 2 pathways are involved in the reorganization of the actin cytoskeleton: Ca^{2+}-dependent activation of myosin light-chain kinase downstream of G_q family members and activation of Rho family members downstream of G_{13}.[21,116] Several proteins having both G_α-interacting domains and GEF domains can link G_{12} family members to Rho family members, including p115RhoGEF.[117] With the exception of ADP, shape change persists in platelets from mice that lack $G_{q\alpha}$[39] but is lost when $G_{13\alpha}$ expression is suppressed, alone or in combination with $G_{12\alpha}$.[40] A combination of inhibitor and genetic approaches suggests that G_{13}-dependent Rho activation leads to shape change via pathways that include the Rho-activated kinase (p160ROCK) and

LIM kinase.[116,118,119] Activation of these kinases results in phosphorylation of myosin light-chain kinase and cofilin, helping to regulate both actin filament formation and myosin. ADP, on the other hand, depends more heavily on G_q-dependent activation of PLC to produce shape change and is able to activate G_{13} only as a consequence of TXA_2 generation; hence, the loss of ADP-induced shape change when G_q signaling is suppressed.

PI3 Kinase Activation

An additional category of critical events needed for robust platelet activation involves activation of the PI3-kinase (PI3K) isoforms expressed in platelets, either by G_i family members (PI3Kγ) or by phosphotyrosine-dependent signaling pathways downstream of collagen receptors (PI3K$\alpha\beta\delta$). PI3-kinases phosphorylate PI-4-P and PI-4,5-P_2 to produce PI-3,4-P_2 and PI-3,4,5-P_3, respectively. Among the best-described consequence of PI3K activation in platelets is the activation of the protein kinase, Akt. Knockout and inhibitor studies show that all 3 Akt isoforms are necessary for normal platelet activation.[120–122] Knockout and inhibitor studies also show a G_i/PI3K-dependent mechanism for activating Rap1b,[85,105] which, given the clinical usefulness of $P2Y_{12}$ antagonists as antiplatelet agents, seems to be a mechanism that is important for stabilizing platelet aggregates. However, aside from Rap1b and GSK3β, a kinase the activity of which is negatively regulated by Akt, little is known about Akt-dependent signaling pathways in platelets. To our knowledge, the Akt-dependent GEF for Rap1b has yet to be identified. PI3Kβ has been proposed as a target for antiplatelet agents.[123]

CONTACT-DEPENDENT AND CONTACT-FACILITATED SIGNALING

As platelet activation proceeds, platelets that were previously mobile come into increasingly stable contact with each other, eventually with sufficient proximity that molecules on the surface of 1 platelet can interact directly with molecules on the surface of adjacent platelets.[124] Although in theory this situation could occur anywhere within the growing hemostatic thrombus, it is likely to occur most readily in the thrombus core, where platelets are most densely packed (see Fig. 1).[8] Stable cohesive contacts between platelets require engagement of $\alpha_{IIb}\beta_3$ with 1 of its ligands, after which inward-directed (ie, outside-in) signaling occurs through the integrin. Inward-directed signaling also occurs through other surface molecules, which can engage their counterparts on the surface of adjoining platelets. Some of these molecules have been shown to affect platelet activation and thrombus stability, either positively or negatively. Others serve primarily to help form contacts between platelets and create a protected space in which soluble molecules, including agonists, can accumulate. In the next section, several examples are considered in which contact-dependent signaling has been studied in platelets and shown to have a meaningful impact.

Outside-In Signaling by Integrins

Activated $\alpha_{IIb}\beta_3$ bound to fibrinogen, fibrin, or VWF provides the dominant cohesive force that holds platelet aggregates together. It also contributes a further impetus for sustained platelet activation by serving as a scaffold for the assembly of signaling molecules.[125–127] The term outside-in signaling refers to the effects of these molecules.[128] Integrin signaling depends in large part on the formation of protein complexes that link to the integrin cytoplasmic domain. Some of the protein-protein interactions that involve the cytoplasmic domains of $\alpha_{IIb}\beta_3$ help regulate integrin activation; others participate in outside-in signaling and clot retraction. Proteins that are reportedly capable of binding directly to the cytoplasmic domains of $\alpha_{IIb}\beta_3$ include β_3-endonexin, CIB1, talin, kindlin, myosin, Shc, and the tyrosine kinases, Src, Fyn, and Syk. As noted earlier, the binding of talin and kindlin is believed to be one of the final events in the allosteric regulation of integrin activation.[129–132] Some other interactions require the phosphorylation of tyrosine residues Y773 and Y785 (Y747 and Y759 in mice) in the β_3 cytoplasmic domain by Src family members. Substitution of Y747 and Y759 with phenylalanine produces mice with platelets that tend to disaggregate and that show impaired clot retraction and a tendency to rebleed from tail bleeding time sites.[133] Fibrinogen binding to the extracellular domain of activated $\alpha_{IIb}\beta_3$ stimulates an increase in the activity of Src family kinases and Syk.[133,134] Studies of platelets from mice lacking these kinases suggest that these events are required for the initiation of outside-in signaling and for full platelet spreading, irreversible aggregation, and clot retraction.[135–138] There is evidence that the ITAM-containing receptor, FcRγIIA, is the link between Src family kinase and Syk activation in human platelets activated by $\alpha_{IIb}\beta_3$, although if so, a different receptor must perform this role in mouse platelets, which do not express FcRγIIA.[139]

Contact-Dependent Ligand-Receptor Interactions

The proximity of 1 platelet to another can also permit the direct binding of cell surface ligands to cell surface receptors on adjacent platelets. Two examples that we have studied are the interactions of ephrinB1 and sema4D with their cognate receptors. Ephrins are cell surface molecules attached by either a GPI anchor (ephrin [Eph] A family members) or a single transmembrane domain (ephrin B family members) that serve as ligands for cell surface receptor tyrosine kinases in the Eph A and B families. Eph kinases, like Eph B family members, have a single transmembrane domain that includes the catalytic domain and protein/protein interaction motifs. Human platelets express at least 2 Eph kinases, EphA4 and EphB1, and their ligand, ephrinB1.[140] Forced clustering of either EphA4 or ephrinB1 results in cytoskeletal changes leading to platelet spreading, as well as increased adhesion to fibrinogen, Rap1b activation, and granule secretion.[140,141] EphA4 associates with $\alpha_{IIb}\beta_3$ and Eph/ephrin interactions promote phosphorylation of the β_3 cytoplasmic domain. Conversely, blockade of Eph/ephrin interactions impairs clot retraction and causes platelet disaggregation at low agonist concentrations, resulting in impaired thrombus growth.[140,142] It also inhibits platelet accumulation on collagen under flow.[140,142] These observations suggest that close contacts between platelets during the early stages of thrombus formation allow the binding of ephinB1 to EphA4 and EphB1 in *trans* to provide signaling for sustained integrin activation.

Semaphorin 4D (Sema4D, CD100) provides another example of a ligand that is involved in contact-dependent signaling in platelets. Like the ephrins, semaphorins are best known for their role in the developing nervous system,[143] but they have also been implicated in organogenesis, vascularization, and immune cell regulation.[144] The 25 members of the semaphorin family are defined by a large sema domain[145] and divided into 8 classes differing in part by how (and whether) they are anchored to the surface of the cell that expresses them.[146] Sema4D, which has a transmembrane domain, is expressed on the surface of both mouse and human platelets. Platelet activation causes a rapid increase in surface expression, after which there is a gradual decline below the original expression level as the sema4D exodomain is cleaved and shed by the metalloprotease, ADAM17.[147] Inhibiting or deleting ADAM17 blocks this process. Sema4D$^{-/-}$ mouse platelets have a defect in their responses to collagen and convulxin in vitro, and a reduced response to vascular injury in vivo.[147] Responses to thrombin, ADP, and TXA$_2$ mimetics are normal.[147,148] The collagen defect has been mapped to a failure to maximally activate Syk downstream of the collagen receptor, GPVI. Events in the pathway upstream of Syk occur normally in sema4D$^{-/-}$ plate-lets.[147,148] These defects are observed only when platelets come in contact with each other and can be reversed by adding soluble recombinant sema4D. Thus, the evidence suggests that sema4D provides a contact-dependent boost in collagen signaling. The platelets that are most likely to be activated via GPVI are those in con-tact with collagen. If so, then the sema4D signaling is likely most relevant for the plate-lets closest to the vessel wall at the site of injury. Human platelets express at least 2 receptors for sema4D: CD72 and a member of the plexin B family.[147] Mouse platelets express the plexin, but not CD72. However, although the presence of these Sema4D receptors has been established, the extent to which they mediate Sema4D signaling in platelets remains to be determined.

OBTAINING AN OPTIMAL RESPONSE TO INJURY

The molecular mechanisms that drive platelet activation reflect an evolutionary compromise. This compromise can be thought of as establishing a threshold for platelet activation. If the threshold is too high, then platelets become useless for he-mostasis. If too low, then opportunities for unwarranted platelet activation increase (**Fig. 5**). An optimal platelet response to injury can be defined as one in which blood loss is restrained and hemostasis is achieved without the penalty of further tissue damage caused by unwarranted vascular occlusion. The set point is established by balancing the intracellular signaling mechanisms that drive platelet activation in response to injury with regulatory mechanisms that either dampen those responses or prevent their initiation in the first place. The normal environment of the platelet in-cludes the other blood cells, the soluble molecules found in plasma and, most criti-cally, the vascular wall and the endothelial cells that line it, all of which are subject to change in the face of injury, disease, circadian rhythms, and aging. Many of these entities serve as extrinsic regulators of platelet activation. A healthy endothelium

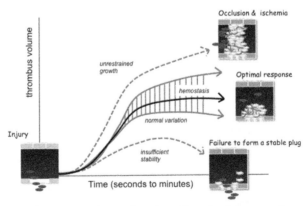

Fig. 5. Formation of an optimal platelet plug. Vascular injury produces a hemostatic response that can be too aggressive (leading to occlusion and ischemia), inadequate (lead-ing to further bleeding), or optimal. This model suggests that an optimal response varies in detail (hence, a range of normal), but is best viewed as a response that results in hemostasis with a minimum of blood loss and an avoidance of unwarranted vascular occlusion. In the setting of a vascular wall disease such as atherosclerosis, the rapid accumulation of platelets on top of a ruptured plaque represents an escape from normal restraints.

provides a physical barrier that limits platelet activation. It also produces inhibitors of platelet activation, including NO,[149] PGI$_2$,[150–152] and the ecto-ADPase, CD39, which hydrolyzes plasma ADP that would otherwise sensitize platelets to activation by other agonists.[153] In addition to these extrinsic regulators, several intrinsic regulators of platelet activation have been identified. A few of them are considered here.

Regulation of G Protein-Dependent Signaling

As noted earlier, most of the platelet agonists act via GPCRs. Because mechanisms exist that can limit the activation of GPCRs, platelet activation can be tightly regulated. The role of RGS proteins in platelets is just beginning to be explored. RGS proteins limit signaling intensity and duration by accelerating the intrinsic hydrolysis of GTP by activated G protein α subunits.[154] As many as 10 RGS proteins have been identified in platelets at the RNA level, but to our knowledge, only RGS10 and RGS18 have been confirmed at the protein level.[155–160] The evidence that RGS proteins are biologically relevant in platelets comes from studies on mice in which glycine 184 in the α subunit of G$_{i2}$ has been replaced with serine, rendering it unable to interact with RGS proteins without impairing the ability of G$_{i2}$ to interact with either receptors or downstream effectors. This substitution produces the predicted gain of platelet function in vitro and in vivo, even in the heterozygous state.[57] At the molecular level, the G$_{i2\alpha}$(G184S) allele causes an attenuated increase in cAMP levels in response to PGI$_2$ and a substantial increase in basal Akt activation, 2 events that occur downstream of G$_{i2}$ in platelets. In contrast, agonist-stimulated increases in [Ca^{2+}]$_i$ and Rap1 activation are unaffected, indicating no crossover into G$_{q\alpha}$-dependent signaling pathways.

These results show that removing the restraining hand of RGS proteins on G$_{i2}$ in platelets is sufficient to produce a pronounced gain of function, arguing that the normal role of the RGS proteins is to limit platelet activation. If so, then the timing of the interaction of RGS proteins with activated G proteins becomes critical as well. If signaling is constrained too early, then platelet activation might never occur, whereas if signaling is shut down too late, more platelets might accumulate than are needed. Two recent studies show that RGS proteins interact with other molecules the role of which may be to regulate RGS protein availability. The first of these proteins is the scaffold protein, spinophilin, which binds RGS10 and RGS18 in resting platelets, and then releases them on platelet activation. Knocking out spinophilin in mice produces a loss of function in platelets, as would be expected if RGS10 and RGS18 interact prematurely with activated G proteins when spinophilin is not present.[161] A second group of RGS protein-interacting proteins in platelets includes members of the 14-3-3 scaffold protein family. 14-3-3 family members can bind to phosphorylated serine residues in RGS18, an interaction that is displaced when cAMP-dependent protein kinase A phosphorylates RGS18.[162] Taken together, these recent observations suggest that spinophilin serves as a critical node within the platelet signaling network.

cAMP and Protein Kinase A

Rising cAMP levels turn off signaling in platelets. Regulatory molecules released from endothelial cells cause G$_{s\alpha}$-mediated increases in adenylyl cyclase activity (PGI$_2$) and inhibit the hydrolysis of cAMP by phosphodiesterases (NO).[163] When added to platelets in vitro, PGI$_2$ can cause a greater than 10-fold increase in the platelet cAMP concentration, but even small increases in cAMP levels (2-fold or less) impair platelet activation.[164] Deletion of either G$_{i2\alpha}$ or G$_{z\alpha}$ causes an increase in the basal cAMP concentration in mouse platelets.[85] cAMP phosphodiesterase inhibitors such as dipyridamole act as antiplatelet agents by raising cAMP levels. Conversely, loss of PGI$_2$ receptor (IP) expression causes a decrease in basal cAMP levels, an enhanced response to agonists, and a predisposition to thrombosis in murine arterial injury models.[85,165] Despite ample evidence that cAMP inhibits platelet activation, the mechanism by which it does this is not fully defined. cAMP-dependent protein kinase A is believed to be involved, but other mechanisms may be as well. Substrates for the kinase in platelets include serine and threonine residues in some GPCRs, IP_3 receptors, GPIbβ, vasodilator-stimulated phosphoprotein, RGS18, and Rap1b, but it remains unclear whether a single substrate or small group of substrates accounts for most of the effect or whether it is the accumulated effect of phosphorylation of many substrates.[162,166–174]

Adhesion/Junction Receptors Contribute to Contact-Dependent Signaling

In addition to amplifying platelet activation, contact-dependent signaling can also help to limit thrombus growth and stability. Examples of this phenomenon include platelet/endothelial cell adhesion molecule-1 (PECAM-1), carcinoembryonic antigen-related cell adhesion molecule 1 (CEACAM1) and at least 2 members of the CTX family of adhesion molecules, ESAM and JAM-A. PECAM-1 is a type 1 transmembrane protein with 6 extracellular domains, the most distal of which can form homophilic interactions in trans.[175] The cytoplasmic domain contains 2 immunoreceptor tyrosine inhibitory motifs (ITIMs) that can bind the tyrosine phosphatase, SHP-2.[176] PECAM-1-deficient platelets show enhanced responses to collagen in vitro and in vivo.[177–179] CEACAM1 is a second ITIM family member expressed on the platelet surface that can form homophilic and heterophilic interactions with other CEACAM superfamily members. In contrast to PECAM-1, the CEACAM1 ITIMs prefer SHP-1 over SHP-2, although either can become bound.[180,181] The CEACAM1 knockout, like the PECAM-1 knockout, produces an enhanced platelet response, showing increased platelet activation in vitro in response to collagen and increased thrombus formation in a $FeCl_3$ injury model.[182] ESAM and JAM-A have 2 extracellular immunoglobulin domains, a single transmembrane region and a cytoplasmic tail of varying length that terminates in a binding site for PDZ domain-containing proteins. ESAM is associated with α-granules in resting platelets, but localizes to junctions during platelet activation.[183] ESAM$^{-/-}$ platelets show increased aggregation in response to low doses of GPCR agonists and are more resistant to disaggregation compared with wild-type platelets. In vivo, ESAM$^{-/-}$ mice form larger and more stable thrombi compared with their wild-type counterparts.[183] Collectively, these studies suggest that ESAM negatively regulates platelet function through contact-dependent homophilic interactions, although the mechanistic basis for these observations remains to be identified. JAM-A$^{-/-}$ mice also show a gain of function phenotype.[184]

SUMMARY

Platelets are part of the initial response to vascular injury intended to resist further blood loss by producing a hemostatic plug or thrombus. Conventional models portray such thrombi as relatively uniform masses of fully activated platelets intermixed with fibrin. Recent observational studies suggest that reality is more complex in at least the microcirculation, with fibrin deposition concentrated close to the vessel wall at the site of injury and the extent of platelet activation varying inversely with distance from the injury such that a hierarchical structure is formed. Underlying platelet activation is flexible signaling network within the platelets that sums the response to multiple platelet agonists, including collagen, thrombin, ADP, TxA_2, and epinephrine. Critical events in this network include the activation of PLC, an increase in cytosolic Ca^{2+}, reorganization of the platelet cytoskeleton, granule secretion, and the steps that link

Ca^{2+} to activation of the platelet fibrinogen receptor, $\alpha_{IIb}\beta_3$, so that platelet aggregates can form. Extrinsic regulators provided by a healthy endothelium dampen platelet responsiveness and resist unwarranted platelet activation, whereas intrinsic regulators such as RGS proteins limit signaling downstream of platelet agonists once it has been initiated. As activated platelets come into increasingly stable contact with each other, molecules on their surface are able to interact directly, generating a wave of contact-dependent signaling events. Such events can amplify platelet activation, but can also help to mold the growing thrombus by limiting the extent of platelet activation.

REFERENCES

1. Kanaji S, Fahs SA, Shi Q, et al. Contribution of platelet versus endothelial VWF to platelet adhesion and hemostasis. J Thromb Haemost 2012;10(8):1646–52.
2. Reininger AJ, Heijnen HF, Schumann H, et al. Mechanism of platelet adhesion to von Willebrand factor and microparticle formation under high shear stress. Blood 2006;107:3537–45.
3. Ruggeri ZM, Orje JN, Habermann R, et al. Activation-independent platelet adhesion and aggregation under elevated shear stress. Blood 2006;108:1903–10.
4. Munnix IC, Cosemans JM, Auger JM, et al. Platelet response heterogeneity in thrombus formation. Thromb Haemost 2009;102:1149–56.
5. Nesbitt WS, Westein E, Tovar-Lopez FJ, et al. A shear gradient-dependent platelet aggregation mechanism drives thrombus formation. Nat Med 2009;15:665–73.
6. Bellido-Martin L, Chen V, Jasuja R, et al. Imaging fibrin formation and platelet and endothelial cell activation in vivo. Thromb Haemost 2011;105:776–82.
7. Nishimura S, Manabe I, Nagasaki M, et al. In vivo imaging visualizes discoid platelet aggregations without endothelium disruption and implicates contribution of inflammatory cytokine and integrin signaling. Blood 2012;119:e45–56.
8. Brass LF, Wannemacher KM, Ma P, et al. Regulating thrombus growth and stability to achieve an optimal response to injury. J Thromb Haemost 2011;9(Suppl 1):66–75.
9. Italiano JE Jr, Richardson JL, Patel-Hett S, et al. Angiogenesis is regulated by a novel mechanism: pro- and antiangiogenic proteins are organized into separate platelet alpha granules and differentially released. Blood 2008;111:1227–33.
10. Peters CG, Michelson AD, Flaumenhaft R. Granule exocytosis is required for platelet spreading: differential sorting of alpha-granules expressing VAMP-7. Blood 2012;120:199–206.
11. Battinelli EM, Markens BA, Italiano JE Jr. Release of angiogenesis regulatory proteins from platelet alpha granules: modulation of physiologic and pathologic angiogenesis. Blood 2011;118:1359–69.
12. Kamykowski J, Carlton P, Sehgal S, et al. Quantitative immunofluorescence mapping reveals little functional coclustering of proteins within platelet alpha-granules. Blood 2011;118:1370–3.
13. Kato K, Martinez C, Russell S, et al. Genetic deletion of mouse platelet glycoprotein Ibbeta produces a Bernard-Soulier phenotype with increased alpha-granule size. Blood 2004;104:2339–44.
14. Brass LF, Vassallo RR Jr, Belmonte E, et al. Structure and function of the human platelet thrombin receptor: studies using monoclonal antibodies against a defined epitope within the receptor N-terminus. J Biol Chem 1992;267:13795–8.
15. Mills DC. ADP receptors on platelets. Thromb Haemost 1996;76:835–56.

16. Gachet C, Hechler B, Léon C, et al. Activation of ADP receptors and platelet function. Thromb Haemost 1997;78:271–5.
17. Daniel JL, Dangelmaier C, Jin JG, et al. Molecular basis for ADP-induced platelet activation I. Evidence for three distinct ADP receptors on human platelets. J Biol Chem 1998;273:2024–9.
18. Jin JG, Daniel JL, Kunapuli SP. Molecular basis for ADP-induced platelet activation II. The P2Y1 receptor mediates ADP-induced intracellular calcium mobilization and shape change in platelets. J Biol Chem 1998;273:2030–4.
19. Hollopeter G, Jantzen HM, Vincent D, et al. Identification of the platelet ADP receptor targeted by antithrombotic drugs. Nature 2001;409:202–7.
20. Motulsky HJ, Insel PA. [3H]Dihydroergocryptine binding to alpha-adrenergic receptors of human platelets. A reassessment using the selective radioligands [3H]prazosin, [3H]yohimbine, and [3H]rauwolscine. Biochem Pharmacol 1982;31:2591–7.
21. Offermanns S. In vivo functions of heterotrimeric G-proteins: studies in Galpha-deficient mice. Oncogene 2001;20:1635–42.
22. Shattil SJ, Kim C, Ginsberg MH. The final steps of integrin activation: the end game. Nat Rev Mol Cell Biol 2010;11:288–300.
23. Brass LF, Bensusan HB. The role of collagen quaternary structure in the platelet: collagen interaction. J Clin Invest 1974;54:1480–7.
24. Santoro SA. Identification of a 160,000 dalton platelet membrane protein that mediates the initial divalent cation-dependent adhesion of platelets to collagen. Cell 1986;46:913–20.
25. Brass LF, Faile D, Bensusan HB. Direct measurement of the platelet: collagen interaction by affinity chromatography on collagen/Sepharose. J Lab Clin Med 1976;87:525–34.
26. Clemetson JM, Polgar J, Magnenat E, et al. The platelet collagen receptor glycoprotein VI is a member of the immunoglobulin superfamily closely related to FcalphaR and the natural killer receptors. J Biol Chem 1999;274:29019–24.
27. Massberg S, Gawaz M, Gruner S, et al. A crucial role of glycoprotein VI for platelet recruitment to the injured arterial wall in vivo. J Exp Med 2003;197:41–9.
28. Kato K, Kanaji T, Russell S, et al. The contribution of glycoprotein VI to stable platelet adhesion and thrombus formation illustrated by targeted gene deletion. Blood 2003;102:1701–7.
29. Poole A, Gibbins JM, Turner M, et al. The Fc receptor gamma-chain and the tyrosine kinase Syk are essential for activation of mouse platelets by collagen. EMBO J 1997;16:2333–41.
30. Nieswandt B, Brakebusch C, Bergmeier W, et al. Glycoprotein VI but not alpha2beta1 integrin is essential for platelet interaction with collagen. EMBO J 2001;20:2120–30.
31. Keely PJ, Parise LV. The alpha2beta1 integrin is a necessary co-receptor for collagen-induced activation of Syk and the subsequent phosphorylation of phospholipase Cgamma2 in platelets. J Biol Chem 1996;271:26668–76.
32. Consonni A, Cipolla L, Guidetti G, et al. Role and regulation of phosphatidylinositol 3-kinase beta in platelet integrin alpha2beta1 signaling. Blood 2012;119:847–56.
33. Nieuwenhuis HK, Akkerman JW, Houdijk WP, et al. Human blood platelets showing no response to collagen fail to express glycoprotein Ia. Nature 1985;318:470–2.

34. Sixma JJ, Van Zanten GH, Huizinga EG, et al. Platelet adhesion to collagen: an update. Thromb Haemost 1997;78:434–8.
35. Kuijpers MJ, Schulte V, Bergmeier W, et al. Complementary roles of glycoprotein VI and alpha2beta1 integrin in collagen-induced thrombus formation in flowing whole blood ex vivo. FASEB J 2003;17:685–7.
36. Schmaier AA, Zou Z, Kazlauskas A, et al. Molecular priming of Lyn by GPVI enables an immune receptor to adopt a hemostatic role. Proc Natl Acad Sci U S A 2009;106:21167–72.
37. Nesbitt WS, Giuliano S, Kulkarni S, et al. Intercellular calcium communication regulates platelet aggregation and thrombus growth. J Cell Biol 2003;160: 1151–61.
38. Kulkarni S, Nesbitt WS, Dopheide SM, et al. Techniques to examine platelet adhesive interactions under flow. Methods Mol Biol 2004;272:165–86.
39. Offermanns S, Toombs CF, Hu YH, et al. Defective platelet activation in Galphaq-deficient mice. Nature 1997;389:183–6.
40. Moers A, Nieswandt B, Massberg S, et al. G13 is an essential mediator of platelet activation in hemostasis and thrombosis. Nat Med 2003;9:1418–22.
41. Barr AJ, Brass LF, Manning DR. Reconstitution of receptors and GTP-binding regulatory proteins (G proteins) in Sf9 cells: a direct evaluation of selectivity in receptor-G protein coupling. J Biol Chem 1997;272:2223–9.
42. Kim S, Foster C, Lecchi A, et al. Protease-activated receptor 1 and 4 do not stimulate G(i) signaling pathways in the absence of secreted ADP and cause human platelet aggregation independently of G(i) signaling. Blood 2002;99: 3629.
43. Vu TK, Hung DT, Wheaton VI, et al. Molecular cloning of a functional thrombin receptor reveals a novel proteolytic mechanism of receptor activation. Cell 1991;64:1057–68.
44. Connolly AJ, Ishihara H, Kahn ML, et al. Role of the thrombin receptor in development and evidence for a second receptor. Nature 1996;381:516–9.
45. Griffin CT, Srinivasan Y, Zheng YW, et al. A role of thrombin receptor signaling in endothelial cells during embryonic development. Science 2001;293:1666–70.
46. Nakanishi-Matsui M, Zheng YW, Sulciner DJ, et al. PAR3 is a cofactor for PAR4 activation by thrombin. Nature 2000;404:609–10.
47. Xu WF, Andersen H, Whitmore TE, et al. Cloning and characterization of human protease-activated receptor 4. Proc Natl Acad Sci U S A 1998;95:6642–6.
48. Kahn ML, Zheng YW, Huang W, et al. A dual thrombin receptor system for platelet activation. Nature 1998;394:690–4.
49. Ishii K, Gerszten R, Zheng YW, et al. Determinants of thrombin receptor cleavage. Receptor domains involved, specificity, and role of the P3 aspartate. J Biol Chem 1995;270:16435–40.
50. Covic L, Gresser AL, Kuliopulos A. Biphasic kinetics of activation and signaling for PAR1 and PAR4 thrombin receptors in platelets. Biochemistry 2000;39: 5458–67.
51. Shapiro MJ, Weiss EJ, Faruqi TR, et al. Protease-activated receptors 1 and 4 are shut off with distinct kinetics after activation by thrombin. J Biol Chem 2000;275: 25216–21.
52. Kahn ML, Nakanishi-Matsui M, Shapiro MJ, et al. Protease-activated receptors 1 and 4 mediate activation of human platelets by thrombin. J Clin Invest 1999;103: 879–87.
53. Sambrano GR, Weiss EJ, Zheng Y-W, et al. Role of thrombin signaling in platelets in hemostasis and thrombosis. Nature 2001;413:74–8.

54. Jin JG, Kunapuli SP. Coactivation of two different G protein-coupled receptors is essential for ADP-induced platelet aggregation. Proc Natl Acad Sci U S A 1998; 95:8070–4.

55. Brass LF, Woolkalis MJ. Dual regulation of cAMP formation by thrombin in HEL cell, a leukemic cell line with megakaryocytic properties. Biochem J 1992;281: 73–80.

56. Brass LF, Woolkalis MJ, Manning DR. Interactions in platelets between G proteins and the agonists that stimulate phospholipase C and inhibit adenylyl cyclase. J Biol Chem 1988;263:5348–55.

57. Signarvic RS, Cierniewska A, Stalker TJ, et al. RGS/Gi2alpha interactions modulate platelet accumulation and thrombus formation at sites of vascular injury. Blood 2010;116:6092–100.

58. De Cristofaro R, De Candia E, Rutella S, et al. The Asp272-Glu282 region of platelet glycoprotein Ibalpha interacts with the heparin-binding site of alpha-thrombin and protects the enzyme from the heparin-catalyzed inhibition by anti-thrombin III. J Biol Chem 2000;275:3887–95.

59. Celikel R, McClintock RA, Roberts JR, et al. Modulation of alpha-thrombin function by distinct interactions with platelet glycoprotein Ibalpha. Science 2003; 301:218–21.

60. De Marco L, Mazzucato M, Masotti A, et al. Function of glycoprotein Ibalpha in platelet activation induced by alpha-thrombin. J Biol Chem 1991;266:23776–83.

61. Harmon JT, Jamieson GA. Platelet activation by thrombin in the absence of the high affinity thrombin receptor. Biochemistry 1988;27:2151–7.

62. Mazzucato M, De Marco L, Masotti A, et al. Characterization of the initial alpha-thrombin interaction with glycoprotein Ibalpha in relation to platelet activation. J Biol Chem 1998;273:1880–7.

63. De Candia E, Hall SW, Rutella S, et al. Binding of thrombin to glycoprotein Ib accelerates hydrolysis of PAR1 on intact platelets. J Biol Chem 2001;276:4692–8.

64. Dörmann D, Clemetson KJ, Kehrel BE. The GPIb thrombin-binding site is essential for thrombin-induced platelet procoagulant activity. Blood 2000;96:2469–78.

65. Tello-Montoliu A, Tomasello SD, Ueno M, et al. Antiplatelet therapy: thrombin receptor antagonists. Br J Clin Pharmacol 2011;72:658–71.

66. Morrow DA, Braunwald E, Bonaca MP, et al. Vorapaxar in the secondary prevention of atherothrombotic events. N Engl J Med 2012;366:1404–13.

67. Tricoci P, Huang Z, Held C, et al. Thrombin-receptor antagonist vorapaxar in acute coronary syndromes. N Engl J Med 2012;366:20–33.

68. Scirica BM, Bonaca MP, Braunwald E, et al. Vorapaxar for secondary prevention of thrombotic events for patients with previous myocardial infarction: a prespecified subgroup analysis of the TRA 2 degrees P-TIMI 50 trial. Lancet 2012; 380(9850):1317–24.

69. Fisher GJ, Bakshian S, Baldassare JJ. Activation of human platelets by ADP causes a rapid rise in cytosolic free calcium without hydrolysis of phosphatidylinositol-4,5-bisphosphate. Biochem Biophys Res Commun 1985;129:958–64.

70. Daniel JL, Dangelmaier CA, Selak M, et al. ADP stimulates IP3 formation in human platelets. FEBS Lett 1986;206:299–303.

71. Léon C, Hechler B, Vial C, et al. The P2Y1 receptor is an ADP receptor antagonized by ATP and expressed in platelets and megakaryoblastic cells. FEBS Lett 1997;403:26–30.

72. Zhang FL, Luo L, Gustafson E, et al. ADP is the cognate ligand for the orphan G protein-coupled receptor SP1999. J Biol Chem 2001;276:8608–15.

73. McKenzie AB, Mahout-Smith MP, Sage SO. Activation of receptor-operated channels via P2X1 not P2T purinoreceptors in human platelets. J Biol Chem 1996;271:2879–81.

74. Vial C, Hechler B, Léon C, et al. Presence of P2X1 purinoceptors in human platelets and megakaryoblastic cell lines. Thromb Haemost 1997;78:1500–4.

75. Sun B, Li J, Okahara K, et al. P2X1 purinoceptor in human platelets–molecular cloning and functional characterization after heterologous expression. J Biol Chem 1998;273:11544–7.

76. Mahaut-Smith MP, Ennion SJ, Rolf MG, et al. ADP is not an agonist at P2X1 receptors: evidence for separate receptors stimulated by ATP and ADP on human platelets. Br J Psychol 2000;131:108–14.

77. Fung CY, Brearley CA, Farndale RW, et al. A major role for P2X1 receptors in the early collagen-evoked intracellular Ca2+ responses of human platelets. Thromb Haemost 2005;94:37–40.

78. Mahaut-Smith MP, Tolhurst G, Evans RJ. Emerging roles for P2X1 receptors in platelet activation. Platelets 2004;15:131–44.

79. Hechler B, Lenain N, Marchese P, et al. A role of the fast ATP-gated P2X1 cation channel in thrombosis of small arteries in vivo. J Exp Med 2003;198:661–7.

80. Tolhurst G, Vial C, Leon C, et al. Interplay between P2Y(1), P2Y(12), and P2X(1) receptors in the activation of megakaryocyte cation influx currents by ADP: evidence that the primary megakaryocyte represents a fully functional model of platelet P2 receptor signaling. Blood 2005;106:1644–51.

81. Soulet C, Hechler B, Gratacap MP, et al. A differential role of the platelet ADP receptors P2Y and P2Y in Rac activation. J Thromb Haemost 2005;3: 2296–306.

82. Nurden P, Savi P, Heilmann E, et al. An inherited bleeding disorder linked to a defective interaction between ADP and its receptor on platelets. Its influence on glycoprotein IIb-IIIa complex function. J Clin Invest 1995;95:1612–22.

83. Foster CJ. Molecular identification and characterization of the platelet ADP receptor targeted by thienopyridine drugs using P2Yac-null mice. J Clin Invest 2001;107:1591–8.

84. Jantzen HM, Milstone DS, Gousset L, et al. Impaired activation of murine platelets lacking Galphai2. J Clin Invest 2001;108:477–83.

85. Yang J, Wu J, Jiang H, et al. Signaling through Gi family members in platelets–redundancy and specificity in the regulation of adenylyl cyclase and other effectors. J Biol Chem 2002;277:46035–42.

86. Yang J, Wu J, Kowalska MA, et al. Loss of signaling through the G protein, Gz, results in abnormal platelet activation and altered responses to psychoactive drugs. Proc Natl Acad Sci U S A 2000;97:9984–9.

87. Cattaneo M, Gachet C. ADP receptors and clinical bleeding disorders. Arterioscler Thromb Vasc Biol 1999;19:2281–5.

88. Fabre JE, Nguyen MT, Latour A, et al. Decreased platelet aggregation, increased bleeding time and resistance to thromboembolism in P2Y1-deficient mice. Nat Med 1999;5:1199–202.

89. Léon C, Hechler B, Freund M, et al. Defective platelet aggregation and increased resistance to thrombosis in purinergic P2Y1 receptor-null mice. J Clin Invest 1999;104:1731–7.

90. Paul BZ, Jin JG, Kunapuli SP. Molecular mechanism of thromboxane A2-induced platelet aggregation–essential role for P2TAC and alpha2A receptors. J Biol Chem 1999;274:29108–14.

91. Nash CA, Severin S, Dawood BB, et al. Src family kinases are essential for primary aggregation by G(i)-coupled receptors. J Thromb Haemost 2010;8: 2273–82.

92. Gerrard JM, Carroll RC. Stimulation of protein phosphorylation by arachidonic acid and endoperoxide analog. Prostaglandins 1981;22:81–94.

93. FitzGerald GA. Mechanisms of platelet activation: thromboxane A2 as an amplifying signal for other agonists. Am J Correct 1991;68:11B–5B.

94. Brass LF, Shaller CC, Belmonte EJ. Inositol 1,4,5-triphosphate-induced granule secretion in platelets. Evidence that the activation of phospholipase C mediated by platelet thromboxane receptors involves a guanine nucleotide binding protein-dependent mechanism distinct from that of thrombin. J Clin Invest 1987;79:1269–75.

95. Hirata T, Ushikubi F, Kakizuka A, et al. Two thromboxane A2 receptor isoforms in human platelets–opposite coupling to adenylyl cyclase with different sensitivity to Arg60 to Leu mutation. J Clin Invest 1996;97:949–56.

96. Gao Y, Tang S, Zhou S, et al. The thromboxane A2 receptor activates mitogen-activated protein kinase via protein kinase C-dependent Gi coupling and Src-dependent phosphorylation of the epidermal growth factor receptor. J Pharmacol Exp Ther 2001;296:426–33.

97. Thomas DW, Mannon RB, Mannon PJ, et al. Coagulation defects and altered hemodynamic responses in mice lacking receptors for thromboxane A2. J Clin Invest 1998;102:1994–2001.

98. Higuchi W, Fuse I, Hattori A, et al. Mutations of the platelet thromboxane A2 (TXA2) receptor in patients characterized by the absence of TXA2-induced platelet aggregation despite normal TXA2 binding activity. Thromb Haemost 1999;82:1528–31.

99. Rao AK, Willis J, Kowalska MA, et al. Differential requirements for platelet aggregation and inhibition of adenylate cyclase by epinephrine. Studies of a familial platelpha2-adrenergic receptor defect. Blood 1988;71:494–501.

100. Tamponi G, Pannocchia A, Arduino C, et al. Congenital deficiency of alpha2-adrenoreceptors on human platelets: description of two cases. Thromb Haemost 1987;58:1012–6.

101. Newman KD, Williams LT, Bishopric NH, et al. Identification of alpha-adrenergic receptors in human platelets by 3H-dihydroergocryptine binding. J Clin Invest 1978;61:395–402.

102. Kaywin P, McDonough M, Insel PA, et al. Platelet function in essential thrombocythemia: decreased epinephrine responsivenesss associated with a deficiency of platelet alpha-adrenergic receptors. N Engl J Med 1978;299:505–9.

103. Siess W, Weber PC, Lapetina EG. Activation of phospholipase C is dissociated from arachidonate metabolism during platelet shape change induced by thrombin or platelet-activating factor. Epinephrine does not induce phospholipase C activation or platelet shape change. J Biol Chem 1984;259: 8286–92.

104. Williams A, Woolkalis MJ, Poncz M, et al. Identification of the pertussis toxin-sensitive G proteins in platelets, megakaryocytes and HEL cells. Blood 1990; 76:721–30.

105. Woulfe D, Jiang H, Mortensen R, et al. Activation of Rap1B by Gi family members in platelets. J Biol Chem 2002;277:23382–90.

106. Heemskerk JW, Willems GM, Rook MB, et al. Ragged spiking of free calcium in ADP-stimulated human platelets: regulation of puff-like calcium signals in vitro and ex vivo. J Physiol 2001;535:625–35.

107. Heemskerk JW, Hoyland J, Mason WT, et al. Spiking in cytosolic calcium concentration in single fibrinogen-bound fura-2-loaded human platelets. Biochem J 1992;283:379–83.
108. Purvis JE, Chatterjee MS, Brass LF, et al. A molecular signaling model of platelet phosphoinositide and calcium regulation during homeostasis and P2Y1 activation. Blood 2008;112:4069–79.
109. Varga-Szabo D, Braun A, Nieswandt B. STIM and Orai in platelet function. Cell Calcium 2011;50:270–8.
110. Crittenden JR, Bergmeier W, Zhang Y, et al. CalDAG-GEFI integrates signaling for platelet aggregation and thrombus formation. Nat Med 2004;10:982–6.
111. Rittenhouse-Simmons S, Deykin D. Release and metabolism of arachidonate in human platelets. In: Gordon JL, editor. Platelets in biology and pathology-2. Elsevier/North-Holland; 1981. p. 349–72.
112. Rittenhouse-Simmons S, Russell FA, Deykin D. Mobilization of arachidonic acid in human platelets. Kinetics and Ca2+ dependency. Biochim Biophys Acta 1977;488:370–80.
113. Börsch-Haubold AG, Ghomashchi F, Pasquet S, et al. Phosphorylation of cytosolic phospholipase A2 in platelets is mediated by multiple stress-activated protein kinase pathways. Eur J Biochem 1999;265:195–203.
114. Börsch-Haubold AG, Kramer RM, Watson SP. Cytosolic phospholipase A2 is phosphorylated in collagen- and thrombin-stimulated human platelets independent of protein kinase C and mitogen-activated protein kinase. J Biol Chem 1995;270:25885–92.
115. Jin JG, Quinton TM, Zhang J, et al. Adenosine diphosphate (ADP)-induced thromboxane A2 generation in human platelets requires coordinated signaling through integrin alphaIIbbeta3 and ADP receptors. Blood 2002;99:193–8.
116. Klages B, Brandt U, Simon MI, et al. Activation of G12/G13 results in shape change and Rho/Rho-kinase-mediated myosin light chain phosphorylation in mouse platelets. J Cell Biol 1999;144:745–54.
117. Fukuhara S, Chikumi H, Gutkind JS. RGS-containing RhoGEFs: the missing link between transforming G proteins and Rho? Oncogene 2001;20:1661–8.
118. Wilde JI, Retzer M, Siess W, et al. ADP-induced platelet shape change: an investigation of the signalling pathways involved and their dependence on the method of platelet preparation. Platelets 2000;11:286–95.
119. Pandey D, Goyal P, Bamburg JR, et al. Regulation of LIM-kinase 1 and cofilin in thrombin-stimulated platelets. Blood 2005;107:575–83.
120. Woulfe D, Jiang H, Morgans A, et al. Defects in secretion, aggregation, and thrombus formation in platelets from mice lacking Akt2. J Clin Invest 2004; 113:441–50.
121. Chen J, De S, Damron DS, et al. Impaired platelet responses to thrombin and collagen in AKT-1-deficient mice. Blood 2004;104:1703–10.
122. O'Brien KA, Stojanovic-Terpo A, Hay N, et al. An important role for Akt3 in platelet activation and thrombosis. Blood 2011;118:4215–23.
123. Jackson SP, Schoenwaelder SM, Goncalves I, et al. PI 3-kinase p110beta: a new target for antithrombotic therapy. Nat Med 2005;11:507–14.
124. Brass LF, Zhu L, Stalker TJ. Minding the gaps to promote thrombus growth and stability. J Clin Invest 2005;115:3385–92.
125. Shattil SJ. The beta3 integrin cytoplasmic tail: protein scaffold and control freak. J Thromb Haemost 2009;7(Suppl 1):210–3.
126. Prevost N, Kato H, Bodin L, et al. Platelet integrin adhesive functions and signaling. Meth Enzymol 2007;426:103–15.

127. Stegner D, Nieswandt B. Platelet receptor signaling in thrombus formation. J Mol Med 2011;89:109–21.

128. Shattil SJ, Newman PJ. Integrins: dynamic scaffolds for adhesion and signaling in platelets. Blood 2004;104:1606–15.

129. Calderwood DA, Ginsberg MH. Talin forges the links between integrins and actin. Nat Cell Biol 2003;5:694–7.

130. Calderwood DA, Zent R, Grant R, et al. The talin head domain binds to integrin beta subunit cytoplasmic tails and regulates integrin activation. J Biol Chem 1999;274:28071–4.

131. Tadokoro S, Shattil SJ, Eto K, et al. Talin binding to integrin beta tails: a final common step in integrin activation. Science 2003;302:103–6.

132. Ratnikov BI, Partridge AW, Ginsberg MH. Integrin activation by talin. J Thromb Haemost 2005;3:1783–90.

133. Law DA, DeGuzman FR, Heiser P, et al. Integrin cytoplasmic tyrosine motif is required for outside-in alphaIIbbeta3 signalling and platelet function. Nature 1999;401:808–11.

134. Law DA, Nannizzi-Alaimo L, Ministri K, et al. Genetic and pharmacological analyses of Syk function in alphaIIbbeta3 signaling in platelets. Blood 1999;93: 2645–52.

135. Payrastre B, Missy K, Trumel C, et al. The integrin alphaIIb/beta3 in human platelet signal transduction. Biochem Pharmacol 2000;60:1069–74.

136. Philips DR, Prasad KS, Manganello J, et al. Integrin tyrosine phosphorylation in platelet signaling. Curr Opin Cell Biol 2001;13:546–54.

137. Phillips DR, Nannizzi-Alamio L, Prasad KS. Beta3 tyrosine phosphorylation in alphaIIbbeta3 (platelet membrane GP IIb-IIIa) outside-in integrin signaling. Thromb Haemost 2001;86:246–58.

138. Obergfell A, Eto K, Mocsai A, et al. Coordinate interactions of Csk, Src and Syk kinases with alphaIIbbeta3 initiate integrin signaling to the cytoskeleton. J Cell Biol 2002;157:265–75.

139. Boylan B, Gao C, Rathore V, et al. Identification of FcgammaRIIa as the ITAM-bearing receptor mediating alphaIIbbeta3 outside-in integrin signaling in human platelets. Blood 2008;112:2780–6.

140. Prevost N, Woulfe D, Tanaka T, et al. Interactions between Eph kinases and ephrins provide a mechanism to support platelet aggregation once cell-to-cell contact has occurred. Proc Natl Acad Sci U S A 2002;99:9219–24.

141. Prevost N, Woulfe DS, Tognolini M, et al. Signaling by ephrinB1 and Eph kinases in platelets promotes Rap1 activation, platelet adhesion, and aggregation via effector pathways that do not require phosphorylation of ephrinB1. Blood 2004;103:1348–55.

142. Prevost N, Woulfe DS, Jiang H, et al. Eph kinases and ephrins support thrombus growth and stability by regulating integrin outside-in signaling in platelets. Proc Natl Acad Sci U S A 2005;102:9820–5.

143. Pasterkamp RJ, Giger RJ. Semaphorin function in neural plasticity and disease. Curr Opin Neurobiol 2009;19:263–74.

144. Roth L, Koncina E, Satkauskas S, et al. The many faces of semaphorins: from development to pathology. Cell Mol Life Sci 2009;66:649–66.

145. Gherardi E, Love CA, Esnouf RM, et al. The sema domain. Curr Opin Struct Biol 2004;14:669–78.

146. Negishi M, Oinuma I, Katoh H. Plexins: axon guidance and signal transduction. Cell Mol Life Sci 2005;62:1363–71.

147. Zhu L, Bergmeier W, Wu J, et al. Regulated surface expression and shedding support a dual role for semaphorin 4D in platelet responses to vascular injury. Proc Natl Acad Sci U S A 2007;104:1621–6.

148. Wannemacher KM, Zhu L, Jiang H, et al. Diminished contact-dependent reinforcement of Syk activation underlies impaired thrombus growth in mice lacking Semaphorin 4D. Blood 2010;116:5707–15.

149. Furlong B, Henderson AH, Lewis MJ, et al. Endothelium-derived relaxing factor inhibits in vitro platelet aggregation. Br J Pharmacol 1987;90:687–92.

150. Whittle BJ, Moncada S. Pharmacological interactions between prostacyclin and thromboxanes. Br Med Bull 1983;39:232–8.

151. Weksler BB. Prostacyclin. Prog Hemost Thromb 1982;6:113–38.

152. Yuhki K, Kojima F, Kashiwagi H, et al. Roles of prostanoids in the pathogenesis of cardiovascular diseases: novel insights from knockout mouse studies. Pharmacol Ther 2011;129:195–205.

153. Marcus AJ, Broekman MJ, Drosopoulos JH, et al. The endothelial cell ecto-ADPase responsible for inhibition of platelet function is CD39. J Clin Invest 1997;99:1351–60.

154. Abramow-Newerly M, Roy AA, Nunn C, et al. RGS proteins have a signalling complex: interactions between RGS proteins and GPCRs, effectors, and auxiliary proteins. Cell Signal 2006;18:579–91.

155. Yowe D, Weich N, Prabhudas M, et al. RGS18 is a myeloerythroid lineage-specific regulator of G-protein-signalling molecule highly expressed in megakaryocytes. Biochem J 2001;359:109–18.

156. Nagata Y, Oda M, Nakata H, et al. A novel regulator of G-protein signaling bearing GAP activity for Galphai and Galphaq in megakaryocytes. Blood 2001;97:3051–60.

157. Kim SD, Sung HJ, Park SK, et al. The expression patterns of RGS transcripts in platelets. Platelets 2006;17:493–7.

158. Gagnon AW, Murray DL, Leadley RJ. Cloning and characterization of a novel regulator of G protein signalling in human platelets. Cell Signal 2002;14:595–606.

159. Garcia A, Prabhakar S, Hughan S, et al. Differential proteome analysis of TRAP-activated platelets: involvement of DOK-2 and phosphorylation of RGS proteins. Blood 2004;103:2088–95.

160. Berthebaud M, Riviere C, Jarrier P, et al. RGS16 is a negative regulator of SDF-1-CXCR4 signaling in megakaryocytes. Blood 2005;106:2962–8.

161. Ma P, Cierniewska A, Signarvic R, et al. A newly-identified complex of spinophilin and the tyrosine phosphatase, SHP-1, modulates platelet activation by regulating G protein-dependent signaling. Blood 2012;119:1935–45.

162. Gegenbauer K, Elia G, Blanco-Fernandez A, et al. Regulator of G-protein signaling protein 18 integrates activating and inhibitory signaling in platelets. Blood 2012;119(16):3799–807.

163. Haslam RJ, Dickinson NT, Jang EK. Cyclic nucleotides and phosphodiesterases in platelets. Thromb Haemost 1999;82:412–23.

164. Keularts IM, Van Gorp RM, Feijge MA, et al. Alpha2A-adrenergic receptor stimulation potentiates calcium release in platelets by modulating cAMP levels. J Biol Chem 2000;275:1763–72.

165. Murata T, Ushikubi F, Matsuoka T, et al. Altered pain perception and inflammatory response in mice lacking prostacyclin receptor. Nature 1997;388:678–82.

166. Quinton TM, Dean WL. Cyclic AMP-dependent phosphorylation of the inositol-1,4,5-trisphosphate receptor inhibits Ca2+ release from platelet membranes. Biochem Biophys Res Commun 1992;184:893–9.
167. Grunberg B, Kruse HJ, Negrescu EV, et al. Platelet rap1B phosphorylation is a sensitive marker for the action of cyclic AMP- and cyclic GMP-increasing platelet inhibitors and vasodilators. J Cardiovasc Pharmacol 1995;25:545–51.
168. Grunberg B, Negrescu E, Siess W. Synergistic phosphorylation of platelet rap1B by SIN-1 and iloprost. Eur J Pharmacol 1995;288:329–33.
169. Smolenski A. Novel roles of cAMP/cGMP dependent signaling in platelets. J Thromb Haemost 2011;10(2):167–76.
170. Margarucci L, Roest M, Preisinger C, et al. Collagen stimulation of platelets induces a rapid spatial response of cAMP and cGMP signaling scaffolds. Mol Biosyst 2011;7:2311–9.
171. Wangorsch G, Butt E, Mark R, et al. Time-resolved in silico modeling of fine-tuned cAMP signaling in platelets: feedback loops, titrated phosphorylations and pharmacological modulation. BMC Syst Biol 2011;5:178.
172. Gambaryan S, Kobsar A, Rukoyatkina N, et al. Thrombin and collagen induce a feedback inhibitory signaling pathway in platelets involving dissociation of the catalytic subunit of protein kinase A from an NFkappaB-IkappaB complex. J Biol Chem 2010;285:18352–63.
173. Hayashi H, Sudo T. Effects of the cAMP-elevating agents cilostamide, cilostazol and forskolin on the phosphorylation of Akt and GSK-3beta in platelets. Thromb Haemost 2009;102:327–35.
174. Zahedi RP, Lewandrowski U, Wiesner J, et al. Phosphoproteome of resting human platelets. J Proteome Res 2008;7:526–34.
175. Newman PJ, Newman DK. Signal transduction pathways mediated by PECAM-1: new roles for an old molecule in platelet and vascular cell biology. Arterioscler Thromb Vasc Biol 2003;23:953–64.
176. Jackson DE, Kupcho KR, Newman PJ. Characterization of phosphotyrosine binding motifs in the cytoplasmic domain of platelet/endothelial cell adhesion molecule-1 (PECAM-1) that are required for the cellular association and activation of the protein-tyrosine phosphatase, SHP-2. J Biol Chem 1997;272: 24868–75.
177. Moraes LA, Barrett NE, Jones CI, et al. PECAM-1 regulates collagen-stimulated platelet function by modulating the association of PI3 Kinase with Gab1 and LAT. J Thromb Haemost 2010;8:2530–41.
178. Patil S, Newman DK, Newman PJ. Platelet endothelial cell adhesion molecule-1 serves as an inhibitory receptor that modulates platelet responses to collagen. Blood 2001;97:1727–32.
179. Falati S, Patil S, Gross PL, et al. Platelet PECAM-1 inhibits thrombus formation in vivo. Blood 2006;107:535–41.
180. Huber M, Izzi L, Grondin P, et al. The carboxyl-terminal region of biliary glycoprotein controls its tyrosine phosphorylation and association with protein-tyrosine phosphatases SHP-1 and SHP-2 in epithelial cells. J Biol Chem 1999; 274:335–44.
181. Beauchemin N, Kunath T, Robitaille J, et al. Association of biliary glycoprotein with protein tyrosine phosphatase SHP-1 in malignant colon epithelial cells. Oncogene 1997;14:783–90.
182. Wong C, Liu Y, Yip J, et al. CEACAM1 negatively regulates platelet-collagen interactions and thrombus growth in vitro and in vivo. Blood 2009;113: 1818–28.

183. Stalker TJ, Wu J, Morgans A, et al. Endothelial cell specific adhesion molecule (ESAM) localizes to platelet-platelet contacts and regulates thrombus formation in vivo. J Thromb Haemost 2009;7:1886–96.
184. Naik MU, Stalker TJ, Brass LF, et al. JAM-A protects from thrombosis by suppressing integrin alphaIIbbeta3-dependent outside-in signaling in platelets. Blood 2012;119:3352–60.

Testing Platelet Function

Paul Harrison, BSc, PhD, FRCPath[a],*, Marie Lordkipanidzé, BPharm, PhD[b]

KEYWORDS

- Platelets • Platelet function • Bleeding time • Platelet aggregation
- Antiplatelet drugs

KEY POINTS

- Platelet function testing immediately presents a series of unique problems to any laboratory or clinic. Platelet function testing assesses the dynamics of living cells in contrast to tests that determine a defined quantity or measurement of a clinical biomarker (eg, cholesterol or blood pressure).
- Most platelet function tests have traditionally been used for the diagnosis and management of patients presenting with bleeding problems rather than thrombosis.
- Platelet function testing is poorly standardized and normal quality control measures are often difficult to implement.
- Platelet function tests are increasingly used for monitoring the efficacy of antiplatelet drugs, with the aim of predicting bleeding or thrombosis.
- Current guidelines advise against routine monitoring of antiplatelet therapy with platelet function tests.

INTRODUCTION

It is becoming increasingly clear that platelets are multitalented, with many recently discovered new functions (inflammation, host defense, fetal vascular remodeling, tumor growth and metastasis, and so forth).[1–4] Nevertheless, the best established role of platelets remains that of maintaining normal hemostasis, with any imbalance resulting in pathologic bleeding or thrombosis.[5] Most platelet function tests have traditionally been used for the diagnosis and management of patients presenting with bleeding problems rather than thrombosis.[6] Because platelets are implicated in the development of atherothrombosis, however, which is responsible for considerable mortality and morbidity in the Western world,[7,8] new and existing platelet function

Disclosure Statement: P. Harrison is a consultant for Sysmex UK and has received funding from Siemens Diagnostics and Eli Lilly. His wife is an employee of Instrumentation Laboratory UK. M. Lordkipanidzé has received speaker honoraria from Eli Lilly.
[a] School of Immunity and Infection, University of Birmingham Medical School, Birmingham B15 2TT, UK; [b] Centre for Cardiovascular Sciences, Institute of Biomedical Research, College of Medical and Dental Sciences, University of Birmingham, Edgbaston, Birmingham B15 2TT, UK
* Corresponding author.
E-mail address: P.Harrison.1@bham.ac.uk

Hematol Oncol Clin N Am 27 (2013) 411–441
http://dx.doi.org/10.1016/j.hoc.2013.03.003
0889-8588/13/$ – see front matter © 2013 Elsevier Inc. All rights reserved.

hemonc.theclinics.com

tests are increasingly used for monitoring the efficacy of antiplatelet drugs to treat these conditions and/or to try to identify patients at risk of arterial disease. Conversely, as increasing numbers of patients are being treated with antiplatelet drugs, there is an associated increased risk of bleeding, especially during trauma and surgical procedures. Platelet function tests are, therefore, also increasingly proposed as presurgical/ perioperative tools to aid in the prediction of bleeding and for monitoring the efficacy of various types of prohemostatic therapies. The enhanced clinical need coupled with the development of new, simpler tests and point-of-care (POC) instruments, has resulted in an increasing tendency of platelet function testing to be performed away from specialized clinical or research hemostasis laboratories, where the more traditional and complex tests are still performed.[9,10]

This article discusses currently available clinical tests of platelet function. Although some assays study global hemostasis as a whole, most platelet function assays target a specific phase of platelet function. **Table 1** provides a detailed summary of currently available platelet function and hemostatic tests that depend to some extent on platelets, coupled with their clinical utility, advantages, and disadvantages.

QUALITY CONTROL, BLOOD SAMPLING, AND ANTICOAGULATION

Platelet function testing presents many challenges in ensuring that accurate and meaningful results are obtained. Firstly, unlike with coagulation tests, there are no widely available internal or external quality control materials available. Most assays are performed on fresh blood, so many laboratories either establish normal ranges using control blood obtained from healthy volunteers or assay samples known to be normal in parallel to ensure that each test/reagent is viable.

Many platelet function tests, including the historical gold standard, light transmission aggregometry (LTA), remain poorly standardized. Among the variables, the most commonly cited are the range of agonists and agonist concentrations used, the choice of anticoagulant, and the method used to process the samples. The quality, handling, temperature, and age of a blood sample can cause significant artifacts in platelet analysis. For this reason, most laboratories test platelet function within a narrow time window (<2 hours), although some studies have shown that storage of blood up to 6 hours after drawing had a minimal effect on responses to all agonists, with the exception of ADP.[11] Although the use of citrate is convenient within a coagulation laboratory, because citrate tubes are also used for clotting tests, anticoagulation of a blood sample through calcium chelation can immediately present a problem for platelet function testing because normal platelet function is largely calcium dependent. This problem can be overcome by use of nonchelating anticoagulants (eg, direct thrombin inhibitors, such as hirudin or lepirudin, or D-phenylalanyl-L-prolyl-L-arginine chloromethyl ketone [PPACK]). Because most platelet tests have been traditionally performed with citrated blood samples, however, it is often difficult to compare results between different studies using other anticoagulants. Handling of blood samples can also introduce artifactual activation or desensitization. Tests performed in whole blood present with immediate advantages but also with subtle differences compared with those that use platelet-rich plasma (PRP), which has to be prepared by centrifugation. Artifactual variables should be minimized during phlebotomy, anticoagulation, sample transit, and handling within a laboratory. There are several published guidelines that can help minimize platelet activation and platelet aggregation.[12] These include using a light tourniquet, using a needle of at least 21 gauge, a nontraumatic venipuncture with smooth blood flow, discarding the first few milliliters of blood drawn, using polypropylene or siliconized glass tubes/syringes, ensuring immediate gentle mixing with anticoagulant,

Table 1
An alphabetical list of many of the currently used tests of platelet function and global hemostatic tests with a significant dependence on platelet number and function

Name of Test	Principle	Advantages	Disadvantages	Frequency of Use	Clinical Applications
Adenine nucleotides	Measurement of total and released nucleotides by HPLC or luminescence	Sensitive	Sample preparation, assay calibration, extra equipment	Widely used in specialized laboratories, usually in conjunction with LTA	Diagnosis of storage and release defects
AspirinWorks	Immunoassay of urinary 11-dehydrothromboxane B_2	Measures stable thromboxane metabolite, dependent on COX-1 activity	Indirect assay, not platelet specific, renal function dependent	Increasing use	Monitoring aspirin therapy and identifying poor responders at increased risk of thrombosis
Bleeding time	In vivo cessation of blood flow	In vivo test, physiologic POC	Insensitive, invasive, scarring, high CV	Was widely used, now less popular	Screening test
Blood smear	Microscopic analysis of blood cell on glass slide	Diagnostic	Artifacts can occur	Widely used	Detection of abnormalities in platelet size, number and granules, and leukocyte inclusion bodies
Clot retraction	Measures platelet interaction with fibrin	Simple	Nonspecific	Not widely used	Detection of abnormalities in integrin $\alpha IIb\beta 3$ and fibrinogen

(continued on next page)

Table 1
(continued)

Name of Test	Principle	Advantages	Disadvantages	Frequency of Use	Clinical Applications
Combined aggregometry and luminescence	Combined WBA or LTA and nucleotide release	Monitors release reaction with secondary aggregation	Semiquantitative	Widely used in specialized laboratories, although less than LTA	Diagnosis of a wide variety of acquired and inherited platelet defects, diagnosis of storage and release defects
Electron microscopy	Ultrastructural analysis of platelets	Diagnostic. Whole mount technique useful for dense granular imaging	Expensive, specialized equipment	Only available in special units	Detection of granular and ultrastructural defects, whole mount method can detect dense granular defects
Flow cytometry	Measurement of platelet glycoproteins and activation markers by fluorescence	Whole blood test, small blood volumes, wide variety of tests	Specialized operator, expensive, samples prone to artifact unless carefully prepared	Widely used	Diagnosis of platelet glycoprotein defects, quantification of glycoproteins, detection of platelet activation in vivo or in response to agonists, monitoring antiplatelet therapy (eg, VASP phosphorylation to monitor P2Y$_{12}$ inhibition)
Full blood count	Automated impedance and/or flow cytometry–based analysis of cells	Rapid, precise, provides platelet distribution and MPV	Less accuracy and precision at $<20 \times 10^9$/L	Widely used	Abnormalities in platelet number, size, and distribution; immature platelet fraction now available

Ichor Plateletworks	Platelet counting preactivation and postactivation	Rapid, simple, POC, small blood volume	Indirect test measuring count after aggregation	Used in surgery and cardiology	Monitoring antiplatelet drugs, prediction of bleeding
Impact cone and plate(let) analyzer	Quantification of high shear platelet adhesion/aggregation onto surface	Small blood volume required, high shear, rapid, simple, research (variable) and fixed versions available POC	Dependent on fibrinogen and VWF for adhesion of platelets	Mainly research but increasing use	Detection of inherited and acquired defects in primary hemostasis, detection of platelet hyperfunction, monitoring antiplatelet therapy
Kinetic aggregometer	Monitoring fluorescent platelet accumulation within a thrombus forming in a collagen-coated capillary	Sensitive to amplification pathways	Specialized laboratories only	Mainly Research	Monitoring antiplatelet therapy, detection of defects in primary hemostasis
Laser platelet aggregometer (PA-200)	Monitoring aggregation using a laser	Detection of microaggregates, sensitive	Little widespread experience	Little widespread experience	Detection of platelet hyperfunction
LTA	Low shear platelet-to-platelet aggregation in response to classic agonists	Gold standard	Time-consuming, sample preparation, poorly standardized	Widely used in specialized laboratories	Diagnosis of a wide variety of acquired and inherited platelet defects
96 Well plate LTA (Optimul assay)	Similar to LTA but in 96 well plate	Lower blood/PRP volumes than LTA. Many replicates and dose response curves possible	Little widespread experience	Little widespread experience	Detection of defects in primary hemostasis
Microfluidic devices	Miniaturized multichannel devices	Whole blood, real-time thrombus formation	Little widespread experience	Research only at present	Detection of defects in primary hemostasis

(continued on next page)

Table 1
(continued)

Name of Test	Principle	Advantages	Disadvantages	Frequency of Use	Clinical Applications
PFA-100/200	High shear platelet adhesion and aggregation during formation of a platelet plug	Whole blood test, high shear, small blood volumes, simple, rapid, POC	Inflexible, VWF-dependent, Hct-dependent, insensitive to clopidogrel	Widely used	Detection of inherited and acquired defects in primary hemostasis, monitoring aspirin, monitoring DDAVP therapy
PlaCor PRT	High shear thrombus formation in duplicate channels Blood oscillates through a narrowed channel with a spring to hold the thrombus	POC; finger prick blood	Little widespread experience	Little widespread experience	Rapid detection of SNPs and gene defects
Platelet genome or transcriptome analysis	Total mRNA content by microarray technology	Detection of all mRNAs in platelets and MKs	Instability of mRNA, possible impurity of starting material	Research only at present	Detection of novel gene mutations or transcription defects
Proteomic analysis	Measures total individual protein content	Sensitivity increasing	Loss of some membrane glycoproteins, possible impurity of starting material	Research only at present	Detection of protein deficiencies
Serum thromboxane B_2	Immunoassay	Dependent on COX-1 activity	Prone to artifact, not platelet specific	Widespread use	Monitoring aspirin therapy, detection of thromboxane production defects
Soluble platelet release markers and sheddome (eg, PF4, βTG, sCD40L, sCD62P, GPV and GPVI)	Usually by ELISA	Relatively simple	Prone to artifact during blood collection and processing	Fairly widely used in research	Detection of in vivo platelet activation

Sonoclot analyzer	Impedance detection of changes of viscoelastic properties of celite-activated blood sample	Global test, POC, platelet count and function dependent	Measures clot properties only	Widely used in surgery and anesthesiology	Prediction of surgical bleeding, aid to blood product usage
Thromboelastography (TEG or ROTEM)	Monitoring rate and quality of clot formation	Global whole blood test, POC	Measures clot properties only, largely platelet independent unless platelet activators are used	Widely used in surgery and anesthesiology	Prediction of surgical bleeding, aid to blood product usage, monitoring rFVIIa therapy, new platelet mapping system can be used to monitor antiplatelet therapy (eg, aspirin or clopidogrel)
ThromboLUX	Dynamic light scattering of platelet quality	Simple, measures size and light intensity of platelets and microvesicles	Designed for platelet concentrates only	Little Widespread experience	Assessment of platelet concentrates
VASP	Flow cytometric measurement of vasodilator stimulated phosphoprotein	Measurement of $P2Y_{12}$ occupancy	Requires flow cytometer Insensitive to intermediate inhibition of $P2Y_{12}$	Increasing use	Monitoring $P2Y_{12}$ receptor activity
VerifyNow	Fully automated platelet aggregometer to measure antiplatelet therapy	Simple, POC, 3 test cartridges (aspirin, $P2Y_{12}$, and GP IIb-IIIa)	Inflexible, cartridges can only be used for single purpose	Increasing use	Monitoring antiplatelet therapy
WBA	Monitors changes in impedance in response to classic agonists	Whole blood test, multichannel version available.	Older instruments require electrodes to be cleaned and recycled	Widely used in specialized laboratories, although less than LTA	Diagnosis of a wide variety of acquired and inherited platelet defects

Abbreviations: βTG, β-thromboglobulin; CV, coefficient of variation; DDAVP, desmopressin; ELISA, enzyme-linked immunoassay; Hct, hematocrit; MK, megakaryocytes; MPV, mean platelet volume; mRNA, messenger RNA; PF4, platelet factor 4; rFVIIa, recombinant activated factor VII; sCD40L, soluble CD40 ligand; sCD62P, soluble CD62P (P-selectin); SNP, single-nucleotide polymorphism.

minimizing delays from sampling to analysis, keeping all tubes at room temperature, checking that blood tubes are not overfilled or underfilled, and avoiding unnecessary manipulation of the sample.[12] These measures are most often used when performing the sensitive technique of measuring platelet activation by flow cytometry, but it could be argued that they should also be implemented when performing any platelet function testing. Many potential problems with samples are commonly overlooked and this may explain the wide interlaboratory variability reported for platelet function testing. Therefore, ensuring sample quality is of utmost importance before any platelet function testing is performed.

THE IN VIVO BLEEDING TIME

Platelet function testing began with the application of in vivo bleeding time by Duke in 1910.[13] The technique consists of inflicting a small incision in the skin of the forearm or the earlobe and recording the time required for a clot to form at the site of the incision and to stop the flow of blood. The bleeding time was further refined by the Ivy technique and the availability of commercial spring-loaded template disposable devices containing sterile blades (eg, Simplate II, Organon Teknika) (**Fig. 1**). It was regarded as the most useful screening test of platelet function until the early 1990s.[6,14,15]

Advantages and Limitations of the Assay

The bleeding time test is simple; it measures physiologic hemostasis, including the role of the vessel wall components and does not require expensive equipment or a specialized laboratory. Despite its simplicity, the bleeding time is poorly reproducible, invasive,

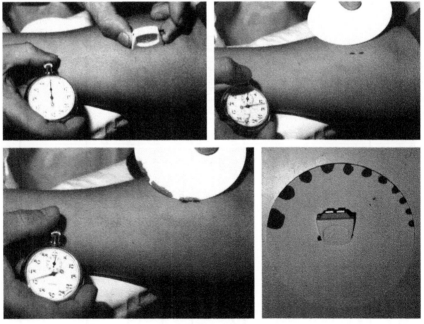

Fig. 1. The in vivo bleeding time test performed with a Simplate II device. Horizontal cuts are made into a cleaned area of forearm skin, excess blood blotted onto filter paper, and the time to cessation of bleeding recorded. (*Courtesy of* Professor Sam Machin, Department of Haematology, University College Hospital, London, UK; with permission.)

insensitive to many mild platelet defects, and time-consuming. In addition, the bleeding time fails to correlate with the bleeding tendency, and an accurate bleeding history is a more valuable screening test.[16–18] As a consequence of these limitations, the widespread use of the bleeding time test has rapidly declined over the past 15 to 20 years, to be replaced by other less-invasive platelet function assays.[16–18] Although a recent UK survey demonstrated that the bleeding time test is widely used in some centers,[19] recent guidelines recommend that it should not be used as a screening test.[12]

LIGHT TRANSMISSION AGGREGOMETRY

LTA, also known as turbidimetric or optical aggregometry, was invented in the 1960s and soon revolutionized the identification and diagnosis of primary hemostatic defects.[20,21] LTA is still regarded as the gold standard of platelet function testing and remains among the most used in specialized laboratories for the identification and diagnosis of many platelet defects.[9,22,23] Briefly, platelet aggregation is measured by analysis of the transmission of light through a sample of PRP obtained by centrifuging anticoagulated whole blood at low g-force.[24] By definition, PRP is a turbid suspension of cells, which significantly reduces light transmission. After addition of a platelet agonist, formation of aggregates reduces the turbidity of the suspension, resulting in increased light transmission (100% light transmission is set with platelet-poor plasma [PPP]). The dynamics of platelet aggregation (expressed as a percentage) are, therefore, measured in real time as platelets aggregate. In recent years, commercial aggregometers have become easier to use with multichannel capability, simple automatic setting of 100% and 0% baselines, and computer operation and storage of results (**Fig. 2**). Some lumiaggregometers can also measure the secretion of nucleotides during aggregation by simultaneously measuring luminescence.[25]

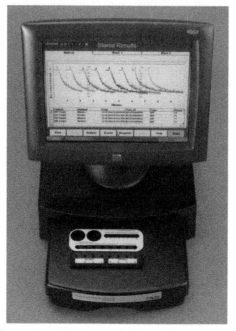

Fig. 2. An example of a modern 8-channel platelet aggregometer. The model shown is the Bio/Data PAP-8E. (*Courtesy of* Biodata, Horsham, PA; with permission.)

Advantages and Limitations of the Assay

Platelet activation and ensuing aggregation measured by LTA can be induced by many agonists and agonist concentrations.[26,27] As a result, LTA offers the possibility of studying platelet activation pathways in detail and has been the preferred platelet function assay in most specialized clinical laboratories over the past 50 years because it correlates with bleeding and ischemic outcomes.[23,28]

Although considered the most useful diagnostic and research tool, LTA is nonphysiologic, because separated platelets are usually stirred under low shear conditions during the test and only form aggregates after addition of agonists, conditions that do not accurately mimic platelet adhesion, activation, and aggregation on vessel wall damage.[9,22,23] As with most platelet function assays, results are influenced by platelet count, making it unsuitable in severely thrombocytopenic patients.[23] Also, conventional LTA using a full panel of agonists requires large blood volumes and significant expertise to perform the tests and to interpret the tracings, triggering the development of new, easier-to-use platelet function assays (see **Table 1**).

Clinical Applications

Most laboratories perform LTA with a panel of different concentrations of classical agonists (eg, ADP, collagen, epinephrine, arachidonic acid, and ristocetin) and sometimes an extended panel of agonists (thrombin receptor activating peptide [TRAP], collagen-related peptide, calcium ionophore, thromboxane mimetics, such as U46619, and so forth), although the exact range of agonists and their concentrations remain poorly standardized between laboratories.[27,29,30] Nonetheless, LTA is still regarded as the gold standard for platelet function testing and remains the most useful technique for diagnosing a wide variety of platelet defects as well as monitoring antiplatelet therapy. Recent efforts to standardize LTA have been published and are available online from the International Society on Thrombosis and Haemostasis Platelet Physiology Subcommittee of the Scientific and Standardization Committee.[12,27,31,32]

MODIFIED 96 WELL PLATE ASSAY FOR PLATELET AGGREGATION

In an attempt to reduce the blood volume necessary for assessment of platelet aggregation yet retain the flexibility of LTA derived from testing multiple platelet activation pathways with specific agonists, several laboratories have developed a modified technique based on light transmission principles but applied to standard 96 well plates.[33–37] The technique requires the same preparatory steps as LTA (ie, isolation of PRP and PPP from whole blood by centrifugation) and, therefore, has similar applications and restrictions. Addition of PRP to wells with platelet agonists either precoated onto the plate or in solution triggers platelet activation and aggregation when the plate is stirred, which changes the absorbance of light passing through the 96 well plate assay. The assessment of platelet function is, therefore, simply assessed by measuring absorbance in a conventional plate reader, which most laboratories possess. Absorbance can be measured either kinetically or as an endpoint (eg, after 5 minutes) and is then converted into percentage of aggregation in similar fashion to LTA based on measuring both control PRP and PPP samples.[36,37]

Advantages and Limitations of the Assay

Just as for LTA, platelet activation and ensuing aggregation can be induced by numerous agonists at varying concentrations, which allows for extensive testing of the different platelet activation pathways. The major advantage of this assay, however, is a drastic reduction in the volume of blood/PRP required and the time required to run the test. Because all agonists are studied simultaneously in up to 96 wells, this technique can provide a rapid assessment of most platelet activation pathways within minutes, including detailed dose-response curves (with replicates), which are rarely obtainable from LTA due to blood volume restrictions, the number of channels available, and time. The availability of standardized lyophilized 96 well plates with a range of agonists at standard concentrations available from a central source could also improve the interlaboratory variation of this assay.[37] Results also can potentially be uploaded to a central server to check quality control of each assay and calculate the results online.

The assay remains experimental and clinical experience with this assay is limited.[34,36,37] As a consequence, how the 96 well plate assay compares with classical LTA is not known. Because of the similarities between the 2 assays, the limitations of LTA also apply to the 96 well plate assay, except the time requirement for an experienced operator.

Clinical Applications

In theory, clinical applications for the 96 well plate assay would be similar to LTA; however, this has not yet been tested in large clinical studies. In a research setting, the assay seems promising for the clinical diagnosis of bleeding disorders as well as for monitoring antiplatelet therapy.[33,34,36–39]

WHOLE BLOOD AGGREGOMETRY

Whole blood aggregometry (WBA) provides a means to study platelet function within anticoagulated whole blood without any sample processing.[40] The test measures the change in resistance or impedance between 2 electrodes as platelets adhere and aggregate in response to classical agonists.[9,22,23,28] The original Chrono-Log instrument was a 2-channel device with luminescence capability, which has been updated to become a fully computerized 2-channel or 4-channel instrument (**Fig. 3**). Although

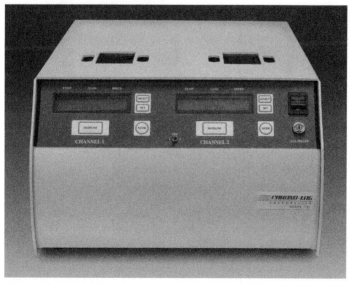

Fig. 3. The Chrono-log Model 700 whole blood/optical 2-channel lumiaggregometer. (*Courtesy of* Chrono-log, Havertown, PA; with permission.)

the earlier versions of this apparatus required electrodes to be carefully cleaned to remove platelet aggregates after each use, the technology now allows for disposable single-use electrodes.

In recent years, a new 5-channel, computerized WBA instrument (Multiplate, Verum Diagnostica) (**Fig. 4**) has gained general favor in clinical laboratories, because it is fully automated and uses disposable cuvettes/electrodes with a range of diverse agonists for different applications, including diagnosis of bleeding and monitoring antiplatelet therapy.[41–45] Although the basic methodologies are similar, the way results are reported are different between the Chrono-Log (in Ω, the maximal amplitude of impedance achieved) and Multiplate (in arbitrary units, as area under the curve achieved over 6 minutes of aggregation).

Advantages and Limitations of the Assay

WBA has many significant advantages, including analysis of platelets in their more natural milieu, the use of smaller sample volumes, and the immediate analysis of samples without manipulation, loss of time, or potential loss of platelet subpopulations or platelet activation during centrifugation. Like LTA, WBA allows for multiple agonists and agonist concentrations, thus allowing for a detailed study of various platelet activation pathways. The manufacturer of Multiplate also offers a full range of standardized agonists for different purposes.

WBA is, however, influenced by several factors, which include the delay between blood sampling and platelet function testing, the anticoagulant used, the platelet count, the hematocrit, and the temperature of the blood.[46–48] Samples also require the addition of a 1:1 ratio of saline, which introduces a significant dilution factor. Furthermore, within each donor, variation tends to be slightly higher than LTA, the test requires technical expertise, and it is expensive.[9] Perhaps most importantly, WBA correlates poorly with LTA and its ability to predict clinical outcomes is debated.[28,48–53]

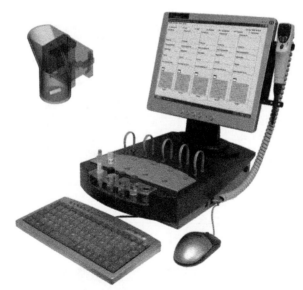

Fig. 4. The Multiplate multiple platelet function 5-channel impedance analyzer. The inset illustrates the disposable cuvettes with electrodes and stir bar. (*Courtesy of* Roche Diagnostics, Burgess Hill, West Sussex, UK; with permission.)

Clinical Applications

WBA has been used to detect and identify congenital and acquired platelet receptor defects as well as monitoring antiplatelet therapy.[48] There is growing interest in using the Multiplate system for near-patient whole blood platelet analysis and antiplatelet therapy monitoring and in identifying patients at increased risk of perioperative bleeding.[41–45,52,54–57]

VERIFYNOW

The VerifyNow (Accumetrics, San Diego, CA) instrument is a whole blood, fully automated POC test specifically developed to monitor antiplatelet therapy.[58] The basis of the VerifyNow assay is that fibrinogen-coated polystyrene beads agglutinate in whole blood in proportion to the number of glycoprotein (GP) IIb-IIIa receptors activated by a specific stimulus, which can be blocked by antiplatelet agents (**Fig. 5**).[58] The VerifyNow system has 3 types of single-use, disposable cartridges that can be used to monitor different antiplatelet drugs: aspirin, clopidogrel, and GPIIb-IIIa antagonists.[58] In the case of aspirin, the agonist used is arachidonic acid, whereas a combination of adenosine diphosphate (ADP) and prostaglandin E_1 is used to monitor the antiplatelet effect of clopidogrel, and TRAP is used to monitor GPIIb-IIIa antagonists.

Blood samples anticoagulated with sodium citrate are inserted into a disposable plastic cartridge containing a lyophilized preparation of human fibrinogen-coated beads, a platelet agonist, buffer, and preservative. Because agglutination of beads occurs after stimulation with the platelet agonist, light transmission through the sample is increased and is converted into aspirin response units for the aspirin cartridge; $P2Y_{12}$ response units and percent inhibition (calculated by comparing the test channel with a TRAP reference channel) for the $P2Y_{12}$ cartridge; and platelet aggregation units for the GPIIb-IIIa cartridge, via a proprietary algorithm.[58,59]

Advantages and Limitations of the Assay

The VerifyNow instrument is a considerable advance, because the test is a fully automated, POC test without the requirements of sample transport, time delays, or a specialized laboratory and it can provide immediate information. The assay can

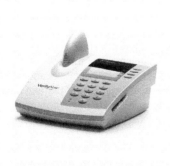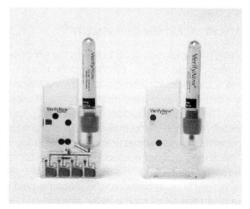

Fig. 5. The VerifyNow instrument. (*Courtesy of* Accumetrics, San Diego, CA; with permission.)

predict future adverse cardiovascular events in patients requiring dual antiplatelet therapy with aspirin and clopidogrel, although the incremental value of platelet function testing on top of classical clinical predictors of worse prognosis was only minimal.[52,57]

Factors influencing performance of the assay include time from blood sampling to testing, platelet count, hematocrit, blood triglyceride, and fibrinogen levels.[58,60] Also, the VerifyNow assay is expensive.

Clinical Applications

The VerifyNow system was specifically designed for monitoring 3 different classes of antiplatelet drugs (ie, aspirin, clopidogrel, and GPIIb-IIIa antagonists). The assay cannot currently be used for any other purpose.

PLATELET COUNT RATIO

It is also possible to monitor platelet aggregometry in whole blood by a simple platelet counting technique. After addition of an agonist to anticoagulated stirred whole blood, platelets aggregate, and the number of free platelets decreases compared with a control tube.[61–65] The Plateletworks aggregation kits and Ichor full blood counter (Helena Biosciences) are simply based on comparing platelet counts within a control EDTA tube and after aggregation with platelet agonists within citrated tubes.[61,66–69]

Advantages and Limitations of the Assay

The main advantage of this assay is its ease of use and wide availability in clinical laboratories, because only a cell counter is required.[9,28,61] As the assay is carried out in whole blood, no sample preparation is required, and platelet interactions with other blood cells are preserved.

Factors influencing this assay remain for the most part unknown, because the assay is seldom used in clinical laboratories despite its apparent advantages. Many laboratories prefer to use their in-house version of the assay.[62,65]

Clinical Applications

Clinical experience with this assay is limited. Plateletworks has been shown, however, to correlate with adverse cardiovascular events in patients requiring dual antiplatelet therapy with aspirin and clopidogrel.[52,57] As for the VerifyNow assay, the incremental value of platelet function testing on top of classical clinical predictors of worse prognosis was only minimal.[52,57]

PLATELET SECRETION ASSESSMENT

Platelet degranulation contributes to the process of platelet activation. Because platelet granules contain various prothrombotic molecules, assessment of the level of some of these substances in plasma or blood can also provide an estimate of platelet activation.[70] The most frequently used assay of platelet secretion is assessment of platelet nucleotides. The simplest approach to measuring nucleotides is to use a lumiaggregometer. Alternatively, high-performance liquid chromatography (HPLC) or bioluminescent measurement of lysed platelet preparations at standardized counts offer 2 other approaches to measuring platelet nucleotides. Flow cytometric analysis of mepacrine uptake and release from granules can also been used.[71,72] Release reactions can also be measured by a variety of tests based on the measurement of platelet granule constituents (eg, uptake and release of radiolabeled serotonin, platelet factor 4, β-thromboglobulin, and ADP/ATP) before and after degranulation with a strong platelet agonist.

Advantages and Limitations of the Assay

LTA is not 100% sensitive to storage pool and release defects. Therefore, studying stored and released nucleotides simultaneously with platelet aggregation increases the diagnostic accuracy of the assay.[73]

Platelet secretion must be normalized to a standardized platelet count to be comparable between individuals. There is, however, no common standard for evaluation of platelet secretion, which requires each laboratory to set up its own standard reference ranges.

Clinical Applications

Many laboratories do not routinely assess release reactions and, if relying on LTA alone, may, therefore, not always detect all release defects, which, according to some investigators, may be surprisingly common.[30,74,75] Some aggregometers are particularly useful because they can provide simultaneous measurement of ATP luminescence during the aggregation response and, as expected, demonstrate the release reaction during secondary aggregation. Thus, any defects in storage or release can be simultaneously determined along with the LTA tracing.[73,76]

THROMBOXANE METABOLITES

Thromboxane A_2 (TXA_2) is a short-lived, lipid mediator synthesized by platelets from arachidonic acid and released from the phospholipid membrane on platelet activation.[77,78] Its main role is in amplification of platelet activation and recruitment of additional platelets to the site of injury.[79] Derived by the sequential action of cyclooxygenase (COX)-1 and thromboxane synthase on arachidonic acid, TXA_2 activates the thromboxane receptor on surrounding platelets and is rapidly degraded in plasma to inactive metabolites within 30 seconds.[77,78] Because of its short half-life, TXA_2 cannot be easily measured in biologic samples; however, stable metabolites of TXA_2 are measurable in both blood and urine. The most commonly studied metabolites are TXB_2 and 11-dehydro-TXB_2.[80,81]

Quantitation of TXB_2 is usually carried out by immunoassays or mass spectrometry, either in serum derived from whole blood allowed to clot at 37°C for 30 to 60 minutes[82] or in PRP after platelet activation and aggregation.[83] TXB_2 is rapidly cleared from the circulation (half-life 7 minutes) and is further converted to stable metabolites, including 11-dehydro-TXB_2, the half-life of which is approximately 60 minutes.[84] Whereas only approximately 2.5% of TXB_2 is excreted unchanged in the urine,[85] 11-dehydro-TXB_2 is the major form found in urine and thus can be measured noninvasively.[81,85]

Advantages and Limitations of the Assay

Measurements of TXA_2 metabolites in either blood or urine provide a direct assessment of the COX pathway in vivo. There is a large discrepancy, however, between the capacity (300–400 ng/mL) and the endogenous biosynthesis of TXA_2 (1–2 pg/mL) by platelets.[84,86] For this reason, the measurement of TXB_2 in either serum or plasma is believed to be prone to artifactual platelet activation during sampling.[81]

Clinical Applications

Because this assay measures directly the formation of TXA_2 metabolites, it is particularly useful for evaluating the efficacy of drugs inhibiting the COX pathway. It is, therefore, used to assess the efficacy of aspirin to inhibit its pharmacologic target.

The assay can also be used in patients with bleeding disorders. In the presence of an abnormal platelet response to arachidonic acid, measurement of TXA_2 metabolites can be used to differentiate an anomaly in the platelet's ability to produce TXA_2 from a lack of response from the thromboxane receptor.

ASSESSMENT OF THE PLATELET SHEDDOME

The platelet plasma membrane harbors many of the proteins required for platelet function, supporting the different phases leading to platelet aggregation. In recent years, evidence suggests that the protein content of the platelet plasma membrane is not static and that platelets that undergo activation can dynamically regulate the proteins present on their surface, either by incorporating new proteins (eg, P-selectin from α-granules),[87] by internalizing certain proteins (such as the adenosine receptors),[88] or by proteolytically cleaving certain surface proteins.[89] The platelet sheddome encompasses a growing list of these protein fragments released from the platelet surface by proteinases, such as ADAM17 or ADAM10.[90,91] In a recent study, Fong and colleagues[89] have identified 1048 proteins in the supernatant of activated platelets, 69 of which are possibly platelet-shed proteins. The best-characterized examples of proteins shed from activated platelets are GPIbα, soluble CD62P, soluble CD40L, and GPVI.[89,90,92]

Advantages and Limitations of the Assay

Accurate measurement of in vivo circulating platelet-released proteins is challenging, because any ex vivo platelet activation may lead to artifactual protein shedding. The majority of published studies of shed glycoproteins levels were performed in serum obtained after letting blood clot, which requires platelet activation, and thus releases large amounts of shed proteins ex vivo.[93] This can be circumvented by using plasma instead of serum, but plasma preparation needs to be performed carefully so as not to activate platelets during their removal from plasma.[94]

Clinical Applications

Although many of the shed markers have been shown to play important roles in platelet and vascular biology, the full implications of this shedding process are largely unknown.[89] Nevertheless, measurement of components of the sheddome may prove useful as sensitive and specific biomarkers of platelet activation in vivo. Clinical experience with assessing new markers of the platelet sheddome remains, however, limited.[90,94,95] Soluble P-selectin is historically the most widely used shed platelet activation marker and has been shown to increase in various pathologic conditions.[96,97] Soluble P-selectin is, however, in part derived from endothelial cells.[96]

FLOW CYTOMETRIC ANALYSIS OF PLATELET FUNCTION

In the past 20 years, flow cytometric analysis of platelets has developed into a powerful and popular means to study many aspects of platelet biology and function.[98] Preferred modern methods use diluted anticoagulated whole blood incubated with a variety of reagents, including antibodies and dyes that bind specifically to individual platelet proteins, granules, and lipid membranes.[99–101] The most common platelet activation markers assessed by flow cytometry are P-selectin expression on the platelet surface (as a marker of α-granule secretion), the conformational change in integrin αIIbβ3 into its active state (measured with monoclonal antibody PAC-1), platelet-leukocyte conjugates, and phosphorylation of vasodilator-stimulated phosphoprotein (VASP), as a marker of $P2Y_{12}$ receptor activation-dependent signaling.

Advantages and Limitations of the Assay

Measurements of platelet markers by flow cytometry can be carried out in a small volume of whole blood, thus avoiding sample preparation steps and allowing for a physiologic milieu for platelet interactions.[100,101] Moreover, the test can be performed independently of platelet count, making the assay useful in patients with thrombocytopenia.[100]

Among the disadvantages of the assay, the cost and the requirement for a specialized technician are the most important.[101] The necessity to study platelet function within 45 minutes of blood collection can be bypassed by fixation of the blood sample.[100] The interpretation of results remains somewhat subjective, which makes the results of this assay difficult to compare from one laboratory to another; however, efforts have been made to standardize the use of flow cytometry for platelet function testing.[100,102]

Clinical Applications

Briefly, flow cytometric analysis of platelets is commonly used to measure platelet count, to determine the state of activation of platelets, to diagnose anomalies in number or function of platelet receptors, to monitor efficacy of antiplatelet drugs, and to assess platelet turnover.

PLATELET FUNCTION ANALYZER (PFA-100/200)

The platelet function analyzer (PFA)-100 device has been available for several years and is in widespread use in many clinical and research laboratories.[103,104] The test was originally developed by Kratzer and Born[105] as a prototype instrument, the Thrombostat 4000, and further developed into the PFA-100 and the PFA-200 (Siemens).[106,107] The PFA-200 is a modern update of the original PFA-100 device first released in the mid-1990s (**Fig. 6**). The update of the instrument should not affect the test results because this is a cartridge-based assay, in which a small volume of blood

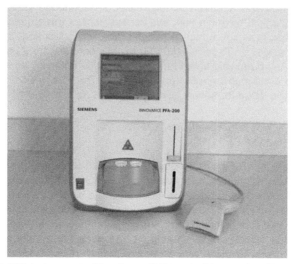

Fig. 6. The PFA-200 instrument. (*Courtesy of* Siemens Diagnostics, New York, NY; with permission.)

is aspirated through an aperture (150 μm in diameter) in a membrane coated with collagen and ADP (CADP cartridge) or collagen and epinephrine (CEPI cartridge).[108] These platelet activators combine with the high shear conditions induced by aspiration of blood through the cartridge to activate platelets, resulting in platelet plug formation, which eventually occludes the aperture. The instrument monitors the drop in flow rate and the time required to obtain full occlusion of the aperture is reported as closure time (CT), up to a maximum of 300 seconds. Because these 2 cartridges have been shown to be largely insensitive to $P2Y_{12}$ receptor inhibitors, a third INNOVANCE PFA P2Y cartridge is now available for detecting this class of drugs.[109–111] The cartridge contains a smaller aperture of 100 μm and the membrane is coated with a combination of ADP and prostaglandin E_1 supplemented with calcium.

Advantages and Limitations of the Assay

This global test of platelet function is simple and rapid, does not require substantial specialist training, and only requires 0.8 mL of blood per cartridge.[23] It is a whole blood assay and, therefore, avoids any sample preparation. The CT is influenced by platelet count and hematocrit and results need to be carefully interpreted in patients with a platelet count or hematocrit below 50 × 10^9/L or 25%, respectively.[9,22,23,112] Due to the high shear conditions within the cartridge capillary and aperture, the test is highly dependent on von Willebrand factor (VWF) levels, which makes it suitable for screening of von Willebrand disease (VWD) but makes it unsuitable for platelet function testing in this cohort.[113] Because the PFA-100 is also often insensitive to the detection of mild platelet function defects, including secretion and release defects, it offers an optional but limited screening tool for detecting platelet function disorders.[12,114] The CT is also influenced by the nature of the anticoagulant used, in particular the concentration of sodium citrate used as anticoagulant, with 3.8% giving greater stability in CT readings.[115]

Clinical Applications

Clinical applications of PFA-100/200 are numerous and have been recently reviewed.[104,114] They include screening for VWD and its treatment monitoring, identification of inherited and acquired platelet defects, monitoring antiplatelet therapy, assessment of surgical bleeding risk, and assessment of thrombotic risk. The PFA-100/200, however, is a global test of platelet (and VWF) function; it is not specific for any platelet defect.[104] The PFA-100/200 might, therefore, be a useful but limited screening test. Any putative platelet function defect detected by prolongation of the CT needs to be confirmed by more specific tests. The PFA-100/200 offers a good negative predictive value for severe platelet function defects and type II and type III VWD.[12,114]

THROMBOELASTOGRAPHY

Thromboelastography (TEG) was developed more than 50 years ago.[116–118] The older instrument has been significantly upgraded to the modern TEG analyzer 5000 series (**Fig. 7**). Anticoagulated whole blood is incubated in a heated sample cup in which a pin is suspended that is connected to a computer.[119] The cup oscillates 5° in each direction. In normal anticoagulated blood, the pin is unaffected, but as the blood clots, any impediment in motion of the cup is then transmitted to the pin. Whole blood or recalcified plasma can be used, with or without activators of the tissue factor or contact factor pathways.[119] Rotational TEG (ROTEM) is an adaptation of the TEG in which the cup is stationary and the pin oscillates (**Fig. 8**).[117–119]

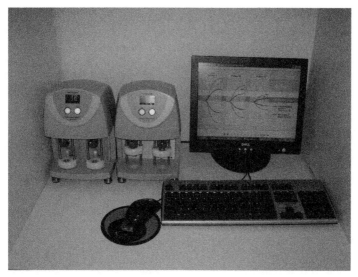

Fig. 7. The Haemoscope TEG instrument.

TEG provides various data relating to clot formation and fibrinolysis (the lag time before the clot starts to form, the rate at which clotting occurs, the maximal amplitude of the trace or clot strength, and the extent and rate of amplitude reduction). With the PlateletMapping system, arachidonic acid and ADP can be used as agonists to pre-activate platelets within the TEG system, thus making the assay theoretically suitable to monitor antiplatelet drugs, although the test lacks sensitivity to detect moderate changes in platelet function.[64,119,120]

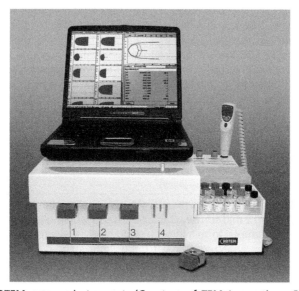

Fig. 8. The ROTEM gamma instrument. (*Courtesy of* TEM Innovations GmbH, Munich, Germany; with permission.)

Advantages and Limitations of the Assay

TEG/ROTEM tests are rapid to perform (<30 minutes) and have traditionally been used as POC tests in surgical departments. Their main advantage is to provide a complete profile of clot formation, including the kinetics of clotting, clot strength, and fibrinolysis. Both tests thus provide a global portrait of clot formation within whole blood and allow for interactions between whole blood elements, including platelets and the coagulation system.

In an attempt to show reproducibility and consistency using TEG/ROTEM, a group of investigators from different countries have formed the TEG-ROTEM Working Group.[121] Their initial observations suggest that there is significant interlaboratory variation. Also, both tests exhibit relative insensitivity to various aspects of platelet function and they are, therefore, not routinely recommended for platelet function testing.

Clinical Applications

Unlike more-specific platelet function tests, these instruments have been traditionally used within surgical and anesthesiology departments as POC tests for determining the risk of bleeding and as a guide to transfusion requirements.[119,122] Despite their widespread clinical use, interlaboratory variation can be problematic. The TEG Platelet-Mapping system has been used to monitor antiplatelet therapy.

CONE AND PLATE(LET) ANALYZER (IMPACT)

The cone and plate(let) analyzer was originally developed by Varon to monitor platelet adhesion to a plate coated with collagen or extracellular matrix under high shear conditions of 1800 s^{-1}.[123–125] Further refinements of the analyzer have introduced a polystyrene surface to which plasma proteins, in particular fibrinogen and VWF, are immobilized and form a thrombogenic surface.[126] The commercial version of the device, the Impact R (Matis Medical), is composed of a mobile cone and a stationary plate in which a small volume of blood (0.13 mL) is introduced manually (**Fig. 9**). The shear created by the rotating cone stimulates platelets to adhere to the plate over a fixed time interval. Excess blood is then washed away before adhered platelets are stained and visualized by a microscope and image analysis software that takes a series of successive images of the plate. The software calculates several parameters, including surface coverage and average size, and provides a distribution histogram of adhered platelets. There is also a recently released fully automated version of the instrument called the Impact (Matis Medical). There is a range of research instruments available, including the Impact RS (with shear rate between 25 s^{-1} and 400 s^{-1}), the Impact RHS (with high shear rates between 1930 s^{-1} to 13,000 s^{-1}), and the Impact RP (that mimics pulsatile blood flow).

Advantages and Limitations of the Assay

The assay is fully automated, requires a small blood volume and no blood processing, and is simple and rapid to use. Because it uses whole blood at variable shear rates, the system attempts to mimic a physiologically relevant milieu for platelets. When normal blood is analyzed, platelet deposition is shear dependent and time dependent, reaching maximal levels within 2 minutes at high shear rate (1800 s^{-1}).[126]

The assay is, however, dependent on hematocrit levels, with a sharp decrease in platelet deposition at hematocrit levels below 30%.[127] The assay is also dependent on platelet count, with close to linear reduction in platelet deposition with decreases

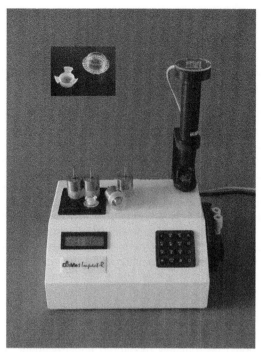

Fig. 9. The DiaMed Impact-R device. The cone and plate are shown in the inset. (*Courtesy of* Matis Medical, Inc, Beersel, Belgium; with permission.)

in platelet numbers.[127] As a result, the assay may be of limited use in patients with thrombocytopenia.

Clinical Applications

Clinical experience with this device is limited and there are few publications using this instrument in large patient cohorts. The assay has been reported as a predictor of bleeding in patients with thrombocytopenia,[124,128] and in patients undergoing cardiopulmonary bypass surgery.[129] The assay has been used to screen children with a positive history of bleeding for platelet defects but was found of little use when clinical variables were taken into account.[130] With a modified technique requiring priming of platelets with specific agonists prior to shear induction, the assay has been tested in patients taking antiplatelet agents but has been shown to be of limited use in this context.[123,131]

SUMMARY AND THE FUTURE OF PLATELET FUNCTION TESTING

Up until the late 1980s, the only clinical platelet function tests that were available were the bleeding time, LTA, and various biochemical assays.[6] These were mainly performed within specialized research and clinical laboratories. Around this time, many researchers began to use flow cytometry to study various aspects of platelet biology and this soon led to the widespread commercial availability of reagents (antibodies and dyes). In a short space of time, flow cytometry has, therefore, become an important tool both in the clinical and research laboratory. With the recent convergence of flow cytometric and impedance principles within many commercial full blood counters, an increasing number of fully automated platelet parameters can be determined within these analyzers without the need of a specialized operator. These parameters include immunologic platelet counting,[132,133] measurement of platelet activation, and determination of the immature platelet fraction.[134,135]

In the early 1990s, it was realized that the bleeding time was unreliable as a screening test despite its widespread use. Although LTA has become an indispensable gold standard test for the diagnosis of many platelet-related disorders, it is well recognized that it does not accurately simulate all aspects of platelet function and its utility is significantly limited outside of specialized laboratories. Although many researchers were already using flow chambers and microscopy to study platelet behavior under conditions that simulate in vivo conditions more accurately, these tests were restricted to specialized laboratories and were, therefore, not ideally suitable for routine clinical applications. This, coupled with the limitations of both LTA and the bleeding time, paved the way for the development of several easy-to-use, prototype PFAs. Not surprisingly, there has been a high casualty rate among the first generation of these instruments, because commercialization requires a large capital investment to overcome many hurdles in the development of a reliable clinical test. Nevertheless, several different prototypes have been fully developed into commercial instruments that are widely available to both clinical and research laboratories. These include the PFA-100/200, VerifyNow, Impact, Plateletworks, and modifications of the TEG. Some of these instruments have Food and Drug Administration approval for a variety of different applications. Although many of these tests have potential clinical utility, more research is required to determine whether routine testing will provide clinically relevant data and whether antiplatelet therapy should be routinely monitored and treatment adapted or titrated based on the result of a platelet function test. Monitoring $P2Y_{12}$ inhibition could offer the potential of tailoring therapy by identifying poor responders to clopidogrel and optimizing the levels of platelet inhibition using alternative drugs, such as prasugrel or ticagrelor.[136] In 2010, the Food and Drug Administration added a boxed warning to clopidogrel to alert prescribers to the possibility of CYP genetic polymorphisms resulting in poor metabolism and poor clopidogrel responsiveness[137] but without giving any guidance on how to manage such patients. The American Heart Association and the American College of Cardiology Foundation have recently published a consensus document giving a class IIb recommendation (level of evidence C) for the use of platelet function or genetic testing by recommending a selective and limited approach to testing until better evidence exists.[138] This debate has also recently been thoroughly reviewed in 2 articles for and against testing under the common theme, "Do platelet function testing and genotyping improve outcome in patients treated with antithrombotic agents."[139,140] Whether these tests can reliably predict thrombosis or bleeding and monitor prohemostatic therapy in various settings also needs to be determined. Large randomized controlled trials are required to determine the true prognostic and therapeutic value of any existing or new platelet function test.

It is ironic that intravital microscopy of platelets, originally described by Bizzozero in 1882, has become a powerful research tool for studying the role of platelets in thrombosis.[141] With significant advances in microscopy and digital imaging/processing, it is now possible to perform real-time imaging of fluorescently labeled platelets and hemostatic system components during thrombus formation within animal models.[142] This has already resulted in many exciting discoveries about platelets and their dynamic interactions with the vessel wall and coagulation system. Future platelet function instruments could, therefore, be based on studying the interaction of fluorescently tagged platelets with subendothelial matrix protein-coated surfaces under flow conditions that closely mimic in vivo conditions. One such potential

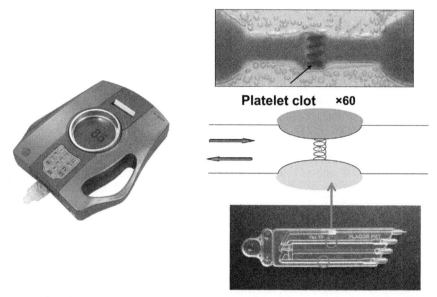

Fig. 10. The PlaCor PRT device. Nonanticoagulated blood from a finger prick is taken up into a disposable cartridge, which contains 2 microfluidic channels containing a narrowed aperture and a spring. The blood is oscillated back and forward through the reaction channels and the high shear conditions activate the platelets resulting in thrombus formation, which is held in position by the spring. The instrument measures the time to occlusion of the 2 channels in seconds. (*Courtesy of* PlaCor, Inc, Plymouth, MN; with permission.)

example is a kinetic platelet aggregometer that provides sensitive information about the rate of fluorescent platelet adhesion and thrombus stabilization in real time.[143] This type of technology could potentially be developed into multichannel and miniaturized microfluidic versions (eg, the Cellix VenaFlux platform using various biochips and the Fluxion BioFlux platform).[144-151]

There will be increasing development of more POC assays (eg, the PlaCor PRT), which use a small volume of nonanticoagulated finger prick blood within a disposable cartridge (**Fig. 10**).[152] Advances in the definition of both the platelet genome and proteome have led to many recent discoveries in platelet biology. Use of these technologies within specifically designed arrays or chips (covering just the key genes/proteins that are known to be defective in a range of disorders) could potentially revolutionize not only the diagnosis of inherited defects in platelet function but also also the rapid identification of individuals with increased risk of bleeding or thrombosis. The availability of cheaper deep-sequencing technology in the near future will also open up the possibility of mass screening of patients with both bleeding and thrombotic disorders.[153] Platelet function testing is, therefore, at a particularly interesting stage, because the development of new technologies and new instruments may have future utility in a variety of different clinical and laboratory settings.

REFERENCES

1. Feng W, Madajka M, Kerr BA, et al. A novel role for platelet secretion in angiogenesis: mediating bone marrow-derived cell mobilization and homing. Blood 2011;117(14):3893–902.

2. Nurden AT. Platelets, inflammation and tissue regeneration. Thromb Haemost 2011;105(Suppl 1):S13–33.
3. Bertozzi CC, Hess PR, Kahn ML. Platelets: covert regulators of lymphatic development. Arterioscler Thromb Vasc Biol 2010;30(12):2368–71.
4. Watson SP, Herbert JM, Pollitt AY. GPVI and CLEC-2 in hemostasis and vascular integrity. J Thromb Haemost 2010;8(7):1456–67.
5. George JN. Platelets. Lancet 2000;355(9214):1531–9.
6. The British Society for Haematology BCSH, Thrombosis Task F. Guidelines on platelet function testing. J Clin Pathol 1988;41(12):1322–30.
7. Gawaz M, Langer H, May AE. Platelets in inflammation and atherogenesis. J Clin Invest 2005;115(12):3378–84.
8. Ruggeri ZM. Platelets in atherothrombosis. Nat Med 2002;8(11):1227–34.
9. Harrison P. Progress in the assessment of platelet function. Br J Haematol 2000; 111(3):733–44.
10. Harrison P. Platelet function analysis. Blood Rev 2005;19(2):111–23.
11. Dawood BB, Wilde J, Watson SP. Reference curves for aggregation and ATP secretion to aid diagnose of platelet-based bleeding disorders: effect of inhibition of ADP and thromboxane A(2) pathways. Platelets 2007;18(5): 329–45.
12. Harrison P, Mackie I, Mumford A, et al. Guidelines for the laboratory investigation of heritable disorders of platelet function. Br J Haematol 2011; 155(1):30–44.
13. Duke WW. The relation of blood platelets to hemorrhagic disease. Description of a method for determining the bleeding time and the coagulation time and report of three cases of hemorrahagic disease relieved by blood transfusion. JAMA 1910;55:1185–92.
14. Harker LA, Hanson SR, Wilcox JN, et al. Antithrombotic and antilesion benefits without hemorrhagic risks by inhibiting tissue factor pathway. Haemostasis 1996; 26(Suppl 1):76–82.
15. Nilsson IM, Magnusson S, Borchgrevink C. The Duke and Ivy methods for determination of the bleeding time. Thromb Diath Haemorrh 1963;10:223–34.
16. Rodgers RP, Levin J. A critical reappraisal of the bleeding time. Semin Thromb Hemost 1990;16(1):1–20.
17. Lind SE. The bleeding time does not predict surgical bleeding. Blood 1991; 77(12):2547–52.
18. Peterson P, Hayes TE, Arkin CF, et al. The preoperative bleeding time test lacks clinical benefit: College of American Pathologists' and American Society of Clinical Pathologists' position article. Arch Surg 1998;133(2):134–9.
19. Jennings I, Woods TA, Kitchen S, et al. Platelet function testing: practice among UK National External Quality Assessment Scheme for Blood Coagulation participants, 2006. J Clin Pathol 2008;61(8):950–4.
20. Born GV. Aggregation of blood platelets by adenosine diphosphate and its reversal. Nature 1962;194:927–9.
21. O'Brien JM. Platelet Aggregation. II. Some results from a new method of study. J Clin Pathol 1962;15:452–81.
22. Michelson AD. Platelet function testing in cardiovascular diseases. Circulation 2004;110(19):e489–93.
23. Rand ML, Leung R, Packham MA. Platelet function assays. Transfus Apheresis Sci 2003;28(3):307–17.
24. Born GV, Cross MJ. The aggregation of blood platelets. J Physiol 1963;168: 178–95.

25. Pai M, Wang G, Moffat KA, et al. Diagnostic usefulness of a lumi-aggregometer adenosine triphosphate release assay for the assessment of platelet function disorders. Am J Clin Pathol 2011;136(3):350–8.
26. Zhou L, Schmaier AH. Platelet aggregation testing in platelet-rich plasma: description of procedures with the aim to develop standards in the field. Am J Clin Pathol 2005;123(2):172–83.
27. Hayward CP, Moffat KA, Raby A, et al. Development of North American consensus guidelines for medical laboratories that perform and interpret platelet function testing using light transmission aggregometry. Am J Clin Pathol 2010;134(6):955–63.
28. Nicholson NS, Panzer-Knodle SG, Haas NF, et al. Assessment of platelet function assays. Am Heart J 1998;135(5 Pt 2 Su):S170–8.
29. Cattaneo M, Hayward CP, Moffat KA, et al. Results of a worldwide survey on the assessment of platelet function by light transmission aggregometry: a report from the platelet physiology subcommittee of the SSC of the ISTH. J Thromb Haemost 2009;7(6):1029.
30. Moffat KA, Ledford-Kraemer MR, Nichols WL, et al. Variability in clinical laboratory practice in testing for disorders of platelet function: results of two surveys of the North American Specialized Coagulation Laboratory Association. Thromb Haemost 2005;93(3):549–53.
31. Christie DJ, Avari T, Carrington LR, et al. Platelet function testing by aggregometry: approved guideline. Wayne (PA): Clinical and Laboratory Standards Institute; 2008;28(31):1–45.
32. Cattaneo M, Cerletti C, Harrison P, et al. Recommendations for the standardization of light transmission aggregometry: A consensus of the working party from the Platelet Physiology Subcommittee of SSC/ISTH. J Thromb Haemost, in press.
33. Sun B, Tandon NN, Yamamoto N, et al. Luminometric assay of platelet activation in 96-well microplate. Biotechniques 2001;31(5):1174, 1176, 1178 passim.
34. Armstrong PC, Dhanji AR, Truss NJ, et al. Utility of 96-well plate aggregometry and measurement of thrombi adhesion to determine aspirin and clopidogrel effectiveness. Thromb Haemost 2009;102(4):772–8.
35. Moran N, Kiernan A, Dunne E, et al. Monitoring modulators of platelet aggregation in a microtiter plate assay. Anal Biochem 2006;357(1):77–84.
36. Chan MV, Armstrong PC, Papalia F, et al. Optical multichannel (optimul) platelet aggregometry in 96-well plates as an additional method of platelet reactivity testing. Platelets 2011;22(7):485–94.
37. Chan MV, Warner TD. Standardised optical multichannel (optimul) platelet aggregometry using high-speed shaking and fixed time point readings. Platelets 2012;23(5):404–8.
38. Mylotte D, Peace AJ, Tedesco AT, et al. Clopidogrel discontinuation and platelet reactivity following coronary stenting. J Thromb Haemost 2011;9(1):24–32.
39. Peace AJ, Tedesco AF, Foley DP, et al. Dual antiplatelet therapy unmasks distinct platelet reactivity in patients with coronary artery disease. J Thromb Haemost 2008;6(12):2027–34.
40. Cardinal DC, Flower RJ. The electronic aggregometer: a novel device for assessing platelet behavior in blood. J Pharmacol Methods 1980;3(2):135–58.
41. Seyfert UT, Haubelt H, Vogt A, et al. Variables influencing Multiplate(TM) whole blood impedance platelet aggregometry and turbidimetric platelet aggregation in healthy individuals. Platelets 2007;18(3):199–206.
42. Mueller T, Dieplinger B, Poelz W, et al. Utility of whole blood impedance aggregometry for the assessment of clopidogrel action using the novel Multiplate

analyzer—comparison with two flow cytometric methods. Thromb Res 2007; 121(2):249–58.

43. Paniccia R, Antonucci E, Maggini N, et al. Assessment of platelet function on whole blood by multiple electrode aggregometry in high-risk patients with coronary artery disease receiving antiplatelet therapy. Am J Clin Pathol 2009;131(6):834–42.

44. Valarche V, Desconclois C, Boutekedjiret T, et al. Multiplate whole blood impedance aggregometry: a new tool for von Willebrand disease. J Thromb Haemost 2011;9(8):1645–7.

45. Solomon C, Traintinger S, Ziegler B, et al. Platelet function following trauma. A Multiple Electrode Aggregometry study. Thromb Haemost 2011;106(2): 322–30.

46. Haubelt H, Anders C, Hellstern P. Can platelet function tests predict the clinical efficacy of aspirin? Semin Thromb Hemost 2005;31(4):404–10.

47. Stissing T, Dridi NP, Ostrowski SR, et al. The influence of low platelet count on whole blood aggregometry assessed by multiplate. Clin Appl Thromb Hemost 2011;17(6):E211–7.

48. McGlasson DL, Fritsma GA. Whole blood platelet aggregometry and platelet function testing. Semin Thromb Hemost 2009;35(2):168–80.

49. Storey RF, May JA, Wilcox RG, et al. A whole blood assay of inhibition of platelet aggregation by glycoprotein IIb/IIIa antagonists: comparison with other aggregation methodologies. Thromb Haemost 1999;82(4):1307–11.

50. Lordkipanidzé M, Pharand C, Nguyen T, et al. Comparison of four tests to assess inhibition of platelet function by clopidogrel in stable coronary artery disease patients. Eur Heart J 2008;29:2877–85.

51. Lordkipanidzé M, Pharand C, Schampaert E, et al. A comparison of six major platelet function tests to determine the prevalence of aspirin resistance in patients with stable coronary artery disease. Eur Heart J 2007;28(14):1702–8.

52. Breet NJ, van Werkum JW, Bouman HJ, et al. Comparison of platelet function tests in predicting clinical outcome in patients undergoing coronary stent implantation. JAMA 2010;303(8):754–62.

53. Sibbing D, Braun S, Morath T, et al. Platelet reactivity after clopidogrel treatment assessed with point-of-care analysis and early drug-eluting stent thrombosis. J Am Coll Cardiol 2009;53(10):849–56.

54. Ranucci M, Baryshnikova E, Soro G, et al. Multiple electrode whole-blood aggregometry and bleeding in cardiac surgery patients receiving thienopyridines. Ann Thorac Surg 2011;91(1):123–9.

55. Hofer CK, Zollinger A, Ganter MT. Perioperative assessment of platelet function in patients under antiplatelet therapy. Expert Rev Med Devices 2010;7(5): 625–37.

56. Sibbing D, Steinhubl SR, Schulz S, et al. Platelet aggregation and its association with stent thrombosis and bleeding in clopidogrel-treated patients: initial evidence of a therapeutic window. J Am Coll Cardiol 2010;56(4):317–8.

57. Breet NJ, van Werkum JW, Bouman HJ, et al. High on-aspirin platelet reactivity as measured with aggregation-based, cyclooxygenase-1 inhibition sensitive platelet function tests is associated with the occurrence of atherothrombotic events. J Thromb Haemost 2010;8(10):2140–8.

58. van Werkum JW, Harmsze AM, Elsenberg EH, et al. The use of the VerifyNow system to monitor antiplatelet therapy: a review of the current evidence. Platelets 2008;19(7):479–88.

59. Michelson AD, Frelinger AL III, Furman MI. Current options in platelet function testing. Am J Cardiol 2006;98(10A):4N–10N.

60. Wang JC, Aucoin-Barry D, Manuelian D, et al. Incidence of aspirin nonresponsiveness using the Ultegra Rapid Platelet Function Assay-ASA. Am J Cardiol 2003;92(12):1492–4.
61. Campbell J, Ridgway H, Carville D. Plateletworks: a novel point of care platelet function screen. Mol Diagn Ther 2008;12(4):253–8.
62. Fox SC, Burgess-Wilson M, Heptinstall S, et al. Platelet aggregation in whole blood determined using the Ultra-Flo 100 Platelet Counter. Thromb Haemost 1982;48(3):327–9.
63. Heptinstall S, Fox S, Crawford J, et al. Inhibition of platelet aggregation in whole blood by dipyridamole and aspirin. Thromb Res 1986;42(2):215–23.
64. Blais N, Pharand C, Lordkipanidzé M, et al. Response to aspirin in healthy individuals. Cross-comparison of light transmission aggregometry, VerifyNow system, platelet count drop, thromboelastography (TEG) and urinary 11-dehydrothromboxane B(2). Thromb Haemost 2009;102(2):404–11.
65. Lordkipanidzé M, Pharand C, Schampaert E, et al. Evaluation of the platelet count drop method for assessment of platelet function in comparison with "gold standard" light transmission aggregometry. Thromb Res 2009;124(4):418–22.
66. Carville DG, Schleckser PA, Guyer KE, et al. Whole blood platelet function assay on the ICHOR point-of-care hematology analyzer. J Extra Corpor Technol 1998;30(4):171–7.
67. Craft RM, Chavez JJ, Snider CC, et al. Comparison of modified Thrombelastograph and Plateletworks whole blood assays to optical platelet aggregation for monitoring reversal of clopidogrel inhibition in elective surgery patients. J Lab Clin Med 2005;145(6):309–15.
68. White MM, Krishnan R, Kueter TJ, et al. The use of the point of care Helena ICHOR/Plateletworks and the Accumetrics Ultegra RPFA for assessment of platelet function with GPIIB-IIIa antagonists. J Thromb Thrombolysis 2004;18(3):163–9.
69. Lennon MJ, Gibbs NM, Weightman WM, et al. A comparison of Plateletworks and platelet aggregometry for the assessment of aspirin-related platelet dysfunction in cardiac surgical patients. J Cardiothorac Vasc Anesth 2004;18(2):136–40.
70. Yardumian DA, Mackie IJ, Machin SJ. Laboratory investigation of platelet function: a review of methodology. J Clin Pathol 1986;39(7):701–12.
71. Wall JE, Buijs-Wilts M, Arnold JT, et al. A flow cytometric assay using mepacrine for study of uptake and release of platelet dense granule contents. Br J Haematol 1995;89(2):380–5.
72. Gordon N, Thom J, Cole C, et al. Rapid detection of hereditary and acquired platelet storage pool deficiency by flow cytometry. Br J Haematol 1995;89(1):117–23.
73. Cattaneo M. Light transmission aggregometry and ATP release for the diagnostic assessment of platelet function. Semin Thromb Hemost 2009;35(2):158–67.
74. Cattaneo M. Inherited platelet-based bleeding disorders. J Thromb Haemost 2003;1(7):1628–36.
75. Hayward CP. Diagnostic evaluation of platelet function disorders. Blood Rev 2011;25(4):169–73.
76. White MM, Foust JT, Mauer AM, et al. Assessment of lumiaggregometry for research and clinical laboratories. Thromb Haemost 1992;67(5):572–7.
77. Nakahata N. Thromboxane A2: physiology/pathophysiology, cellular signal transduction and pharmacology. Pharmacol Ther 2008;118(1):18–35.

78. Hamberg M, Svensson J, Samuelsson B. Thromboxanes: a new group of biologically active compounds derived from prostaglandin endoperoxides. Proc Natl Acad Sci U S A 1975;72(8):2994–8.

79. FitzGerald GA. Mechanisms of platelet activation: thromboxane A2 as an amplifying signal for other agonists. Am J Cardiol 1991;68(7):11B–5B.

80. FitzGerald GA, Oates JA, Hawiger J, et al. Endogenous biosynthesis of prostacyclin and thromboxane and platelet function during chronic administration of aspirin in man. J Clin Invest 1983;71(3):676–88.

81. Catella F, Healy D, Lawson JA, et al. 11-Dehydrothromboxane B2: a quantitative index of thromboxane A2 formation in the human circulation. Proc Natl Acad Sci U S A 1986;83(16):5861–5.

82. Cox D, Maree AO, Dooley M, et al. Effect of enteric coating on antiplatelet activity of low-dose aspirin in healthy volunteers. Stroke 2006;37(8):2153–8.

83. Cornelissen J, Kirtland S, Lim E, et al. Biological efficacy of low against medium dose aspirin regimen after coronary surgery: analysis of platelet function. Thromb Haemost 2006;95(3):476–82.

84. Patrono C, Ciabattoni G, Pugliese F, et al. Estimated rate of thromboxane secretion into the circulation of normal humans. J Clin Invest 1986;77(2):590–4.

85. Roberts LJ 2nd, Sweetman BJ, Oates JA. Metabolism of thromboxane B2 in man. Identification of twenty urinary metabolites. J Biol Chem 1981;256(16):8384–93.

86. Patrono C, Ciabattoni G, Pinca E, et al. Low dose aspirin and inhibition of thromboxane B2 production in healthy subjects. Thromb Res 1980;17(3–4):317–27.

87. Furie B, Furie BC, Flaumenhaft R. A journey with platelet P-selectin: the molecular basis of granule secretion, signalling and cell adhesion. Thromb Haemost 2001;86(1):214–21.

88. Mundell S, Kelly E. Adenosine receptor desensitization and trafficking. Biochim Biophys Acta 2011;1808(5):1319–28.

89. Fong KP, Barry C, Tran AN, et al. Deciphering the human platelet sheddome. Blood 2011;117(1):e15–26.

90. Gardiner EE, Karunakaran D, Shen Y, et al. Controlled shedding of platelet glycoprotein (GP)VI and GPIb-IX-V by ADAM family metalloproteinases. J Thromb Haemost 2007;5(7):1530–7.

91. Qiao JL, Shen Y, Gardiner EE, et al. Proteolysis of platelet receptors in humans and other species. Biol Chem 2010;391(8):893–900.

92. Bergmeier W, Piffath CL, Cheng G, et al. Tumor necrosis factor-alpha-converting enzyme (ADAM17) mediates GPIbalpha shedding from platelets in vitro and in vivo. Circ Res 2004;95(7):677–83.

93. Conde ID, Kleiman NS. Soluble CD40 ligand in acute coronary syndromes. N Engl J Med 2003;348(25):2575–7 [author reply: 2575–7].

94. Al-Tamimi M, Mu FT, Moroi M, et al. Measuring soluble platelet glycoprotein VI in human plasma by ELISA. Platelets 2009;20(3):143–9.

95. Blann AD, Lanza F, Galajda P, et al. Increased platelet glycoprotein V levels in patients with coronary and peripheral atherosclerosis–the influence of aspirin and cigarette smoking. Thromb Haemost 2001;86(3):777–83.

96. Chong BH, Murray B, Berndt MC, et al. Plasma P-selectin is increased in thrombotic consumptive platelet disorders. Blood 1994;83(6):1535–41.

97. Ikeda H, Takajo Y, Ichiki K, et al. Increased soluble form of P-selectin in patients with unstable angina. Circulation 1995;92(7):1693–6.

98. Linden MD, Frelinger AL III, Barnard MR, et al. Application of flow cytometry to platelet disorders. Semin Thromb Hemost 2004;30(5):501–11.

99. Michelson AD, Furman MI. Laboratory markers of platelet activation and their clinical significance. Curr Opin Hematol 1999;6(5):342–8.
100. Schmitz G, Rothe G, Ruf A, et al. European Working Group on Clinical Cell Analysis: consensus protocol for the flow cytometric characterisation of platelet function. Thromb Haemost 1998;79(5):885–96.
101. Michelson AD. Flow cytometry: a clinical test of platelet function. Blood 1996; 87(12):4925–36.
102. Matzdorff A. Platelet function tests and flow cytometry to monitor antiplatelet therapy. Semin Thromb Hemost 2005;31(4):393–9.
103. Harrison P. The role of PFA-100 testing in the investigation and management of haemostatic defects in children and adults. Br J Haematol 2005;130(1): 3–10.
104. Favaloro EJ. Clinical Utility of the PFA-100. Semin Thromb Hemost 2008;34(8): 709–33.
105. Kratzer MA, Born GV. Simulation of primary haemostasis in vitro. Haemostasis 1985;15(6):357–62.
106. Kundu SK, Heilmann EJ, Sio R, et al. Description of an in vitro platelet function analyzer—PFA-100. Semin Thromb Hemost 1995;21(Suppl 2):106–12.
107. Kundu SK, Heilmann EJ, Sio R, et al. Characterization of an in vitro platelet function analyzer—PFA-100. Clin Appl Thromb Hemost 1996;2:241–9.
108. Favaloro EJ. Utility of the PFA-100 for assessing bleeding disorders and monitoring therapy: a review of analytical variables, benefits and limitations. Haemophilia 2001;7(2):170–9.
109. Koessler J, Kobsar AL, Rajkovic MS, et al. The new INNOVANCE PFA P2Y cartridge is sensitive to the detection of the P2Y12 receptor inhibition. Platelets 2011;22:19–25.
110. Linnemann B, Schwonberg J, Rechner AR, et al. Assessment of clopidogrel non-response by the PFA-100 system using the new test cartridge INNOVANCE PFA P2Y. Ann Hematol 2010;89(6):597–605.
111. Edwards A, Jakubowski JA, Rechner AR, et al. Evaluation of the INNOVANCE PFA P2Y test cartridge: sensitivity to P2Y(12) blockade and influence of anticoagulant. Platelets 2012;23(2):106–15.
112. Carcao MD, Blanchette VS, Stephens D, et al. Assessment of thrombocytopenic disorders using the Platelet Function Analyzer (PFA-100). Br J Haematol 2002; 117(4):961–4.
113. Favaloro EJ. Clinical application of the PFA-100. Curr Opin Hematol 2002;9(5): 407–15.
114. Hayward CP, Harrison P, Cattaneo M, et al. Platelet function analyzer (PFA)-100 closure time in the evaluation of platelet disorders and platelet function. J Thromb Haemost 2006;4(2):312–9.
115. Jilma B. Platelet function analyzer (PFA-100): a tool to quantify congenital or acquired platelet dysfunction. J Lab Clin Med 2001;138(3):152–63.
116. Hartert H. Thrombelastography, a method for physical analysis of blood coagulation. Z Gesamte Exp Med 1951;117(2):189–203.
117. Luddington RJ. Thrombelastography/thromboelastometry. Clin Lab Haematol 2005;27(2):81–90.
118. Salooja N, Perry DJ. Thrombelastography. Blood Coagul Fibrinolysis 2001;12(5): 327–37.
119. Chen A, Teruya J. Global hemostasis testing thromboelastography: old technology, new applications. Clin Lab Med 2009;29(2):391–407.

120. Scharbert G, Auer A, Kozek-Langenecker S. Evaluation of the Platelet Mapping Assay on rotational thromboelastometry ROTEM. Platelets 2009;20(2): 125–30.
121. Chitlur M, Sorensen B, Rivard GE, et al. Standardization of thromboelastography: a report from the TEG-ROTEM working group. Haemophilia 2011; 17(3):532–7.
122. Afshari A, Wikkelso A, Brok J, et al. Thrombelastography (TEG) or thromboelastometry (ROTEM) to monitor haemotherapy versus usual care in patients with massive transfusion. Cochrane Database Syst Rev 2011;(3):CD007871.
123. Spectre G, Brill A, Gural A, et al. A new point-of-care method for monitoring antiplatelet therapy: application of the cone and plate(let) analyzer. Platelets 2005; 16(5):293–9.
124. Kenet G, Lubetsky A, Shenkman B, et al. Cone and platelet analyser (CPA): a new test for the prediction of bleeding among thrombocytopenic patients. Br J Haematol 1998;101(2):255–9.
125. Varon D, Lashevski I, Brenner B, et al. Cone and plate(let) analyzer: monitoring glycoprotein IIb/IIIa antagonists and von Willebrand disease replacement therapy by testing platelet deposition under flow conditions. Am Heart J 1998; 135(5):S187–93.
126. Shenkman B, Savion N, Dardik R, et al. Testing of platelet deposition on polystyrene surface under flow conditions by the cone and plate(let) analyzer: role of platelet activation, fibrinogen and von Willebrand factor. Thromb Res 2000; 99(4):353–61.
127. Varon D, Dardik R, Shenkman B, et al. A new method for quantitative analysis of whole blood platelet interaction with extracellular matrix under flow conditions. Thromb Res 1997;85(4):283–94.
128. Misgav M, Shenkman B, Budnik I, et al. Differential roles of fibrinogen and von Willebrand factor on clot formation and platelet adhesion in reconstituted and immune thrombocytopenia. Anesth Analg 2011;112(5):1034–40.
129. Gerrah R, Snir E, Brill A, et al. Platelet function changes as monitored by cone and plate(let) analyzer during beating heart surgery. Heart Surg Forum 2004; 7(3):E191–5.
130. Revel-Vilk S, Varon D, Shai E, et al. Evaluation of children with a suspected bleeding disorder applying the Impact-R [Cone and Plate(let) Analyzer]. J Thromb Haemost 2009;7(12):1990–6.
131. van Werkum JW, Bouman HJ, Breet NJ, et al. The Cone-and-Plate(let) analyzer is not suitable to monitor clopidogrel therapy: a comparison with the flowcytometric VASP assay and optical aggregometry. Thromb Res 2010;126(1):44–9.
132. Harrison P, Ault KA, Chapman S, et al. An interlaboratory study of a candidate reference method for platelet counting. Am J Clin Pathol 2001;115(3):448–59.
133. Kunz D, Kunz WS, Scott CS, et al. Automated CD61 immunoplatelet analysis of thrombocytopenic samples. Br J Haematol 2001;112(3):584–92.
134. Abe Y, Wada H, Tomatsu H, et al. A simple technique to determine thrombopoiesis level using immature platelet fraction (IPF). Thromb Res 2006;118(4): 463–9.
135. Briggs C, Kunka S, Hart D, et al. Assessment of an immature platelet fraction (IPF) in peripheral thrombocytopenia. Br J Haematol 2004;126(1):93–9.
136. Bonello L, Tantry US, Marcucci R, et al; Working Group on High On-Treatment Platelet Reactivity. Consensus and future directions on the definition of high on-treatment platelet reactivity to adenosine diphosphate. J Am Coll Cardiol 2010;56(12):919–33.

137. Smock KJ, Saunders PJ, Rodgers GM, et al. Laboratory evaluation of clopidogrel responsiveness by platelet function and genetic methods. Am J Hematol 2011;86(12):1032–4.

138. Wright RS, Anderson JL, Adams CD, et al. 2011 ACCF/AHA Focused Update of the Guidelines for the Management of Patients With Unstable Angina/Non-ST-Elevation Myocardial Infarction (Updating the 2007 Guideline): a report of the American College of Cardiology Foundation/American Heart Association Task Force on Practice Guidelines. Circulation 2011;123(18):2022–60.

139. Krishna V, Diamond GA, Kaul S. The role of platelet reactivity and genotype testing in the prevention of atherothrombotic cardiovascular events remains unproven. Circulation 2012;125(10):1288–303.

140. Gurbel PA, Tantry US. Platelet function testing and genotyping improve outcome in patients treated with antithrombotic agents. Circulation 2012; 125(10):1276–87.

141. de Gaetano G. A new blood corpuscle: an impossible interview with Giulio Bizzozero. Thromb Haemost 2001;86(4):973–9.

142. Furie B, Furie BC. Thrombus formation in vivo. J Clin Invest 2005;115(12): 3355–62.

143. Phillips DR, Conley PB, Sinha U, et al. Therapeutic approaches in arterial thrombosis. J Thromb Haemost 2005;3(8):1577–89.

144. Tovar-Lopez FJ, Rosengarten G, Westein E, et al. A microfluidics device to monitor platelet aggregation dynamics in response to strain rate microgradients in flowing blood. Lab Chip 2010;10(3):291–302.

145. Hosokawa K, Ohnishi T, Kondo T, et al. A novel automated microchip flow-chamber system to quantitatively evaluate thrombus formation and antithrombotic agents under blood flow conditions. J Thromb Haemost 2011;9:2029–37.

146. Kent NJ, O'Brien S, Basabe-Desmonts L, et al. Shear-mediated platelet adhesion analysis in less than 100 mul of blood: toward a POC platelet diagnostic. IEEE Trans Biomed Eng 2011;58(3):826–30.

147. Basabe-Desmonts L, Meade G, Kenny D. New trends in bioanalytical microdevices to assess platelet function. Expert Rev Mol Diagn 2010;10(7):869–74.

148. Lincoln B, Ricco AJ, Kent NJ, et al. Integrated system investigating shear-mediated platelet interactions with von Willebrand factor using microliters of whole blood. Anal Biochem 2010;405(2):174–83.

149. Gutierrez E, Petrich BG, Shattil SJ, et al. Microfluidic devices for studies of shear-dependent platelet adhesion. Lab Chip 2008;8(9):1486–95.

150. Neeves KB, Maloney SF, Fong KP, et al. Microfluidic focal thrombosis model for measuring murine platelet deposition and stability: PAR4 signaling enhances shear-resistance of platelet aggregates. J Thromb Haemost 2008;6(12):2193–201.

151. Conant CG, Nevill JT, Zhou Z, et al. Using well-plate microfluidic devices to conduct shear-based thrombosis assays. J Lab Autom 2011;16(2):148–52.

152. Würtz M, Hvas AM, Wulff LN, et al. Shear-induced platelet aggregation in aspirin-treated patients: initial experience with the novel PlaCor PRT device. Thromb Res 2012;130(5):753–8.

153. Watson SP, Lowe GC, Lordkipanidzé M, et al; The GAPP consortium. Genotyping and phenotyping of platelet function disorders. J Thromb Haemost 2013. http://dx.doi.org/10.1111/jth.12199.

Genetic Dissection of Platelet Function in Health and Disease Using Systems Biology

Wadie F. Bahou, MD

KEYWORDS

- Gene profiling • Thrombosis • Hemostasis • Megakaryocytopoiesis • Proteomics

KEY POINTS

- Technological advances in protein and genetic analysis have altered the means by which platelet disorders can be characterized and studied in health and disease.
- When integrated into a single analytical framework, these collective technologies are referred to as systems biology, a unified approach that links platelet function with genomic/proteomic studies to provide insight into the role of platelets in broad human disorders such as cardiovascular and cerebrovascular disease.
- Analyzing and comparing genetic expression data with sophisticated proteomic identification technologies has altered the landscape for delineating gene/protein networks regulating functional platelet responses.

INTRODUCTION
Relevance of Platelet Functional Disorders in Health and Disease

Molecular platelet disorders cause bleeding syndromes of varying severity, best characterized for cell-surface receptor defects involving $\alpha_{IIb}\beta_3$ and the GPIb-IX-V complex, and less frequently known to involve distinct signaling pathways or defects of granule formation.[1] By contrast, there is a paucity of information on the molecular etiology of the "prothrombotic" platelet, despite long-standing evidence for the role of activated platelets in the development of focal ischemia.[2,3] The latter observation is clearly supported by clinical studies of platelet activation markers during transitory and thrombotic vascular events.[4–10] Causal evidence for the critical influence of platelets in

Conflict of Interest: The author is a consultant to Stony Brook Biotechnology, which focuses on identification, development, and commercialization of genetic biomarkers for platelet disorders.
Funding: Research encompassed by this article is supported by grants from the NIH (HL 091939) and the New York State Stem Cell Board (NYSTEM: C024317 and N08G-021).
Department of Medicine, Health Sciences Center, Stony Brook University, T15-040, 101 Nicolls Road, Stony Brook, NY 11794-8151, USA
E-mail address: wadie.bahou@sbumed.org

Hematol Oncol Clin N Am 27 (2013) 443–463
http://dx.doi.org/10.1016/j.hoc.2013.03.002
0889-8588/13/$ – see front matter © 2013 Elsevier Inc. All rights reserved.

human vascular events is highlighted by the efficacy of antiplatelet agents as therapeutic and prophylactic modalities in the setting of cerebrovascular ischemia,[11–13] as established by observations of fewer nonfatal strokes in patients with prior stroke or transient ischemic attack, and fewer nonfatal strokes among patients treated for completed stroke.[14,15] Comparable cardiovascular data exist demonstrating that interventions with antiplatelet agents offer therapeutic efficacy as interventional strategies for coronary artery disease (CAD), acute coronary syndromes, and percutaneous transluminal coronary angioplasty, either in acute settings or as prophylactic modalities.[4–7,11,16,17] Antiplatelet agents, however, are not without toxicity, and "breakthrough" thromboembolic episodes remain prevalent.[18] Thus the development of risk stratification strategies and/or platelet phenotypic/genotypic assays ("biomarkers") able to predict responsiveness or adverse events have emerged as a research direction of the biopharmaceutical industry, and have the potential for widespread clinical application.

CLINICAL FEATURES
Genetic Risk Factors for Platelet-Associated Cerebrovascular/Cardiovascular Diseases

Research designed to identify genetic risk factors in patients with thrombophilia have shown the strongest association in venous thromboembolic disease, with less consistent results in subjects with cerebrovascular or cardiovascular disease.[19] Evidence exists that abnormal expression of platelet proteins may favor platelet activation and thrombus formation, data best developed for platelet cell-surface glycoprotein receptors studied within the context of patients with CAD. For example, quantitative expression of the platelet integrin $\alpha_2\beta_1$ is variable, and platelets expressing higher levels have an increased ability to bind collagen.[20,21] Similarly, the 807T/873A $\alpha_2\beta_1$ polymorphism is known to increase the surface density of receptors on platelets, and is associated with an increased risk of ischemic heart disease in homozygotes. This genetic risk is enhanced in the background of subjects who smoke,[22] and may also represent a risk factor for stroke in young patients.[23] Similarly, it has been suggested that the PL^{A1} GPIIIa ($\beta3$) polymorphism is associated with stroke in patients younger than 50 years,[24] and that a Kozak T/C polymorphism within the GPIb gene is associated with stroke.[25,26] Nonetheless, other studies have been unable to demonstrate a risk between common platelet single-nucleotide polymorphisms (SNPs) and thrombotic risk.[27–31] Many of the initial attempts to dissect out genetic risk factors were largely case-control studies in which subjects were grouped based on known SNPs of well-characterized platelet protein receptors (eg, PL^{A1} vs PL^{A2}); that is, candidate genetic studies. Indeed, an emerging paradigm is that platelet-associated vascular risk is regulated by a large number of genetic loci each exerting small effects; this concept is not dissimilar to highly heritable quantitative traits such as height.[32]

Genetics of Functional Platelet Responses

Data using multiple activation models clearly demonstrate that platelet responses to the majority (if not all) agonists is highly variable within the population.[33–37] By contrast, the extent of platelet responsiveness within individuals is consistent over time, unrelated to agonist or quantitative outcome measures.[33–35,38–40] These observations are consistent with those that demonstrate high levels of platelet function heritability in siblings,[41] twins,[42] and families with a history of premature CAD.[43] Platelets retain megakaryocyte-derived mRNA[44,45] and an abundant and diverse array of microRNAs (miRNAs),[46–48] and have evolved unique adaptive signals for maintenance of genetic and protein diversity.[47] Quiescent platelets generally display minimal translational activity, although maximally activated platelets retain the capacity for protein synthesis.[46] Newly formed "reticulated" platelets retain larger quantities of mRNAs and have been associated with enhanced thrombotic risk in patients with thrombocytosis.[49] Approaches to study platelet functional responses as quantitative trait loci linked to overall platelet responsiveness is a logical extension of these collective observations, designed to integrate transcriptomic and genomic information to variability in platelet activation and disease outcome.[18,41] Indeed, in the only study reported to date focusing on a 97-member candidate gene subset to analyze adenosine diphosphate (ADP) and collagen responses, the combined effects of multiple SNPs accounted for 38% to 46% (collagen) and 13% to 16% (ADP) of the platelet variability in a healthy cohort. This variability appears to be considerably less than that predicted by the Framingham Heart Study[41]; furthermore, no data have been provided for variability in other activation-restricted signaling pathways. Recently, approaches have been developed that adapt nonbiased candidate gene lists for more robust analyses incorporating genetic expression studies with genotyping as a more extensive approach to define the genetic basis of platelet phenotypic variability. These approaches are generally referred to as systems biology.

ETIOLOGY AND PATHOGENESIS: MOLECULAR GENETICS OF PLATELET FUNCTION
Platelet Molecular Machinery

Platelets contain as little as 2×10^{-3} fg mRNA/cell (approximately 3–4 logs less RNA than a typical nucleated cell[50]), although younger platelets contain relatively larger amounts of mRNA.[49] Platelets contain rough endoplasmic reticulum and polyribosomes, and retain the ability for protein biosynthesis from cytoplasmic mRNA.[46,51] Quiescent platelets generally display minimal translational activity, although newly formed platelets synthesize various α-granule and membrane glycoproteins such as GPIb and GPIIb/IIIa ($\alpha_{IIb}\beta_3$). Historically the platelet mRNA content was considered static and invariant, although recent evidence has been presented for signal-dependent pre-mRNA splicing in platelets,[47] suggesting a model whereby activation-dependent fluctuations of the mRNA pool could result in a dynamically altered platelet proteome. Furthermore, stimulation of quiescent platelets by agonists such as α-thrombin increases protein synthesis of various platelet proteins including the regulatory protein Bcl-3,[46] the proinflammatory cytokine interleukin-1β,[47] and the clot stabilizer plasminogen activator inhibitor 1.[52] These data provide an evolutionary dynamism consistent with an adaptability to modify the genetic and proteomic composition in real time. This novel paradigmatic shift reinforces the need to comprehensively dissect the structural genomic/proteomic components to fully appreciate the dynamic nature of platelet responses in normal and diseased conditions.

LABORATORY FEATURES: INTEGRATED SYSTEMS APPROACHES TO DISSECT PLATELET FUNCTION

Theoretically, the integration of informational databases provides for opportunities to comprehensively analyze platelet function. Utilization of genetic, functional, and proteomic datasets provides a highly innovative dissection of the entire platelet functional repertoire within a systems biology framework, an approach considerably broader (with greater implications) than simple analyses of limited differences identified using transcriptomic or proteomic profiling strategies.

As shown in **Fig. 1**, comprehensive systems biology should take into account genetic and proteomic datasets to iteratively analyze platelet function as a predictor of clinical phenotype (referred to as the platelet thrombohemorrhagic balance). Extensive

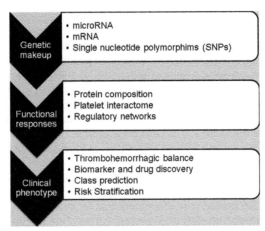

Fig. 1. Generalized schema delineating a systems biology approach for platelet analysis. The schema demonstrates how iterative and integrated analysis of various databases can be adapted for sequential studies linking genetic and protein composition of platelets to the penultimate characteristics linked to a clinical phenotype. Note that the model end points are all relevant to disease-risk stratification, personalized medicine diagnostic, and treatment options.

efforts have gone into applying state-of-the-art technologies to comprehensively define the genetic and protein composition of platelets in normal and diseased states. This information provides the foundation for integrated analytical studies relevant to platelet function and thrombosis risk. The availability of miRNA, genotypic, and proteomic data provide unique opportunities to dissect integrated networks regulating platelet function, information that can be extracted using powerful resources currently being assembled by the platelet research community. Details of some of these databases are provided in **Table 1**.

Outlined here are the various technological approaches that have provided the framework for comprehensive approaches designed to gradually gather platelet

Table 1
Platelet databases

Name	Web Site	Information
Swiss-PROT	http://ca.expasy.org	Platelet proteome on a 2-dimensional gel
Reactome	http://www.reactome.org	Functional platelet complex pathways
Human Protein Reference Database	http://www.hprd.org	PhosphoMotif Finder
PlateletWeb	http://plateletweb.bioapps.biozentrum.uni-wuerzburg.de	Centralized resource for platelet proteome, interactome, and phosphorylation
HaemAtlas	http://t1dbase.org/page/HaemAtlasHome	mRNA expression profiles of hematopoietic cells

function into a clinically relevant framework. Note that the information provided is presented as an overview and is not intended to be comprehensive in scope.

Transcriptomic Analyses Focusing on Platelet mRNAs

Development of global platelet transcript profiling technologies such as microarray and serial analysis of gene expression (SAGE) in conjunction with completion of the Human Genome project led to understanding of the complex processes of gene interactions within a living cell. Unlike microarray, SAGE represents an "open transcript profiling system," which can detect any transcript. "Classical" SAGE[53] relies on the observation that short (<10 bp) sequences ("tags") within 3'-mRNAs can stringently discriminate among the approximately 30,000 genes comprising the human genome, assuming a random nucleotide distribution along a 9-bp stretch (4^9 bp = 262,244 random nucleotide combinations). The sequence of each tag, along with its positional location, uniquely identifies the gene from which it is derived, and differentially expressed genes can be identified in a quantitative manner because the frequency of tag detection reflects the steady-state mRNA level of the cellular transcriptome (www.sagenet.org).[53,54] With relatively deep sampling (>50,000 tags), genes expressed at low levels (<0.01% of total mRNA) can be readily identified, although reliable identification of splice-variant forms still represents a scientific challenge. Several modifications to the original protocols have been devised for (1) generation of longer tags as a means of providing more definitive "tag-to-gene" identification, (2) efficient identification of low-abundant transcripts using subtractive SAGE techniques, and (3) amplification techniques to circumvent small mRNA starting material.[55–57]

Initial successful characterization of platelet-derived mRNA transcripts have been achieved using construction of platelet-specific cDNA libraries[58] and single-gene polymerase chain reaction (PCR)[59] technology. A limited number of published microarray studies using platelet-derived mRNAs have been described, with generally concordant agreements on transcript quantitation and gene-expression patterns.[44,45,60–62] Furthermore, it has become clear that this approach provides an efficient means to identify novel genes and proteins functionally expressed in human platelets.[44] Not surprisingly, platelets retain fewer transcripts than those found in nucleated cells, ranging from approximately 1600 to 3000 mRNAs.[44,45,60,62] The small number of platelet-expressed transcripts reflects the lack of ongoing transcription in the anucleate platelet.

The combination of the complementary transcript profiling techniques microarray and SAGE allowed validation of most abundant platelet transcripts.[44] Initial studies of the limited platelet SAGE library (2033 tags) demonstrated that 89% of platelet RNA tags are mitochondrial (mt) transcripts, presumably related to persistent mt-transcription in the absence of nuclear-derived transcripts. Microarray alone does not detect mitochondrial transcripts because specific probes for human mitochondrion are generally not present on the microarray chip. Recently, analysis of a more comprehensive platelet SAGE library (25,000 tags) revealed that approximately 50% (12,609 tags) of platelet SAGE tags are nucleus derived, whereas the remaining 50% are of mitochondrial origin.[63] However, the overrepresentation of mitochondrial transcripts in platelets is considerably greater than that of its closest cell type, skeletal muscle, in which mitochondrial SAGE tags constitute 20% to 25%.[64]

Platelet MicroRNA Transcriptomic Studies

miRNAs are a special group of short RNA species consisting of 21 to 24 nucleotides, and known to interact with target mRNAs to affect their translational efficacy.[65] miRNA regulation represents an important posttranscriptional control to the primary cellular regulatory pathway through which gene expression defines final protein synthesis. Recent data have demonstrated that both megakaryocytes and platelets retain an abundant and diverse array of miRNAs, and have suggested an extensive regulatory role of hematopoietic-specific miRNAs in the megakaryocytic proliferation and differentiation process.[66–70] Examples include interaction between miR-10a and its direct target HOXA-1, miR-150's role in the differentiation process of megakaryocyte-erythrocyte progenitor cells,[71] and miR-130's repression of transcription factor MAFB.[69] Not surprisingly, dysregulated miRNA expression patterns have been described in myeloproliferative disorders,[72,73] further implicating discrete miRNAs in lineage commitment during normal or dysregulated hematopoiesis.

In addition to precursor megakaryocytes, platelets also retain a competent miRNA pathway capable of converting precursor miRNAs through functional Dicer/Argonaute 2 (Ago2) complexes.[48] Furthermore, evidence has been provided that Ago2–miRNA-223 complexes specifically regulate expression of the functionally important platelet purinergic $P2Y_{12}$ ADP receptor. Additional data suggest that miRNAs (miR-28) can modulate expression of the c-mpl thrombopoietin platelet receptor[74] and that miR-96-mediated regulation of endobrevin/VAMP8 (vesicle-associated membrane protein 8) affects human platelet functional responsiveness.[75] The potential importance of a functionally competent miRNA pathway is underscored by the unusually high miRNA/mRNA platelet ratios in comparison with other hematopoietic cells such as granulocytes and megakaryocytes,[48] suggesting expanded layers for posttranscriptional regulation in platelets.

Platelet Proteomic Studies

Platelet proteomic studies can be grouped into distinct yet overlapping subcategories: proteomic analyses of quiescent platelets (the static platelet proteome) or of activated platelets. In toto proteomic strategies identified many platelet proteins, although subsequent approaches to dissect the changes that occur with platelet activation subcategorized platelet fractions (ie, membrane proteins) or functional end points (ie, phosphorylation patterns, microparticles, and so forth) in response to external stimuli. Such "subproteome" studies use the same tandem mass-spectroscopic technologies, but provide a more detailed analysis of function over time.

Quiescent platelets

Initial attempts to analyze the platelet proteome focused on characterizing proteins in resting platelets using 2-dimensional gel electrophoresis (2-DE) and in-gel protein detection using monoclonal antibodies.[76–78] Similar techniques have been applied to characterize tyrosine-phosphorylated proteins in resting platelets and to establish a platelet protein map.[79] More detailed profiling of platelet proteins using focused isoelectric gradients (pI range 5–11) identified 760 protein features corresponding to 311 different genes, resulting in the annotation of 54% of the 2-DE proteome map.[80] Newer techniques include combined fractional diagonal chromatography (COFRADIC), a non–gel-based technique whereby peptide sets are sorted in a diagonal reverse-phase chromatographic system through a specific modification of their side chains.[81,82] Modifications of this technology identified a core set of 641 platelet proteins,[83] and classification using Gene Ontology demonstrated that 16% were membrane proteins, and 64% were classified as members of cytoskeleton, endoplasmic reticulum, mitochondria, cytosol, or Golgi apparatus. Somewhat unexpectedly, nearly 20% were classified as nucleus restricted; because platelets are anucleate, this observation would suggest that these proteins are megakaryocyte remnants.

Membrane proteins
Progressive, highly sophisticated proteomic methodologies have been applied to study platelet membrane receptors. In general, the study of platelet integral membrane proteins and surface receptors using 2-DE has limitations: (1) the low solubility of these proteins, (2) their association with the platelet membrane, (3) their high molecular weight, and (4) the presence of highly abundant cytoskeleton actin. By applying COFRADIC technologies, studies predicted the presence of 87 putative helix-spanning membrane proteins.[83] A more focused analysis was pursued by enriching membrane proteins before protein identification using microcapillary liquid chromatography systems coupled to tandem mass spectrometry (referred to as μLC-MS/MS). Two distinct solubilization methods were used to reduce the overrepresentation of cytoskeleton proteins, providing for identification of 233 established or putative transmembrane proteins.[84] A more integrated approach combining microarray analysis and mass-spectrometric techniques has been used to identify novel membrane proteins that signal during platelet aggregation, and to characterize tyrosine, threonine, or serine phosphorylated residues on platelet aggregation.[85] Two-phase partitioning and multidimensional protein identification technology (MudPIT) resulted in an assembled dataset of 1282 proteins.[86]

The platelet secretome and its granules
Various proteomic strategies have identified protein subsets that are secreted during platelet activation. Initial studies identified 82 secreted proteins,[45] although a subsequent more robust analysis using thrombin-stimulated platelets expanded this list to more than 300 secreted proteins.[87] Nearly 28% were not known to be released by any cell type, and one-third of the platelet-secreted proteins were previously known. Several of the secreted proteins have previously been described in human atherosclerotic lesions, but are absent in normal vasculature; this approach therefore has the potential to identify putative future targets for drug development in modulating atherosclerosis. Similar approaches have been applied for comprehensive profiling of subfractionated α-granules[88] and dense platelet granules.[89]

Posttranslational studies: the platelet phosphoproteome and glycoproteome
Initial studies to dissect signaling events downstream of thrombin activation used phosphotyrosine antibodies coupled to various proteomic detection technologies including 2-DE. By using the thrombin receptor activating peptide to specifically activate proteinase activated receptor 1, 62 differentially phosphorylated proteins were detected, 41 of which were identified by μLC-MS/MS.[80] Of note, 8 of these appeared to be novel proteins and/or modifications, and the protein repertoire was shown to originate from 31 genes, further highlighting how alternative splicing expands the platelet proteome. Similarly, a novel approach for enrichment of sialylated glycoproteins resulted in the separation of a large number of glycopeptides from the bulk of nonmodified platelet peptides.[90] Recently applied technical advances using phosphopeptide enrichment will likely enhance our understanding of these signal-dependent activation responses.[91]

Platelet microparticles
Platelet activation in vivo causes release of 2 distinct membrane vesicles: microparticles (which bud from the plasma membrane) and exosomes. Microparticles range in size between 0.1 and 1.0 μm, whereas exosomes are smaller (range 40–100 nm). Platelet microparticles retain procoagulant activity, and play hemostatically critical roles in several clinical disorders including heparin-induced thrombocytopenia and immune thrombocytopenic purpura. A recent proteomic study identified 578 proteins

that contain this subcellular proteome,[92] 380 of which had not been previously described in platelet proteomic studies, suggesting these platelet fragments have a unique protein composition.

CLINICAL ANALYSES FOCUSED ON HEALTH AND DISEASE
Platelet Transcriptomics: Essential Thrombocythemia as a Paradigm

Direct analysis of platelet mRNAs has been applied to identify transcriptomic differences between normal platelets and those of patients with essential thrombocythemia (ET).[93] ET represents a myeloproliferative disorder subtype characterized by increased proliferation of megakaryocytes, resulting in elevated circulating platelets.[94] Initial studies designed to establish a proof of principle analyzed platelets from 6 ET patients and 5 healthy controls. Apheresis platelets were used and were purified and analyzed using the Affymetrix HU133A microarray chip, which contains probe sets for 22,283 transcripts. Computational analysis demonstrated distinctly different molecular signatures of normal and ET platelets, and signatures that clearly cosegregated from leukocyte fractions studied in parallel. Collectively, ET platelets demonstrated greater numbers of expressed transcripts in comparison with normal controls, although considerably less than the transcript numbers generally found in nucleated cells and leukocyte fractions.[44] Stringent analyses (ie, marginal or present in all of the arrays within a single group) established the presence of 1840 transcripts expressed in ET platelets versus 1086 transcripts expressed in platelets from healthy controls (P<.03). An unsupervised, hierarchical clustering analysis demonstrated that all ET platelet samples were grouped together on the basis of gene-expression similarities, with only 1 normal sample misclassified as ET. Comparison of leukocyte and platelet transcript profiles allowed delineation of "platelet-restricted genes"; that is, identification of genes whose expression was restricted to platelets (n = 126), an observation that provided unique opportunities to develop platelet class prediction models using a uniquely designed platelet gene chip (see later discussion).

Using a one-way analysis of variance, 170 genes were identified as differentially expressed between normal and ET platelets, most of which were upregulated in ET platelets.[93] Only 29 genes were downregulated in ET platelets, of which a single platelet-restricted gene (HSD17B3) was expressed in all normal platelet arrays, and uniquely underexpressed in ET compared with normal platelets. The HSD17B3 gene encoding the type 3 17β-hydroxysteroid dehydrogenase (17β-HSD3) belongs to the large family of steroid dehydrogenases, and encodes an enzyme that catalyzes conversion of 4-androstenedione to testosterone. Of interest, this enzyme is regarded as testis specific, and molecular defects of the HSD17B3 gene are causally implicated in male pseudohermaphroditism.[95] These data provided the first evidence that HSD17B3 and HSD17B12 are expressed in human platelets and may be involved in ET. Functional 17βHSD3 activity studies demonstrated that platelets retain the capacity to convert testosterone to 4-androstenedione. Furthermore, the high level of expression of HSD17B12 transcript in ET platelets was unassociated with overall enzymatic capabilities in androgen biosynthesis. Collectively, these data provided the first evidence that genome-wide platelet transcript profiling can be adapted to study molecular signatures of platelet-associated diseases. Evidence that platelets retain 17β-HSD3 activity, express distinct subtypes of 17β-HSD enzymes, and demonstrate altered HSD17B expression patterns in a disorder known to be associated with thrombohemorrhagic risk provided novel insights into the interplay between sex hormones, platelet function, and vascular diseases.

Platelet MicroRNA Studies in Human Diseases

Several recent studies have focused on miRNA differences in human hematopoietic stem cell diseases, although studies in human platelets are more limited. Emerging evidence has implicated miRNAs in the control of megakaryocytopoiesis[69] and in progenitor fate during the megakaryocyte-erythroid transition,[71] presumably by modulating expression of key transcriptional regulators.[69,71] Furthermore, distinct patterns of miRNA expression have been seen in differentiated hematopoietic cells[66] and in subsets of patients with myeloproliferative neoplasms,[72,74] further implicating discrete miRNAs in lineage commitment during normal or dysregulated hematopoiesis. To directly extend these studies to human platelets, research from the author's laboratory has analyzed miRNA expression patterns in clinical situations of enhanced platelet production, comparing patterns in ET with those of patients with reactive thrombocytosis (RT). Of note, a nearly identical, unique 21-miRNA signature associated with both conditions was identified. The majority of the differentially expressed miRNAs displayed congruent directional behavior irrespective of the thrombocytosis etiology, supporting a molecular model whereby normal and exaggerated thrombopoiesis represent genetically defined continuums along a convergent pathway, rather than qualitatively distinct genetic entities. Thus, subjects with ET display the most exaggerated expression patterns, whereas those with RT represent an intermediary subset, collectively defined by quantitatively distinct expression patterns of the 21-miRNA signature. These data reinforce and extend to miRNAs the paradigm that quantitative differences involving the genetic fingerprint may be associated with (or confer) distinct phenotypes, that is, a self-limiting phenotype seen in RT rather than the sustained phenotype associated with ET. Given the convergence of *c-mpl*/Tpo and Jak/Stat pathways in normal and myeloproliferative-associated platelet production, it is not unexpected that the 21-miRNA thrombocytosis expression signatures remained concordant, the notable exception being *miR 144/144**, which was specifically upregulated in RT and downregulated in ET. It is interesting that *miR 144* is known to be transcribed with *miR 451* on a single precursor RNA (pri-miRNA),[96] and both are lineage (erythroid)-enriched in hematopoiesis models using zebrafish (*Danio rerio*). The *miR 144/451* locus is a direct GATA1 transcriptional target, although effects on erythropoiesis appear to be restricted to *miR 451*, with no evidence that either miRNA has an effect on thrombopoiesis.[96] Although the orthologous *miR 144/451* locus is conserved on human chromosome 17, the author saw no evidence for dysregulated *miR 451* during thrombocytosis, further supporting the concept that these contiguous genes seem to have divergent effects on the megakaryocyte/erythroid transition. These data imply that distinct pathways of thrombopoiesis may be defined by the lineage-restricted expression patterns (or cognizant transcriptional regulators) of *miR 144*, a direction of research that remains in progress.

Nonplatelet Transcriptomic Studies Designed to Study Thrombotic Risk

The application of gene profiling has been used in clinical diseases associated with thrombosis, using either platelets or peripheral blood mononuclear cells (PBMCs) as the cellular source (**Table 2**). Two studies have reported gene-expression changes associated with ischemic cerebrovascular stroke, differing in the use of PBMCs[97] or neutrophils[98] as the cellular source. Although neutrophil expression patterns appeared to represent more optimal stroke predictors, gene lists could not differentiate between ischemic and hemorrhagic stroke. Another study used leukocytes to identify 108 differentially expressed genes among subjects with CAD in comparison with healthy control subjects.[99] These results were compared with those of gene-expression

Table 2
Human thrombotic diseases studied by global profiling

Transcriptomic Studies	
Disorder	**Cellular Source**
Stroke	PBMC, neutrophils
Coronary artery disease	PBMC, aorta, BM
Acute myocardial infarction	Platelets
Antiphospholipid syndrome	PBMC
Cardiopulmonary bypass	PBMC
Essential thrombocythemia	Platelets
Preeclampsia	2-DE
HELLP	2-DE
Stroke	SELDI
Myocardial infarction	2-DE
Aspirin-resistant coronary artery disease	2-DE
Congenital protein C deficiency	SELDI

Abbreviations: 2- DE, 2-dimensional gel electrophoresis; BM, bone marrow cells; HELLP, hemolysis, elevated liver enzymes, low platelet count syndrome; PBMC, peripheral blood mononuclear cells; SELDI, surface-enhanced laser desorption/ionization.

studies in murine models of atherosclerosis, and their relevance was reinforced by good correlation with human atherosclerotic lesion progression.[100,101] By contrast, cross-species patterns in acute stroke correlated poorly between rats and humans.[98] Studies focusing on cardiopulmonary bypass (CPB) demonstrated a "primed" phenotype of circulating PBMCs in which adhesion and signaling factors were overexpressed.[102] A similar study demonstrated that the CPB coding circuit affected leukocyte gene-expression patterns, specifically demonstrating that heparin caused a more profound alteration in leukocyte gene expression when compared with a non-heparin protein-coating biomaterial.[103] The antiphospholipid antibody syndrome is a strong risk factor for arterial thrombosis, and a recent study demonstrated that PBMC gene-expression patterns predicted an individual's predisposition to developing thrombosis.[104] No attempt was made to subfractionate the starting mononuclear cell population, which also included platelets. This study was limited by its retrospective design, and some of the differences could have been secondary to the primary thrombotic event.

Proteomic Applications in Thrombosis

Surface-enhanced laser desorption/ionization (SELDI)–time of flight mass spectrometry uses protein chips with an affinity matrix (charge, hydrophobicity, or other) and various wash buffers to allow the differential binding of proteins to the chip surface based on binding stringency. In patients with myocardial infarction, a spectral pattern originated from the cleavage of complement C3 α chain to release the C3f peptide and cleavage of fibrinogen to release peptide A.[105] However, ex vivo aminopeptidase activity can confound such findings.[106] Proteomic analysis of plasma samples from a large kindred with type I protein C deficiency was able to discriminate those members who presented with deep vein thrombosis before the age of 40 years from those who did not,[107] suggesting the presence of a gene/protein capable of modifying type I protein C deficiency phenotype of early-onset patients. Although the investigators were unable to identify the individual peaks using SELDI, they noted that higher-resolution instruments are becoming available, such as orthogonal matrix-assisted laser desorption/ionization, which may have the power to produce a fingerprint profile that indicates thrombotic risk. The use of proteomic techniques has led to the identification of potentially useful clinical markers for several disease states (see **Table 2**), such as clusterin for preeclampsia,[108] serum amyloid A for HELLP (*h*emolysis, *e*levated *l*iver enzymes, *l*ow *p*latelet count) syndrome,[109] ApoC-I and ApoC-III for stroke,[110] fatty acid binding protein for stroke,[111] α1-antitrypsin isoform 1 for acute coronary syndrome,[112] and vitamin D binding protein for aspirin resistance in coronary ischemia.[113]

Platelet Proteomics and Cancer

Progressive evidence supports the role for platelets as cancer modulators in general, and in tumor angiogenesis in particular. Platelets contain both stimulators and inhibitors of angiogenesis, with evidence for differential release of either angiogenesis-stimulating proteins or inhibitors.[114] Initially it remained unclear whether protein sequestration by platelets was limited to angiogenesis regulators, although based on comparative patterns in tumor-bearing mice and tumor-free controls it appeared that most differences were restricted to angiogenesis regulators,[115–117] to the exclusion of even more abundant proteins. The uptake of angiogenesis regulators into platelet α-granules was shown to be highly selective.[115,116] For example, albumin levels in platelets of tumor-bearing mice did not differ from those of normal mice, despite the known higher albumin concentrations in plasma. Furthermore, concentrations of angiogenesis regulatory proteins in platelets appear stable under physiologic conditions,[118,119] and appear to parallel early development of murine tumors.[115,116] While small amounts of many of these biomarkers freely circulate in plasma, platelet sequestration and concentration appears exaggerated. Candidate proangiogenic growth factors described to date include vascular endothelial growth factor, basic fibroblast growth factor, and platelet-derived growth factor. Expression levels of platelet factor 4 (PF4) (an inhibitor of angiogenesis) are very similar to those of plasmatic PF4, and levels remains fairly constant under physiologic conditions.[119] However, the changes in PF4 levels (and those of other angiogenesis regulators accompanying tumor growth) are much more robust in platelets than in plasma. Furthermore, the content of α-granules may remain embedded in platelet clots, suggesting a relatively longer-term role in thrombus regulation. Finally, as mirrors for biomarker development, platelet-sequestered angiogenesis regulatory proteins represent dynamic changes despite the relatively short life span of circulating platelets ($\sim$7–10 days in humans and 4–7 days in mice).

THERAPEUTICS AND PROGNOSIS: BIOMARKER DISCOVERY AND CLASS PREDICTION TOOLS RELEVANT TO PLATELET DISORDERS
Biomarker Identification and Phenotypic Prediction

As detailed earlier, global profiling strategies represent highly original tools for biomarker discovery and phenotypic classification. The author's group applied gene-expression profiling to develop discriminatory class prediction models of a benign human disorder (thrombocytosis) as an initial paradigm for molecular classification of platelet disorders. The differentiation of clonal thrombocytosis from RT has important diagnostic and therapeutic implications, because thrombohemorrhagic complications arising in RT are unusual, in contrast to frequent events in patients with clonal disorders, such as ET. Although a cause for thrombocytosis is evident in many patients, its association with occult malignancies, coupled with the fact that ET remains a diagnosis of exclusion (except in the patient subset with the *Jak2*V[617]F mutation), supports the need for well-defined algorithms for platelet class prediction. Discriminatory class prediction models using gene-expression profiling have been developed for various human malignancies, with implications for diagnostics and clinical management. This issue is of considerable importance in developing diagnostic and prognostic genetic biomarkers of platelet function.

As previously reported,[120] the author's group provided the first evidence that gene-expression profiling can be used to molecularly classify platelet phenotypes, using a common human disorder (thrombocytosis) as the paradigmatic proof of principle for study. By applying a novel microarray platform to an extensive cohort of normal and diseased platelet phenotypes, an 11-member gene biomarker subset was identified that effectively predicts phenotypic class in 86% of aggregate platelet samples, with more than 90% classification success when specifically applied to patients with thrombocytosis. The false discovery rate was controlled for using 4 distinct, iterative validation steps: (1) microarray profiling followed by a leave-one-out cross-validation algorithm for the original cohort; (2) application of a confirmatory platform (quantitative reverse transcription–PCR) for the original cohort, again confirmed by a leave-one-out cross-validation algorithm; (3) recruitment of a second independent cohort; and (4) application of the 11-member biomarker subset identified in the original cohort to classify newly recruited patients using quantitative reverse transcription–PCR. The development of computational analyses for platelet phenotypic classification generally follows well-established algorithms, collectively designed to identify small biomarker subsets that classify phenotypes (**Fig. 2**). In theory, comparable

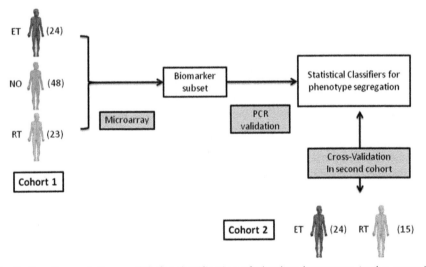

Fig. 2. Genetic prediction models for classification of platelet phenotypes. In the example shown, 3 distinct platelet phenotypes are highlighted: ET (essential thrombocythemia), RT (reactive thrombocytosis), and NO (normal platelet phenotypes as controls). The numbers studied by cohort are shown in parentheses, and are sequentially analyzed by microarray to identify an initial biomarker subset of differentially expressed mRNAs, followed by confirmation of genetic differences using a second methodology (in this case polymerase chain reaction [PCR]). Once confirmed these biomarkers can be used to classify phenotypes (ie, normal, ET, and RT subjects) using statistical discriminant analysis. The final validation step requires recruitment of a second cohort of individuals who are genetically studied by PCR; these genetic quantifications can then be used to predict phenotype (ie, class prediction relevant to thrombocytosis etiology).

approaches should be broadly applicable to platelet-associated genetic abnormalities evident in thrombosis, cancer, and inflammatory diseases, and follow standard iterative approaches as previously described in the author's laboratory.

MicroRNAs as Biomarkers

The author's recent data using miRNA patterns in thrombocytosis have extended these studies and have identified additional miRNAs that may be used as biomarkers for platelet production.[121] Various statistical classifiers were applied to define a limited miRNA subset capable of discriminating normal and thrombocythemic phenotypes. The initial searching algorithm identified 19 distinct combinations of 3 miRNAs demonstrating class prediction accuracy of greater than 90%, although repeat analysis using leave-one-out cross-validation refined this list to 3 miRNAs (*miR 10a*, *miR 148a*, and *miR 490 5p*). The application of this miRNA subset to both the microarray and quantitative PCR data was confirmed using 3 distinct statistical classifiers. Of note, the identical 3-miRNA subset performed less robustly in discriminating RT from healthy controls, results that are entirely consistent with the previously identified limited differences between RT and normal miRNA profiles. Given its aberrant expression during thrombocytosis, these data suggest that *miR 490* represents a unique biomarker of exaggerated megakaryocytopoiesis and/or proplatelet formation, although its physiologic function(s) remains to be precisely elucidated.

Protein Target Identification Using Integrated Platforms

The identification of differentially expressed miRNAs is generally followed by computational methods to identify both mRNA and protein targets. Several computational algorithms are available for identification of mRNA targets of candidate miRNAs, although the algorithms are distinctly developed and inconsistent in their mRNA candidate predictions. For example, the author's miRNA analyses of thrombocytosis identified a novel miRNA *miR 490* (both *5p* and *3p* strands) as an evolutionarily conserved miRNA demonstrating low-level expression during normal thrombopoiesis and exaggerated levels during thrombocytosis. Of the 21-member list, only *miR 490* displayed a generally restricted pattern of expression in megakaryocytes/platelets (relative to leukocytes), with no prior description of this miRNA in myeloproliferative studies,[72–74] and/or models of hematopoiesis[66,96] or megakaryocytic differentiation.[69,71,122] The author's group developed an integrated proteomic/genetic approach to identify putative *miR 490* targets by studying the ET proteome. In some respects, this approach is more powerful and relevant because it uses mRNA genetic target prediction programs, but directly links these data to protein expression, the final denominator in miRNA-mediated translation arrest. **Fig. 3** denotes a generalized workflow model to identify putative *miR 490* targets whose expression could be modulated during thrombocytosis (this schema can be adapted for any differentially expressed miRNA). The author systematically dissected the effects of dysregulated *miRNA 490* expression by incorporating the model linking miRNA, mRNA, and proteomic expression patterns in normal and thrombocytotic states. Previously described mRNA genetic profiles from 6 ET patients and 5 healthy controls were used, and spectral (peptide) counts generated by MudPIT as a semiquantitative means of platelet protein estimation, using samples from 3 healthy controls and 3 ET subjects. If *miRNA 490* modulates protein expression, 2 distinct patterns would be expected: (1) inverse relationship of the miRNA and mRNA/protein pair (ie, an mRNA degradation pathway), or (2) inverse relationship of miRNA and protein without affecting mRNA (ie, translation repression). Detailed integration of the protein profiles with these mRNA/miRNA candidates narrowed the candidate target list from 188 genes (none of which were represented in

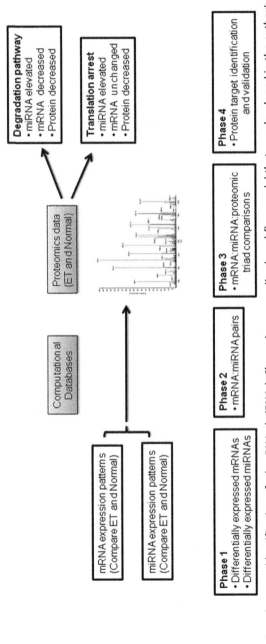

Fig. 3. Protein target identification of microRNAs (miRNAs). Shown is a generalized workflow model that was developed in the author's laboratory to identify protein targets of differentially expressed miRNAs identified in ET (in this example miR 490, although the algorithm can be followed for any miRNA). The analysis follows 4 iterative phases: identification of the mRNAs and miRNAs differentially expressed in ET and normal controls (Phase 1); application of publicly available computational databases to identify miRNA:mRNA pairs using standard target prediction programs (Phase 2); comparison of these miRNA:mRNA pairs with mass spectrometric quantification of whole platelet proteomes by phenotype (ie, ET vs normal) (Phase 3); and protein target identification based on 2 distinct mechanisms of miRNA effects, that is, a degradation pathway whereby the elevated miRNA causes mRNA degradation with concomitant decrease in proteins, or a translation arrest mechanism whereby the elevated miRNA inhibits translation without altering mRNA levels (Phase 4).

the degradation pathway) to a single mRNA/protein pair identified as disheveled-associated activator of morphogenesis 1 (DAAM1). Furthermore, DAAM1 expression appeared as a putative target restricted to translation repression (ie, diminished ET protein expression unrelated to platelet *DAAM1* mRNA levels). Ongoing research is currently being pursued to delineate the role of platelet DAAM1 protein on platelet production.

Future Directions

Proteins seldom act alone in a biological system; they function as part of a network. Analyzing and comparing genetic expression data with sophisticated proteomic identification technologies has altered the landscape for delineating gene/protein networks regulating functional platelet responses. Obviously this new systems biology research requires extensive collaboration with mathematicians and computational biologists, all of whom work synergistically to dissect out new relationships of human diseases. The shared vision is that these integrated approaches will enhance biomarker identification strategies, while developing novel approaches for lead compound development, patient-oriented disease-risk stratification, and optimization of rationale drug treatment for platelet-related disorders.

REFERENCES

1. Bahou WF. Disorders of platelets. In: Kumar D, editor. Genomics and clinical medicine. Oxford: Oxford University Press; 2006. p. 221–48.
2. Denny-Brown D. Recurrent cerebrovascular episodes. Arch Neurol 1960;2: 194–210.
3. Russell RW. Observations on the retinal blood-vessels in monocular blindness. Lancet 1961;2:1422–8.
4. Cella G, Zahavi J, de Haas HA, et al. Beta-thromboglobulin, platelet production time and platelet function in vascular disease. Br J Haematol 1979;43: 127–36.
5. Feinberg WM, Bruck DC, Ring ME, et al. Hemostatic markers in acute stroke. Stroke 1989;20:592–7.
6. Feinberg WM, Pearce LA, Hart RG, et al. Markers of thrombin and platelet activity in patients with atrial fibrillation: correlation with stroke among 1531 participants in the stroke prevention in atrial fibrillation III study. Stroke 1999;30: 2547–53.
7. Zeller JA, Tschoepe D, Kessler C. Circulating platelets show increased activation in patients with acute cerebral ischemia. Thromb Haemost 1999;81:373–7.
8. Uchiyama S, Takeuchi M, Osawa M, et al. Platelet function tests in thrombotic cerebrovascular disorders. Stroke 1983;14:511–7.
9. Uchiyama S, Yamazaki M, Hara Y, et al. Alterations of platelet, coagulation, and fibrinolysis markers in patients with acute ischemic stroke. Semin Thromb Hemost 1997;23:535–41.
10. Konstantopoulos K, Grotta JC, Sills C, et al. Shear-induced platelet aggregation in normal subjects and stroke patients. Thromb Haemost 1995;74:1329–34.
11. Antithrombotic Trialists' Collaboration. Collaborative meta-analysis of randomised trials of antiplatelet therapy for prevention of death, myocardial infarction, and stroke in high risk patients. BMJ 2002;324:71–86.
12. Bousser MG, Eschwege E, Haguenau M, et al. "AICLA" controlled trial of aspirin and dipyridamole in the secondary prevention of athero-thrombotic cerebral ischemia. Stroke 1983;14:5–14.

13. The European Stroke Prevention Study (ESPS). Principal end-points. The ESPS Group. Lancet 1987;2:1351–4.
14. United Kingdom transient ischaemic attack (UK-TIA) aspirin trial: interim results. UK-TIA Study Group. Br Med J (Clin Res Ed) 1988;296:316–20.
15. Diener HC, Cunha L, Forbes C, et al. European Stroke Prevention Study. 2. Dipyridamole and acetylsalicylic acid in the secondary prevention of stroke. J Neurol Sci 1996;143:1–13.
16. Levine G, Ali M, Schafer A. Antithrombotic therapy in patients with acute coronary syndromes. Arch Intern Med 2001;161:937–48.
17. del Zoppo GJ. The role of platelets in ischemic stroke. Neurology 1998;51:S9–14.
18. McKee SA, Sane DC, Deliargyris EN. Aspirin resistance in cardiovascular disease: a review of prevalence, mechanisms, and clinical significance. Thromb Haemost 2002;88:711–5.
19. Federman DG, Kirsner RS. An update on hypercoagulable disorders. Arch Intern Med 2001;161:1051–6.
20. Kunicki TJ, Orchekowski R, Annis D, et al. Variability of integrin alpha2 beta1 activity on human platelets. Blood 1993;82:2693–703.
21. Roest M, Sixma J, Wu Y, et al. Platelet adhesion to collagen in healthy volunteers is influenced by variation of both alpha(2) beta(1) density and von Willebrand factor. Blood 2000;96:1433–7.
22. Moshfegh K, Wiullemin W, Redondo M, et al. Association of two silent polymorphisms of platelet glycoprotein Ia/IIa receptor with risk of myocardial infarction: a case-control study. Lancet 1999;353:351–4.
23. Carlsson L, Santoso S, Spitzer C, et al. The alpha2 gene coding sequence T807/A873 of the platelet collagen receptor integrin alpha2 beta1 might be a genetic risk factor for the development of stroke in younger patients. Blood 1999;93:3583–6.
24. Carter A, Catto A, Bamford J, et al. Platelet GPIIIa PIA and GPIb variable number tandem repeat polymorphisms and markers of platelet activation in acute stroke. Arterioscler Thromb Vasc Biol 1998;18:1124–31.
25. Baker RI, Eikelboom J, Lofthouse E, et al. Platelet glycoprotein Ibalpha Kozak polymorphism is associated with an increased risk of ischemic stroke. Blood 2001;98:36–40.
26. Frank MB, Reiner AP, Schwartz SM, et al. The Kozak sequence polymorphism of platelet glycoprotein Ibalpha and risk of nonfatal myocardial infarction and nonfatal stroke in young women. Blood 2001;97:875–9.
27. Bottiger C, Kastrati A, Koch W, et al. HPA-1 and HPA-3 polymorphisms of the platelet fibrinogen receptor and coronary artery disease and myocardial infarction. Thromb Haemost 2000;83:559–62.
28. Durante-Mangoni E, Davies G, Ahmed N, et al. Coronary thrombosis and the platelet glycoprotein IIIA gene PLA2 polymorphism. Thromb Haemost 1998;80:218–9.
29. Scaglione L, Bergerone S, Gaschino G, et al. Lack of relationship between the P1A1/P1A2 polymorphism of platelet glycoprotein IIIa and premature myocardial infarction. Eur J Clin Invest 1998;28:385–8.
30. Sperr W, Huber KC, Roden M, et al. Inherited platelet glycoprotein polymorphisms and a risk for coronary heart disease in young central Europeans. Thromb Res 1998;90:117–23.
31. Joven J, Simo J, Vilella E, et al. Lipoprotein(a) and the significance of the association between platelet glycoprotein IIIa polymorphisms and the risk of premature myocardial infarction. Atherosclerosis 1998;140:155–9.

32. Weedon MN, Lettre G, Freathy RM, et al. A common variant of HMGA2 is associated with adult and childhood height in the general population. Nat Genet 2007;39:1245–50.
33. Dupont A, Fontana P, Bachelot-Loza C, et al. An intronic polymorphism in the PAR-1 gene is associated with platelet receptor density and the response to SFLLRN. Blood 2003;101:1833–40.
34. Fontana P, Dupont A, Gandrille S, et al. Adenosine diphosphate-induced platelet aggregation is associated with P2Y12 gene sequence variations in healthy subjects. Circulation 2003;108:989–95.
35. Hetherington SL, Singh RK, Lodwick D, et al. Dimorphism in the P2Y1 ADP receptor gene is associated with increased platelet activation response to ADP. Arterioscler Thromb Vasc Biol 2005;25:252–7.
36. Panzer S, Hocker L, Koren D. Agonists-induced platelet activation varies considerably in healthy male individuals: studies by flow cytometry. Ann Hematol 2006;85:121–5.
37. Yee DL, Sun CW, Bergeron AL, et al. Aggregometry detects platelet hyperreactivity in healthy individuals. Blood 2005;106:2723–9.
38. Dale GL. Coated-platelets: an emerging component of the procoagulant response. J Thromb Haemost 2005;3:2185–92.
39. Fontana P, Gandrille S, Remones V, et al. Identification of functional polymorphisms of the thromboxane A2 receptor gene in healthy volunteers. Thromb Haemost 2006;96:356–60.
40. Jones CI, Garner SF, Angenent W, et al. Mapping the platelet profile for functional genomic studies and demonstration of the effect size of the GP6 locus. J Thromb Haemost 2007;5:1756–65.
41. O'Donnell CJ, Larson MG, Feng D, et al. Genetic and environmental contributions to platelet aggregation: the Framingham heart study. Circulation 2001; 103:3051–6.
42. Gaxiola B, Friedl W, Propping P. Epinephrine-induced platelet aggregation. A twin study. Clin Genet 1984;26:543–8.
43. Bray PF, Mathias RA, Faraday N, et al. Heritability of platelet function in families with premature coronary artery disease. J Thromb Haemost 2007;5: 1617–23.
44. Gnatenko DV, Dunn JJ, McCorkle SR, et al. Transcript profiling of human platelets using microarray and serial analysis of gene expression. Blood 2003;101: 2285–93.
45. McRedmond JP, Park SD, Reilly DF, et al. Integration of proteomics and genomics in platelets: a profile of platelet proteins and platelet-specific genes. Mol Cell Proteomics 2004;3:133–44.
46. Weyrich A, Dixon D, Pabla R, et al. Signal-dependent translation of a regulatory protein, Bcl-2, in activated human platelets. Proc Natl Acad Sci U S A 1998;95: 5556–61.
47. Denis MM, Tolley ND, Bunting M, et al. Escaping the nuclear confines: signal-dependent pre-mRNA splicing in anucleate platelets. Cell 2005;122:379–91.
48. Landry P, Plante I, Ouellet DL, et al. Existence of a microRNA pathway in anucleate platelets. Nat Struct Mol Biol 2009;16:961–6.
49. Rinder H, Schuster J, Rinder C, et al. Correlation of thrombosis with increased platelet turnover in thrombocytosis. Blood 1998;91:1288–94.
50. Fink L, Holschermann H, Kwapiszewska G, et al. Characterization of platelet-specific mRNA by real-time PCR after laser-assisted microdissection. Thromb Haemost 2003;90:749–56.

51. Kieffer N, Guichard J, Farcet J, et al. Biosynthesis of major platelet proteins in human blood platelets. Eur J Biochem 1987;164:189–95.
52. Brogren H, Karlsson L, Andersson M, et al. Platelets synthesize large amounts of active plasminogen activator inhibitor 1. Blood 2004;104:3943–8.
53. Velculescu V, Zhang L, Vogelstein B, et al. Serial analysis of gene expression. Science 1995;270:484–7.
54. Zhang L, Zhou W, Velculescu V, et al. Gene expression profiles in normal and cancer cells. Science 1997;276:1268–72.
55. Dunn JJ, McCorkle SR, Praissman LA, et al. Genomic signature tags (GSTs): a system for profiling genomic DNA. Genome Res 2002;12:1756–65.
56. Wang E, Miller L, Ohnmacht G, et al. High-fidelity mRNA amplification for gene profiling. Nat Biotechnol 2000;18:457–9.
57. Peters D, Kassam A, Feingold E, et al. Comprehensive transcript analysis in small quantities of mRNA by SAGE-Lite. Nucleic Acids Res 1999;27:39.
58. Wicki AN, Walz A, Gerber-Huber SN, et al. Isolation and characterization of human blood platelet mRNA and construction of a cDNA library in lambda gt11. Confirmation of the platelet derivation by identification of GPIb coding mRNA and cloning of a GPIb coding cDNA insert. Thromb Haemost 1989;61:448–53.
59. Newman P, Gorski J, White G, et al. Enzymatic amplification of platelet-specific messenger RNA using the polymerase chain reaction. J Clin Invest 1988;82: 739–43.
60. Bugert P, Dugrillon A, Gunaydin A, et al. Messenger RNA profiling of human platelets by microarray hybridization. Thromb Haemost 2003;90:738–48.
61. Mueller A, Dittrich R, Binder H, et al. High dose estrogen treatment increases bone mineral density in male-to-female transsexuals receiving gonadotropin-releasing hormone agonist in the absence of testosterone. Eur J Endocrinol 2005;153:107–13.
62. Sauer S, Lange BM, Gobom J, et al. Miniaturization in functional genomics and proteomics. Nat Rev Genet 2005;6:465–76.
63. Dittrich E, Puttinger H, Schillinger M, et al. Effect of radio contrast media on residual renal function in peritoneal dialysis patients—a prospective study. Nephrol Dial Transplant 2006;21:1334–9.
64. Welle S, Bhatt K, Thornton C. Inventory of high-abundance mRNAs in skeletal muscle of normal men. Genome Res 1999;9:506–13.
65. Bushati N, Cohen SM. microRNA functions. Annu Rev Cell Dev Biol 2007;23: 175–205.
66. Merkerova M, Belickova M, Bruchova H. Differential expression of microRNAs in hematopoietic cell lineages. Eur J Haematol 2008;81:304–10.
67. Yendamuri S, Calin GA. The role of microRNA in human leukemia: a review. Leukemia 2009;23:1257–63.
68. Chen CZ, Li L, Lodish HF, et al. MicroRNAs modulate hematopoietic lineage differentiation. Science 2004;303:83–6.
69. Garzon R, Pichiorri F, Palumbo T, et al. MicroRNA fingerprints during human megakaryocytopoiesis. Proc Natl Acad Sci U S A 2006;103:5078–83.
70. Zhou B, Wang S, Mayr C, et al. miR-150, a microRNA expressed in mature B and T cells, blocks early B cell development when expressed prematurely. Proc Natl Acad Sci U S A 2007;104:7080–5.
71. Lu J, Guo S, Ebert BL, et al. MicroRNA-mediated control of cell fate in megakaryocyte-erythrocyte progenitors. Dev Cell 2008;14:843–53.
72. Bruchova H, Merkerova M, Prchal JT. Aberrant expression of microRNA in polycythemia vera. Haematologica 2008;93:1009–16.

73. Bruchova H, Yoon D, Agarwal AM, et al. Regulated expression of microRNAs in normal and polycythemia vera erythropoiesis. Exp Hematol 2007;35: 1657–67.

74. Girardot M, Pecquet C, Boukour S, et al. miR-28 is a thrombopoietin receptor targeting microRNA detected in a fraction of myeloproliferative neoplasm patient platelets. Blood 2010;116:437–45.

75. Kondkar AA, Bray MS, Leal SM, et al. VAMP8/endobrevin is overexpressed in hyperreactive human platelets: suggested role for platelet microRNA. J Thromb Haemost 2010;8:369–78.

76. Hanash SM, Neel JV, Baier LJ, et al. Genetic analysis of thirty-three platelet polypeptides detected in two-dimensional polyacrylamide gels. Am J Hum Genet 1986;38:352–60.

77. Giometti CS, Anderson NG. Protein changes in activated human platelets. Clin Chem 1984;30:2078–83.

78. Gravel P, Sanchez JC, Walzer C, et al. Human blood platelet protein map established by two-dimensional polyacrylamide gel electrophoresis. Electrophoresis 1995;16:1152–9.

79. Marcus K, Immler D, Sternberger J, et al. Identification of platelet proteins separated by two-dimensional gel electrophoresis and analyzed by matrix assisted laser desorption/ionization-time of flight-mass spectrometry and detection of tyrosine-phosphorylated proteins. Electrophoresis 2000;21:2622–36.

80. Garcia A, Prabhakar S, Brock CJ, et al. Extensive analysis of the human platelet proteome by two-dimensional gel electrophoresis and mass spectrometry. Proteomics 2004;4:656–68.

81. Gevaert K, Ghesquiere B, Staes A, et al. Reversible labeling of cysteine-containing peptides allows their specific chromatographic isolation for non-gel proteome studies. Proteomics 2004;4:897–908.

82. Gevaert K, Goethals M, Martens L, et al. Exploring proteomes and analyzing protein processing by mass spectrometric identification of sorted N-terminal peptides. Nat Biotechnol 2003;21:566–9.

83. Martens L, Van Damme P, Van Damme J, et al. The human platelet proteome mapped by peptide-centric proteomics: a functional protein profile. Proteomics 2005;5:3193–204.

84. Moebius J, Zahedi RP, Lewandrowski U, et al. The human platelet membrane proteome reveals several new potential membrane proteins. Mol Cell Proteomics 2005;4:1754–61.

85. Nanda N, Bao M, Lin H, et al. Platelet endothelial aggregation receptor 1 (PEAR1), a novel epidermal growth factor repeat-containing transmembrane receptor, participates in platelet contact-induced activation. J Biol Chem 2005; 280:24680–9.

86. Lewandrowski U, Wortelkamp S, Lohrig K, et al. Platelet membrane proteomics: a novel repository for functional research. Blood 2009;114:e10–9.

87. Coppinger JA, Cagney G, Toomey S, et al. Characterization of the proteins released from activated platelets leads to localization of novel platelet proteins in human atherosclerotic lesions. Blood 2004;103:2096–104.

88. Maynard DM, Heijnen HF, Horne MK, et al. Proteomic analysis of platelet alpha-granules using mass spectrometry. J Thromb Haemost 2007;5: 1945–55.

89. Hernandez-Ruiz L, Valverde F, Jimenez-Nunez MD, et al. Organellar proteomics of human platelet dense granules reveals that 14-3-3zeta is a granule protein related to atherosclerosis. J Proteome Res 2007;6:4449–57.

90. Lewandrowski U, Sickmann A. N-glycosylation site analysis of human platelet proteins by hydrazide affinity capturing and LC-MS/MS. Methods Mol Biol 2009;534:225–38.

91. Zahedi RP, Lewandrowski U, Wiesner J, et al. Phosphoproteome of resting human platelets. J Proteome Res 2008;7:526–34.

92. Garcia BA, Smalley DM, Cho H, et al. The platelet microparticle proteome. J Proteome Res 2005;4:1516–21.

93. Gnatenko DV, Cupit LD, Huang EC, et al. Platelets express steroidogenic 17beta-hydroxysteroid dehydrogenases. Distinct profiles predict the essential thrombocythemic phenotype. Thromb Haemost 2005;94:412–21.

94. Tefferi A, Thiele J, Orazi A, et al. Proposals and rationale for revision of the World Health Organization diagnostic criteria for polycythemia vera, essential thrombocythemia, and primary myelofibrosis: recommendations from an ad hoc international expert panel. Blood 2007;110:1092–7.

95. Geissler WM, Davis DL, Wu L, et al. Male pseudohermaphroditism caused by mutations of testicular 17 beta-hydroxysteroid dehydrogenase 3. Nat Genet 1994;7:34–9.

96. Dore LC, Amigo JD, Dos Santos CO, et al. A GATA-1-regulated microRNA locus essential for erythropoiesis. Proc Natl Acad Sci U S A 2008;105:3333–8.

97. Moore DF, Li H, Jeffries N, et al. Using peripheral blood mononuclear cells to determine a gene expression profile of acute ischemic stroke: a pilot investigation. Circulation 2005;111:212–21.

98. Tang Y, Xu H, Du X, et al. Gene expression in blood changes rapidly in neutrophils and monocytes after ischemic stroke in humans: a microarray study. J Cereb Blood Flow Metab 2006;26:1089–102.

99. Ma J, Liew CC. Gene profiling identifies secreted protein transcripts from peripheral blood cells in coronary artery disease. J Mol Cell Cardiol 2003;35:993–8.

100. Karra R, Vemullapalli S, Dong C, et al. Molecular evidence for arterial repair in atherosclerosis. Proc Natl Acad Sci U S A 2005;102:16789–94.

101. Seo D, Wang T, Dressman H, et al. Gene expression phenotypes of atherosclerosis. Arterioscler Thromb Vasc Biol 2004;24:1922–7.

102. Tomic V, Russwurm S, Moller E, et al. Transcriptomic and proteomic patterns of systemic inflammation in on-pump and off-pump coronary artery bypass grafting. Circulation 2005;112:2912–20.

103. Seeburger J, Hoffmann J, Wendel HP, et al. Gene expression changes in leukocytes during cardiopulmonary bypass are dependent on circuit coating. Circulation 2005;112:I224–8.

104. Potti A, Bild A, Dressman HK, et al. Gene-expression patterns predict phenotypes of immune-mediated thrombosis. Blood 2006;107:1391–6.

105. Marshall J, Kupchak P, Zhu W, et al. Processing of serum proteins underlies the mass spectral fingerprinting of myocardial infarction. J Proteome Res 2003;2: 361–72.

106. Misek DE, Kuick R, Wang H, et al. A wide range of protein isoforms in serum and plasma uncovered by a quantitative intact protein analysis system. Proteomics 2005;5:3343–52.

107. Svensson AM, Whiteley GR, Callas PW, et al. SELDI-TOF plasma profiles distinguish individuals in a protein C-deficient family with thrombotic episodes occurring before age 40. Thromb Haemost 2006;96:725–30.

108. Watanabe H, Hamada H, Yamada N, et al. Proteome analysis reveals elevated serum levels of clusterin in patients with preeclampsia. Proteomics 2004;4: 537–43.

109. Heitner JC, Koy C, Kreutzer M, et al. Differentiation of HELLP patients from healthy pregnant women by proteome analysis—on the way towards a clinical marker set. J Chromatogr B Analyt Technol Biomed Life Sci 2006;840:10–9.
110. Allard L, Lescuyer P, Burgess J, et al. ApoC-I and ApoC-III as potential plasmatic markers to distinguish between ischemic and hemorrhagic stroke. Proteomics 2004;4:2242–51.
111. Zimmermann-Ivol CG, Burkhard PR, Le Floch-Rohr J, et al. Fatty acid binding protein as a serum marker for the early diagnosis of stroke: a pilot study. Mol Cell Proteomics 2004;3:66–72.
112. Mateos-Caceres PJ, Garcia-Mendez A, Lopez-Farre A, et al. Proteomic analysis of plasma from patients during an acute coronary syndrome. J Am Coll Cardiol 2004;44:1578–83.
113. Lopez-Farre AJ, Mateos-Caceres PJ, Sacristan D, et al. Relationship between vitamin D binding protein and aspirin resistance in coronary ischemic patients: a proteomic study. J Proteome Res 2007;6:2481–7.
114. Italiano JE Jr, Richardson JL, Patel-Hett S, et al. Angiogenesis is regulated by a novel mechanism: pro- and antiangiogenic proteins are organized into separate platelet alpha granules and differentially released. Blood 2008;111:1227–33.
115. Cervi D, Yip TT, Bhattacharya N, et al. Platelet-associated PF-4 as a biomarker of early tumor growth. Blood 2008;111:1201–7.
116. Klement GL, Yip TT, Cassiola F, et al. Platelets actively sequester angiogenesis regulators. Blood 2009;113:2835–42.
117. Pietramaggiori G, Scherer SS, Cervi D, et al. Tumors stimulate platelet delivery of angiogenic factors in vivo: an unexpected benefit. Am J Pathol 2008;173: 1609–16.
118. Larsson A, Skoldenberg E, Ericson H. Serum and plasma levels of FGF-2 and VEGF in healthy blood donors. Angiogenesis 2002;5:107–10.
119. Peterson JE, Zurakowski D, Italiano JE, et al. Normal ranges of angiogenesis regulatory proteins in human platelets. Am J Hematol 2010;85:487–93.
120. Gnatenko DV, Zhu W, Xu X, et al. Class prediction models of thrombocytosis using genetic biomarkers. Blood 2010;115:7–14.
121. Xu X, Gnatenko D, Ju J, et al. Systematic analysis of microRNA fingerprints in thrombocythemic platelets using integrated platforms. Blood 2012;120(17): 3575–85.
122. Opalinska JB, Bersenev A, Zhang Z, et al. MicroRNA expression in maturing murine megakaryocytes. Blood 2010;116:e128–38.

Congenital Thrombocytopenia
Clinical Manifestations, Laboratory Abnormalities, and Molecular Defects of a Heterogeneous Group of Conditions

Riten Kumar, MD, MSc[a], Walter H.A. Kahr, MD, PhD[a,b,c],*

KEYWORDS

- Congenital platelet disorder • Platelet function defects • Thrombocytopenia
- Bleeding disorder

KEY POINTS

- Congenital thrombocytopenias are a heterogeneous group of disorders characterized by a reduction in platelet counts that may or may not be apparent at birth.
- Congenital thrombocytopenias are often accompanied by platelet function abnormalities — depending on the specific defect.
- Bleeding manifestations vary significantly and range from mild to life threatening.
- Certain congenital thrombocytopenias, such as MYH9-related disease (MYH9-RD), Wiskott-Aldrich syndrome (WAS), and thrombocytopenia–absent radius (TAR) syndrome, may be associated with classic phenotypic features that aid in their diagnosis.
- Advances in molecular genetics have greatly improved understanding of the underlying pathogenesis.
- Management depends on the severity of bleeding and presence of associated phenotypic manifestations.

INTRODUCTION

Congenital thrombocytopenias are a rare, heterogeneous group of disorders that result in early-onset thrombocytopenia with marked variability in bleeding

Funding Sources: None.

Conflict of Interest: None.

[a] Division of Haematology/Oncology, Department of Paediatrics, The Hospital for Sick Children, University of Toronto, 555 University Avenue, Toronto, Ontario M5G 1X8, Canada; [b] Program in Cell Biology, Research Institute, The Hospital for Sick Children, 555 University Avenue, Toronto, Ontario M5G 1X8, Canada; [c] Department of Biochemistry, University of Toronto, 1 King's College Circle, Toronto, Ontario M5S 1A8, Canada

* Corresponding author. Program in Cell Biology, Research Institute, The Hospital for Sick Children, 555 University Avenue, Toronto, Ontario M5G 1X8, Canada.

E-mail address: walter.kahr@sickkids.ca

Hematol Oncol Clin N Am 27 (2013) 465–494

http://dx.doi.org/10.1016/j.hoc.2013.02.004

0889-8588/13/$ – see front matter © 2013 Elsevier Inc. All rights reserved.

manifestations ranging from mild to severe, life-threatening bleeds. Although some cases remain unclassifiable, recent advances in molecular genetics have dramatically improved understanding of the underlying pathogenesis of several of these conditions.[1,2] Given the heterogeneity of these syndromes, there are several methods of classification.[3] They may be classified according to the underlying genetic mutation (**Table 1**), size of platelets (**Table 2**), or associated abnormalities of platelet function. In this review, the syndromes have been grouped by the mode of inheritance as autosomal dominant, autosomal recessive, and X-linked.

There are various circumstances under which a patient may be worked up for congenital thrombocytopenias—these include a history of bleeding or easy bruising, family history of thrombocytopenia, or an incidental finding of thrombocytopenia detected on blood count done for an unrelated indication. Given that several congenital thrombocytopenias are associated with only a mild reduction of platelet counts and no hemorrhagic symptoms, a major concern is misdiagnosis of these conditions as the more common immune thrombocytopenia (ITP) and subsequent exposure of patients to unnecessary and often inappropriate therapies, such as splenectomy.

The first step in the work-up of such patients is a thorough bleeding history and family history, which may help differentiate acquired and congenital defects as well as ascertain the inheritance pattern of the bleeding disorder. In the past decade, significant work has been done to develop standardized bleeding questionnaires, which can be used in both adult and pediatric populations.[4,5] Subsequent steps involve performing a complete blood cell count and examination of a peripheral smear. Pseudothrombocytopenia, a common phenomenon caused by platelet clumping in the presence of ethylenediaminetetraacetic acid (EDTA), accounts for 15% to 20% of all cases of isolated thrombocytopenias[3] and is easily ruled out with evaluation of a peripheral smear. The initial inspection of blood smear also helps determine platelet size (small, normal, or large), detect the appearance of agranular platelets, visualize leukocyte inclusions, or detect other red and white cell abnormalities. Further characterization involves bone marrow aspiration and biopsy as well as platelet aggregation studies. Given the emerging data showing a genotype-phenotype correlation for several congenital thrombocytopenias, efforts should be made to refer samples to specialized laboratories that can perform such testing. The purpose of this review is to provide an updated approach to the clinical presentation, laboratory investigation, and management of congenital thrombocytopenias.

AUTOSOMAL DOMINANT THROMBOCYTOPENIAS
MYH9-Related Disease

Introduction
MYH9-RD is an autosomal dominant condition presenting with macrothrombocytopenia and leukocyte inclusion bodies (Döhle-like bodies) present since birth and with a risk of developing nephropathy, sensorineural deafness, and presenile cataracts later in life, secondary to heterozygous mutations in the MYH9 gene encoding for the nonmuscle myosin heavy chain IIA (NMMHC-IIA).[6]

In 1909, Richard May first described the presence of Döhle-like inclusion bodies in the leukocytes of subjects with giant platelets. Subsequently, in 1945, Robert Hegglin described a family in which macrothrombocytopenia and leukocyte inclusion bodies were transmitted in an autosomal dominant fashion.[7] This led to the term, May-Hegglin anomaly, used to describe the triad of thrombocytopenia, giant platelets, and leukocyte inclusion bodies. Over the next 50 years, 3 distinct syndrome complexes, namely Epstein syndrome, Fechtner syndrome, and Sebastian syndrome, described the association of nephritis, sensorineural deafness, and presenile cataracts with dominantly inherited thrombocytopenia and leukocyte inclusion bodies. It was only in the year 2000 that it was shown by 2 independent groups that all these syndromes derive from mutations in the *MYH9* gene, and the term, MYH9-RD, is now preferred.[8,9]

Molecular defect

More than 40 mutations have been identified in *MYH9* gene located on chromosome 22q12–13.[6] They mostly consist of heterozygous missense mutations, suggesting that the pathology is either a dominant negative effect (influencing the function of the normal protein) or haploinsufficiency (inadequate amount of protein).[10] NMMHC-IIA, a 453-kDA protein, is a hetero-hexatetramer that contains 2 heavy chains and 2 pair of light chains, which form a dimer through the interactions between the α-helical tail domains.[6] Each heavy chain contains an N-terminal globular head (exons 1–18), which has ATPase and actin-binding activity, a neck region (exon 19), and a C-terminal α-helical coiled-coil tail domain. NMMHC-IIA plays an important role in several cellular processes requiring force and translocation, such as motility, cytokinesis, phagocytosis, vesicular trafficking, maintenance of stress fibers, and focal adhesions. In addition, 2 recent studies have shown that myosin IIA also has a key role as a negative regulator of platelet formation by inhibition of proplatelet extension via the Rho/ROCK pathway.[11,12] In vitro studies have subsequently shown that the *MYH9* mutation is associated with complete loss of proplatelet extension of megakaryocytes,[13] and it is hypothesized that patients with MYH9-RD have ectopic migration of proplatelets and premature release of platelets into the bone marrow niches, resulting in thrombocytopenia.

Clinical presentation and laboratory evaluation

Bleeding tendency in patients with MYH9-RD tends to be mild to moderate with epistaxis, easy bruising, and menorrhagia being the commonly reported symptoms, though life-threatening bleeds, including intracranial hemorrhage, have also been described.[14,15] It is not unusual, however, for asymptomatic adults to be diagnosed with MYH9-RD after routine blood work. In such situations, an important concern is misdiagnosis of such patients as having ITP and subsequent exposure to inappropriate therapies, including intravenous immunoglobulin (IVIG), steroids, and splenectomy. An absence of family history of macrothrombocytopenia does not rule out MYH9-RD because 35% of the mutations may be sporadic.[6]

Pecci and colleagues,[16] in a seminal study of 108 consecutive patients with gene sequencing–proven MYH9-RD, estimated the prevalence of nephritis, sensorineural hearing loss, and presenile cataracts to be 28%, 60%, and 16%, respectively. Mean age of onset of nephritis and presenile cataracts was 23 (±9) years and 23 (±6) years, respectively, whereas there was homogenous distribution of age of onset for sensorineural hearing loss among all ages. In the same study, the genotype-phenotype correlation of MYH9-RD was elaborated. Mutations in the N-terminal head domain were more likely associated with nephritis ($P<.001$), sensorineural hearing loss ($P<.001$), and more severe thrombocytopenia ($P = .002$) compared with mutations in the tail domain, which usually resulted in hematological manifestations alone.

Mean platelet counts are typically approximately 20×10^9/L to 130×10^9/L with an elevated mean platelet volume (MPV). Automated cell counters can mistake these giant platelets as erythrocytes and may report spuriously low platelet counts, emphasizing the importance of visualizing the blood film. In the study by Pecci and colleagues,[16] mean platelet count of the 108 patients, as measured by automated

Table 1
Congenital thrombocytopenia characterized according to inheritance pattern, genetic mutations, and associated findings

Syndrome (OMIM Entry)	Inheritance Pattern	Gene Involved	Chromosomal Location	Associated Findings
MYH9-RD (multiple)	Autosomal dominant	MYH9	22q12–13	Döhle-like leukocyte inclusion bodies, nephritis, sensorineural hearing loss, and presenile cataracts
Paris-Trousseau (Jacobsen) syndrome (188025; 147791)	Autosomal dominant	FLI1	11q23.3–24	Cognitive and facial abnormalities
PT-VWD (177820)	Autosomal dominant	GP1BA	17p13	Low VWF ristocetin cofactor assay, decrease in HMWVW multimers, increased low-dose RIPA; needs to be differentiated from type IIb VWD.
Radioulnar synostosis with amegakaryocytic thrombocytopenia (605432)	Autosomal dominant	HOXA11	17p15.2	Radioulnar synostosis, clinodactyly, syndactyly, hip dysplasia, sensorineural hearing loss, and progression to pancytopenia
FPD/AML (601399)	Autosomal dominant	RUNX1	22q22	Platelet aggregations shows impaired aggregation to collagen and epinephrine; 35% of the cohort may go on to develop AML.
ANKRD26-related thrombocytopenia (nd)	Autosomal dominant	ANKRD26	10p2	Normal-sized platelets with bone marrow shows dysmegakaryopoiesis; possible increased risk of leukemia

CYCS-related thrombocytopenia (612004)	Autosomal dominant	CYCS	7p15.3	None
TUBB1-related macrothrombocytopenia (nd)	Autosomal dominant	TUBB1	6p21.3	None
BSS (231200)	Autosomal recessive	GP1BA, GP1BB, GP9	17p13, 22q11, 3q21	Platelet aggregation studies show absent ristocetin-induced response.
GPS (139090)	Autosomal recessive (mostly)	NBEAL2	3p21	None
CAMT (604498)	Autosomal recessive	MPL	1p34	Progression to pancytopenia
TAR syndrome (274000)	Autosomal recessive	RBM8A	1q21.1	Bilateral absent radii with thumb present; lower limb, cardiac, gastrointestinal, and renal anomalies
Thrombocytopenia associated with sitosterolemia (210250)	Autosomal recessive	ABCG5, ABCG8	2p21	Stomatocytosis, tendon xanthomas, and premature atherosclerosis
WAS (XLT) (301000)	X-linked	WAS	Xp11.22	Recurrent infections, eczema, with a risk of autoimmunity and lymphoid malignancy
XLT with dyserythropoiesis (300367; 314050)	X-linked	GATA1	Xp11.23	Dyserythropoietic anemia
FLNA-related thrombocytopenia (nd)	X-linked	FLNA	Xq28	Possible association with periventricular nodular heterotopia

Table 2
Classification of inherited thrombocytopenia by platelet size

Small Platelets (MPV <7 fL)	Normal-Sized Platelets (MPV 7–11 fL)	Large Platelets (MPV >11 fL)
WAS	CAMT	MYH9-RD
XLT	TAR	BSS
	Radioulnar synostosis with amegakaryocytic thrombocytopenia	GPS
		VCFS
	FPD/AML	XLT with dyserythropoiesis
	ANKRD26-related thrombocytopenia	PT-VWD
	CYCS-related thrombocytopenia	Paris-Trousseau (Jacobsen) syndrome
		TUBB1-related macrothrombocytopenia
		Thrombocytopenia associated with sitosterolemia

counters, was 31 × 10^9/L; however, the 60 patients who had manual cell counts had a significantly higher mean platelet count at 68 × 10^9/L. Specific diagnostic criteria have been suggested, which combine MPV and mean platelet diameter (MPD) to help distinguish congenital thrombocytopenias from ITP. In a prospective study of 15 patients with MYH9-RD, 20 with Bernard-Soulier syndrome (BSS) and 50 with ITP, MPV, and MPD were significantly higher in patients with congenital thrombocytope-nias.[17] Receiver operating characteristic curves identified that an MPV greater than 12.4 fL had 83% sensitivity and 89% specificity whereas an MPD greater than 3.3 μm had 89% sensitivity and 88% specificity in differentiating congenital thrombo-cytopenia from ITP. Combining the MPV and MPD resulted in sensitivity and speci-ficity of 97% and 89%, respectively.

Döhle-like inclusion bodies in leukocytes can be appreciated on Wright-Geisma–stained blood films in approximately 40% to 80% of patients.[18] These light blue–appearing inclusions are aggregates of NMMHC-IIA observed in the cytoplasm of some neutrophils (**Fig. 1**A). However, since these inclusions are not always present, immunofluorescence staining of blood films using anti–NMMHC-IIA antibody is more sensitive and is able to detect smaller and abnormally localized aggregates (see **Fig. 1**B, C).[6] In a prospective study of a 118 consecutive subjects evaluated for MYH9-RD, using genetic analysis as the gold standard, the sensitivity and specificity of this technique were estimated at 100% and 95%, respectively.[19] Given increasing evidence of genotype-phenotype correlation and its impact on screening for renal dis-ease and hearing loss, whenever possible, gene sequencing of the MYH9 gene should be pursued. Given the clustered distribution of mutations, Balduini and colleagues[6] have suggested a tiered approach with the hot exons, namely, 1, 16, 26, 30, 38, and 40, being sequenced first followed by exons 10, 24, 25, 31, and 37, and, finally, the remaining codons. Patients with confirmed MYH9-RD should be referred to specialized facilities for ongoing screening for nephritis, hearing loss, and cataracts.

Paris-Trousseau (Jacobsen) Syndrome

Paris-Trousseau (Jacobsen) syndrome is an autosomal dominant macrothrombocyto-penia first described in 1993 in a woman and her child.[20,21] It is characterized by mod-erate thrombocytopenia with a subpopulation of platelets demonstrating giant alpha granules (1–2 μm diameter) that stain red on Wright-Giemsa stain (**Fig. 2**). Bone marrow evaluation shows marked dysmegakaryopoiesis with an increase in number of small immature megakaryocytes.[3,10,22] Paris-Trousseau platelets, when stimulated

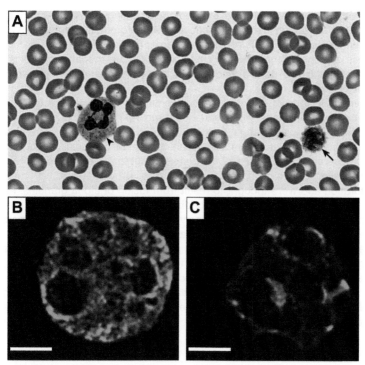

Fig. 1. MYH9-RD. (*A*) Peripheral blood smear (Wright-Giemsa stain) showing a giant platelet (*arrow*) and a Döhle-like (*light blue*) inclusion body in a neutrophil (*arrowhead*) from a patient with MYH9-RD. (*B*) Immunofluorescence microscopy of a blood smear showing normal distribution of cytoplasmic NMMHC-IIA in a normal neutrophil. (*C*) Multiple cytoplasmic clusters of NMMHC-IIA in a neutrophil from a patient with MYH9-RD (scale bars represent 5 μm).

by thrombin, fail to release their alpha granule contents.[20] This syndrome is associated with constitutional deletions of the distal portion of chromosome 11 (11q23.3–24), including the friend leukemia integration (*FLI1*) locus.[20] FLI1, a member of the ETS group of transcription factors, regulates the expression of several genes involved in

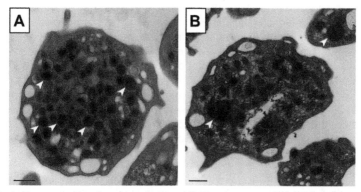

Fig. 2. Paris-Trousseau (Jacobsen) syndrome. (*A*) Platelet transmission electron microscopy image of a control platelet showing normal-sized alpha granules (*arrowheads*). (*B*) Giant alpha granules (*arrowheads*) present in platelets from a patient with Paris-Trousseau (Jacobsen) syndrome (scale bars represent 5 nm).

megakaryocyte differentiation and maturation, including *ITGA2*, *GP9*, *GPIBA*, and *c-MPL,* and its disruption in mice is associated with a dramatic decrease in megakaryocyte number and size.[23–25] Furthermore, overexpression of FLI1 in CD34$^+$ cells from Paris-Trousseau syndrome patients was able to rescue megakaryopoiesis in vitro, thereby confirming this gene's involvement in patient megakaryocyte and platelet abnormalities.[26]

Favier and colleagues[22] reported clinical, hematological, and molecular data on 10 pediatric patients with Paris-Trousseau syndrome. All patients had moderate thrombocytopenia at diagnosis (platelet counts 20–76 × 10^9/L), although there was a trend toward increase in platelet counts a few years after initial diagnosis. Giant alpha granules were observed in 1% to 5% of the platelets, but they were not detected in bone marrow megakaryocytes or those grown in culture. They appeared with megakaryocyte maturation and were thought to result from fusion of alpha granules. Molecular analysis using fluorescence in situ hybridization demonstrated 11q23.3 deletion in all patients, and reverse transcription–polymerase chain reaction confirmed loss of 1 copy of the *FLI1* gene in 9 of 10 patients. Clinically, individuals with Paris-Trousseau have a mild bleeding tendency, although the Jacobsen phenotype, which is thought to result from larger deletions on the long arm of chromosome 11, is more extensive with mental retardation, trigonocephaly, facial dysmorphism, and malformations of the heart, kidney, gastrointestinal tract, genitalia, and skeleton.[27] The *KIRREL3* gene has recently been implicated in the neurocognitive delay associated with Jacobsen syndrome.[28]

Platelet-type von Willebrand Disease

Introduction

Platelet-type von Willebrand disease (PT-VWD) was first described by Weiss and colleagues[29] in 1982, in 4 members of a family presenting with mild bleeding symptoms and intermittent thrombocytopenia. Similar to type 2B von Willebrand disease (VWD), the cohort had increased ristocetin-induced platelet aggregation (RIPA) and loss of high-molecular-weight von Willebrand (HMWVW) multimers. Unlike type 2B VWD, however, the primary defect was thought to exist in the platelets rather than the von Willebrand protein, and Weiss named the condition *pseudo–von Willebrand disease.* Since its initial description, 55 cases of PT-VWD from 23 families have been reported (http://www.pt-vwd.org/).

PT-VWD is an autosomal dominant bleeding diathesis that occurs as a result of gain-of-function mutations in the *GP1BA* gene, coding for the platelet surface glycoprotein, GPIbα. This defect causes spontaneous binding of plasma von Willebrand factor (VWF) to platelets, with subsequent removal of the VWF-platelet complex from circulation, resulting in the thrombocytopenia and bleeding.[30] By contrast, type 2B VWD occurs as a result of gain-of-function mutations in the A1 domain (exon 28) of the *VWF* gene.[10] The phenotypic and laboratory manifestations of both PT-VWD and type 2B VWD are similar. However, given the distinct therapeutic modalities (platelet transfusion for PT-VWD; factor VIII [FVIII]/VWF concentrate for type 2B VWD), it is important to differentiate the 2 conditions.

Molecular defect

To date, 5 mutations causing PT-VWD have been described in the *GP1BA* gene. These include 4 missense mutations, resulting in single amino acid substitutions— Gly233Val,[31] Met239Val,[32] Gly233Ser,[33] and Asp235Tyr[34] —and a novel in-frame deletion of 27bp in the macroglycopeptide region.[35] The amino acid residues, 233, 235, and 239, are situated within a β-hairpin loop in the crystalline structure of

GP1bα, and it is hypothesized that these substitutions stabilize the loop, resulting in an increased affinity to VWF under nonshear conditions.[30,36] A knock-in mouse model of PT-VWD with the Gly233Val mutation not only presents with a bleeding phenotype but also exhibits increase in splenic megakaryocytes, splenomegaly, and increased bone mass.[37]

Clinical presentation and laboratory evaluation

Patients with PT-VWD typically present with mild to moderate mucocutaneous bleeding, which includes easy bruising, frequent epistaxis, menorrhagia, and post-surgical bleeding. Bleeding may become more severe under conditions of stress, pregnancy, and infection due to an increased release in the endogenous VWF under these conditions or after ingestion of aspirin and other drugs with antiplatelet activity.[30,36]

Platelet counts may be normal, although intermittent mild to moderate thrombocytopenia may be appreciated in conditions of stress. Blood films often reveal large platelets (macrothrombocytes) with platelet clumping. FVIII and VWF antigen are typically normal to mildly reduced, with a discordant decrease in von Willebrand functional assays, such as VWF ristocetin cofactor assay and VWF collagen-binding assay, and reduction in HMWVW multimers.[36] The most characteristic finding is enhanced RIPA at concentrations of 0.5 mg/mL or lower.[10] The discrimination of PT-VWD from the more common type 2B VWD is difficult but clinically relevant. It is estimated that PT-VWD is underdiagnosed, with a recent international retrospective/prospective registry demonstrating that 15% of patients diagnosed with type 2B VWD actually had PT-VWD. The following tests may help differentiate the 2 conditions:

1. Cryoprecipitate challenge: patient platelets (platelet-rich plasma or washed platelets) are challenged with cryoprecipitate or a commercial VWF concentrate. Only PT-VWD (and not type 2B VWD) platelets demonstrate aggregation on addition of a concentrated form of VWF.[38] False-positive results have been reported with this technique.[39]
2. RIPA mixing assay: patient platelets (platelet-rich plasma or washed platelets) are mixed with normal plasma, and aggregation is measured in an aggregometer at low-dose (0.5 mg/mL) ristocetin concentration. Platelets from PT-VWD (not type 2B VWD) aggregate under these conditions.[39]
3. Flow cytometry assay: the increased affinity of VWF to platelets induced by ristocetin was recently demonstrated using flow cytometry. Using mixing tests, the investigators were able to differentiate PT-VWD from type 2B VWD.[40]
4. Genetic analysis: gene sequencing of the *GP1BA* gene or the A1 region (exon 28) of the *VWF* gene with identification of mutation remains the gold standard for diagnosis of PT-VWD or type 2B VWD, respectively. This test is only available in specialized centers.[10]

Radioulnar Synostosis with Amegakaryocytic Thrombocytopenia

The association between amegakaryocytic thrombocytopenia and radioulnar synostosis was first reported in 2 unrelated, nonconsanguinous families by Thompson and colleagues.[41,42] Both fathers and 4 affected children presented with proximal fusion of the radius and ulna, resulting in limited pronation and supination of the forearm. Additional phenotypic features included clinodactyly, syndactyly, hip dysplasia, and sensorineural hearing loss. Although the fathers had no hematological manifestations, all 4 children had thrombocytopenia at birth. Initial bone marrow evaluations showed normal cellularity with decreased megakaryocytes, although 3 children eventually progressed to trilineage pancytopenia within 6 months to 6 years, with follow-up bone marrow examinations showing generalized hypocellularity. The fourth child had normalization of platelet counts on follow-up.

Genetic studies identified a single base pair deletion on exon 2 of the *HOXA11* gene, resulting in a translational frameshift followed by a premature stop codon, which was thought to result in the truncation of this transcription factor within its DNA-binding domain. These homeobox (*HOX*) genes encode DNA-binding proteins that regulate gene expression central to bone morphogenesis and hematopoietic cell differentiation.[43] Subsequently, more cases of amegakaryocytic thrombocytopenia in association with radioulnar synostosis have been reported, although *HOXA11* mutations have not been consistently identified.[44,45] The autosomal dominant inheritance, mild deformity of the forearm, and persistent thrombocytopenia progressing to pancytopenia differentiate this condition from TAR syndrome (discussed later).

Familial Platelet Disorder with Propensity for Myeloid Malignancy

The first pedigree of familial platelet disorder with a propensity for myeloid malignancy (FPD/AML) was described by Dowton and colleagues[46] in 1985, in 22 members of a kindred with autosomal dominant thrombocytopenia, 6 of whom went on to develop hematological malignancies. In 1996, Ho and colleagues[47] reported genetic linkage to chromosome 21q22, and, in 1999, the same group identified heterozygous mutations in *RUNX1* located on 21q22.[48] FPD/AML is currently recognized as a rare autosomal dominant disorder characterized by qualitative and quantitative platelet defects, with a predisposition to develop myeloid malignancies later in life, secondary to heterozygous germline mutations in the *RUNX1 gene*.[49,50] FPD/AML is rare with approximately 30 pedigrees reported in the literature.

The *RUNX1* gene spans 260 kilobases (kb) of genomic sequence on chromosome 21, contains 12 exons, and exhibits a complex pattern of regulated expression at the level of transcription.[51] RUNX1, also known as core binding factor A2, complexes with core binding factor beta (CBFB) to form a heterodimeric, core binding transcription factor that regulates many genes important for hematopoiesis.[52] A highly conserved DNA-binding region called the RUNT homology domain, located near the N-terminus of RUNX1, both enables the dimerization with CBFB and directs binding of RUNX1 to DNA sequences of target genes.[49,50] Mutations in the RUNT homology domain are most commonly reported in kindreds with FPD/AML, although large deletions and mutations in the C-terminus are also described.

The clinical presentation of FPD/AML is variable, with most patients presenting with mucocutaneous bleeding symptoms, including easy bruising, epistaxis, and bleeding with dental and minor surgery.[53] Thrombocytopenia is mild (100–150 × 10^9/L) and is associated with normal-sized platelets. The platelet function analyzer-100 (PFA-100) shows prolonged closure times with both collagen-ADP and collagen-epinephrine cartridges, and platelet aggregation typically shows impaired aggregation with collagen and epinephrine.[49,50] Electron microscopy findings in older cohorts have reported dense granule deficiency. The incidence of acute myeloid leukemia and/or myelodysplastic syndrome in patients with FPD/AML is estimated at 35%, with a median age of diagnosis of 33 years.[53]

AUTOSOMAL RECESSIVE THROMBOCYTOPENIAS
Bernard-Soulier Syndrome

Introduction
In 1948, 2 French hematologists, Jean Bernard and Jean Pierre Soulier, described a young man from a consanguineous family presenting with severe bleeding symptoms,

thrombocytopenia, and large platelets.[54] BSS is now recognized as an autosomal recessive macrothrombocytopenia secondary to quantitative deficiency or qualitative defects in the platelet GPIb-IX-V complex, resulting in decreased platelet adhesion to the subendothelium. BSS is rare, with an estimated prevalence of less than 1 in 1,000,000, although this number is thought an underestimation secondary to misdiagnosis and under-reporting.[55] Heterozygous carriers for BSS mutations are usually asymptomatic, although a proportion of them may have mild bleeding symptoms (discussed later).

Molecular defect
The central function of the GPIb-IX-V complex is to ensure normal primary hemostasis by mediating platelet adhesion to the subendothelium at sites of vascular injury, through binding with VWF. GPIb-IX-V is composed of 4 transmembrane polypeptide subunits, synthesized by 4 separate genes: GPIbα (GP1BA), GPIbβ (GP1BB), GPIX (GP9), and GPV (GP5). The products of these genes assemble on the maturing megakaryocyte in the bone marrow to form the GPIb-IX-V complex, which is stabilized via filamin A.[56] Mutation of the GP1BA gene is associated most frequently with BSS, although mutations in GP1BB and GP9 (but not GP5) also are described.[10] More than 50 distinct mutations have been identified that affect the biosynthesis and/or trafficking of the GPIb-IX-V complex through the Golgi apparatus and endoplasmic reticulum of the megakaryocytes.[57] No correlation between the type of mutation and bleeding phenotypes is observed.

Murine models have shown that the bleeding defect in BSS is predominantly due to loss of the adhesive function of GPIbα of the GPIb-IX-V complex.[58] GPIbα contains the VWF-binding site and 2 thrombin-binding sites. In addition, it also binds to P-selectin, thrombospondin-1, FVIIa, FXI, FXII, αMβ2, and high-molecular-weight kininogen.[56,58] Thus, abnormal bleeding in BSS is thought to result from impairment of GPIbα-VWF interaction at the site of vessel wall damage, although VWF-mediated high shear, platelet-platelet interaction has also been implicated.[59] Additionally, abnormal membrane development during megakaryocyte maturation and impaired proplatelet formation may also contribute to the phenotype.[60,61]

Clinical presentation and laboratory evaluation
Although there is marked heterogeneity in the severity and frequency of bleeding between individuals, most patients with BSS develop significant mucocutaneous hemorrhage in early childhood.[55] Common bleeding manifestations include petechiae, epistaxis, gingival bleeding, menorrhagia, and hemorrhage with trauma or surgery. Angiodysplasia in patients with BSS resulting is severe gastrointestinal bleeding has been described.[62] Often, bleeding and bruising are more significant, as expected from the degree of thrombocytopenia.

Characteristic laboratory findings include moderate thrombocytopenia, giant platelets (Fig. 3), and absent RIPA. Platelet counts range from low ($<$30 $\times$ 10^9/L) to normal,[63] with presence of a small number of giant platelets with a rounded shape (MPV 11–16 fL; diameter 4–10 μm).[55] Automated cell counters can mistake these giant platelets for lymphocytes and may report spuriously low platelet counts, thereby emphasizing the importance of visualizing the blood film. Similar to MYH9-RD, major concerns are misdiagnosis of patients having ITP and subsequent exposure to inappropriate therapies, including splenectomy (discussed earlier).[64] Platelet aggregation studies classically show deficient RIPA, which does not correct with addition of normal plasma, as is the case in VWD. PFA-100 reveals a prolonged closure time ($>$300 seconds) with both the collagen-ADP and collagen-epinephrine cartridges.[65] Flow cytometry

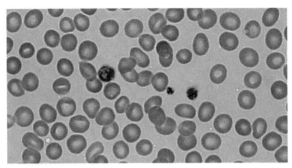

Fig. 3. BSS. Peripheral blood smear (Wright-Giemsa stain) from a patient with BSS showing giant platelets.

analysis, using a panel of specific monoclonal antibodies (anti–CD42a-d) measuring components of the GPIb-IX-V complex, confirms the diagnosis.[55] Electron microscopy, although not necessary for diagnosis, shows increased cytoplasmic vacuoles and membrane complexes in giant platelets and megakaryocytes.[66]

Mediterranean Macrothrombocytopenia

In southern Europe, a common and mild form of macrothrombocytopenia, characterized by absence of severe bleeding and preserved platelet function, has been described.[3,67] A proportion of these cases has since been shown to occur secondary to Ala156Val missense mutation in GPIbα (Bolzano variant).[68] In a recent prospective study from Italy of 216 patients presenting with nonsyndromic autosomal dominant macrothrombocytopenia, 42 (19%), were found heterozygous for the Bolzano mutation. The cohort presented with mild macrothrombocytopenia (mean platelet count 81×10^9/L), reduced expression of GPIb-IX-V, and normal platelet aggregation results. Mild bleeding symptoms were appreciated in 42% of the cohort, although rare cases of postpartum and traumatic intracranial hemorrhage were also described.[69] Therefore, the phenotype and genotype of many families with Mediterranean macrothrombocytopenia is equivalent to carriers of BSS.

Velocardiofacial Syndrome

Velocardiofacial syndrome (DiGeorge/22q11 deletion syndrome) (VCFS) is a common genetic syndrome-complex that occurs secondary to microdeletions on the long arm of chromosome 22 (del22q11) and manifests with a wide range of abnormalities, including cardiac defect, immunodeficiency, hypocalcemia, cleft lip and/or palate, and developmental delay. The deleted chromosome region in more than 90% of patients with VCFS includes the *GP1BB* gene. *GP1BB* encodes for one subunit of the platelet GPIb-V-IX receptor, complete loss of which results in the severe bleeding disorder, BSS. Thus, patients with VCFS may be considered heterozygous BSS patients.

In 1998, Van Geet and colleagues[70] described 3 patients with VCFS who had mild macrothrombocytopenia with preserved platelet function and no bleeding tendency. More recently, however, in a prospective study of 21 patients with VCFS, 16 patients reported increased bruising, epistaxis, and menorrhagia.[71] All 21 patients had undergone surgical interventions, but the investigators were unable to determine, retrospectively, if there was increased perioperative bleeding. Mean platelet count in the patients (175×10^9/L) was significantly lower than unaffected family members (289.5×10^9/L), and MPV (10.6 fL) was significantly higher. Semiquantitative Western blot and flow cytometry documented an expected 50% reduction in the expression of platelet GPIbβ. Platelet function analyzed using PFA-100 revealed prolonged closure time in 70% of the cohort and platelet aggregation to ristocetin was reduced in 50%. In summary, patients with VCFS may have mild macrothrombocytopenia with platelet function defects and a bleeding phenotype that is more subtle than in BSS patients. Patients with VCFS, however, can develop a severe bleeding phenotype if they have mutations on the single *GP1BB* gene on the unaffected chromosome,[72] resulting in compound heterozygous BSS.

Gray Platelet Syndrome

Introduction

Gray platelet syndrome (GPS) was first recognized in 1971 by Raccuglia,[73] who described an 11-year-old boy with a history of petechiae and ecchymosis since birth, who was noted to have thrombocytopenia and gray-appearing agranular platelets on peripheral smear. GPS is a moderate bleeding disorder characterized by the appearance of large platelets lacking alpha granules and their contents.[74] The diagnosis is suspected on visualizing large gray-appearing platelets on a Wright-Giemsa–stained blood film (**Fig. 4**A) and confirmed by thin-section transmission electron microscopy

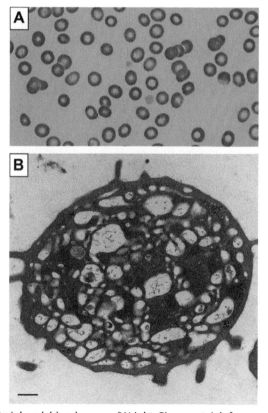

Fig. 4. GPS. (*A*) Peripheral blood smear (Wright-Giemsa stain) from a patient with GPS demonstrating large gray-appearing platelets. (*B*) Platelet transmission electron micrograph from a patient with GPS showing complete absence of alpha granules with increased vacuoles. See transmission electron microscopy of normal platelet in **Fig. 2**A for comparison (scale bar represents 5 nm).

showing complete absence of alpha granules, with normal dense granules and other platelet organelles (see **Fig. 4**B). Studies have shown that platelets and megakaryocytes of GPS patients have rudimentary alpha granule precursors[75] and the basic defect in GPS is thought to be the inability of megakaryocytes to pack endogenously synthesized proteins into developing alpha granules.[76] Immunoblots of platelet lysates show a marked reduction of proteins synthesized in the megakaryocytes, such as platelet factor 4, β-thromboglobulin, and VWF, as well as those endocytosed by megakaryocytes and developing platelets, such as immunoglobulin, albumin, and fibrinogen. The inheritance pattern of GPS is thought to be predominantly autosomal recessive, although autosomal dominant, and at least 1 kindred with X-linked inheritance have been described.[77]

Molecular defect
Using genome-wide linkage analysis in 25 GPS patients from 14 families, the gene for autosomal recessive GPS was initially mapped to a 9.4-Mb interval on 3p21.[76] Homozygosity mapping with single-nucleotide polymorphism arrays from 6 different GPS patients narrowed this interval on 3p21.[78] Subsequently, 3 different groups identified mutations in *NBEAL2* as the cause of GPS.[79–81] NBEAL2 encodes a protein containing a BEACH (Beige and Chediak-Higashi syndrome [CHS]) domain that is predicted to be involved in vesicular trafficking and is likely critical for the development of alpha granules in megakaryocytes and platelets.[81] There is 1 report of X-linked GPS secondary to a *GATA1* Arg216Gln mutation, although some experts think that this should be termed, *X-linked thrombocytopenia with thalassemia*, rather than GPS.[77,82]

Clinical presentation and laboratory evaluation
Understanding of the phenotypic manifestation of GPS has been significantly advanced by a recent review of 21 patients (13 women and 8 men) from 14 unrelated families.[76] The average age of onset of symptoms was 2.6 ($\pm$2.2) years and the average age of diagnosis was 11.8 ($\pm$10.7) years. There was marked heterogeneity in the bleeding tendency, ranging from epistaxis, easy bruising, and postoperative hemorrhage in most patients to severe, fatal metromenorrhagia in 2 patients. Splenomegaly was detected in 88% (15/17) patients.

Thrombocytopenia was moderate and negatively correlated with age, such that mean platelet counts of subjects older than 12 years (46 [$\pm$18] $\times$ 10^9/L) was significantly lower than those seen in younger patients (113 [$\pm$45] $\times$ 10^9/L; $P<.0001$). Platelet aggregation studies were normal in most patients tested and, furthermore, did not correspond with the severity of bleeding. Myelofibrosis was seen in 88% (7/8) of the cohort tested and was thought to be progressive on serial bone marrow evaluations. Myelofibrosis has been described in other series as well[74] and is thought to be secondary to the continual release of growth factors that are not packaged into the alpha granules from the megakaryocytes into the bone marrow. The series also demonstrated high levels of serum vitamin B$_{12}$ in 12 of the 13 patients tested and recommended using vitamin B$_{12}$ levels as a biochemical marker in patients with suspected GPS to reinforce the indication for platelet electron microscopy.

Congenital Amegakaryocytic Thrombocytopenia

Introduction
Since its first description in 1929 by Greenwald and Sherman, approximately 100 cases of congenital amegakaryocytic thrombocytopenia (CAMT) have been described in the literature.[83] CAMT is an autosomal recessive bone marrow failure syndrome that is characterized by severe thrombocytopenia present at birth, an almost complete

lack of megakaryocytes in the bone marrow, and progression to pancytopenia/aplastic anemia within the first few years of life.

Differential diagnoses of severe thrombocytopenia in otherwise healthy newborns include TAR syndrome, radioulnar synostosis with amegakaryocytic thrombocytopenia, and neonatal autoimmune and alloimmune thrombocytopenia. TAR syndrome and radioulnar synostosis with amegakaryocytic thrombocytopenia can usually be identified based on the accompanying congenital anomalies. Neonatal autoimmune thrombocytopenia occurs secondary to the passive transfer of maternal autoantibodies and can be identified by doing a blood count on the mother. Neonatal alloimmune thrombocytopenia occurs secondary to maternal IgG alloantibodies and may be difficult to differentiate from CAMT. With an incidence of 1:1000 to 1:2000 live births, it is more common than CAMT, usually responds to therapy with steroids and IVIG, and resolves within 2 to 4 weeks. Serologic assays using patient or maternal serum can detect platelet specific alloantibodies and help diagnose neonatal alloimmune thrombocytopenia.[84]

Molecular defect

Most cases of CAMT occur secondary to homozygous or compound heterozygous mutations in c-MPL (myeloproliferative leukemia virus oncogene) on 1p34, resulting in abnormal expression or function of the thrombopoietin (TPO) receptor c-MPL.[85] Megakaryocytes lacking a functional c-MPL cannot be stimulated by TPO and, therefore, cannot proliferate. In TPO-null and c-MPL–null mice, platelet numbers are reduced to less than 10% of normal.[86] In addition, hematopoietic progenitors and stem cells were also significantly reduced in these mice, thereby partially explaining the progression to pancytopenia in children with CAMT. Since the first description of c-MPL mutation in a CAMT patient,[87] more than 40 mutations have been described in the 12 coding exons of this gene[88]; 75% of these mutations have been described in the first 5 exons, which encode the first cytokine receptor homology domain, with 60% of the mutations described in exons 1 and 2.

Clinical presentation and laboratory evaluation

A systematic review of 96 patients with CAMT reported marked heterogeneity in bleeding manifestations.[88] Although most patients had epistaxis, easy bruising, and petechiae, 30% (17/57) patients were reported to have serious hemorrhages, with 19% (11/57) developing intracranial bleeds. Thrombocytopenia was diagnosed at birth in 70% (55/77) of patients and within the first year of life in approximately 90% (69/77). The median platelet count at diagnosis was $16 \times 10^9/L$. Based on the clinical course, Germeshausen and colleagues[89] have divided CAMT into 2 subgroups. Patients with persistently low platelet counts after birth and rapid progression to aplastic anemia were classified as CAMT I. These patients predominantly had nonsense or frameshift mutations, which resulted in a complete loss of c-MPL receptor protein. Patients classified as CAMT II had transient improvement and stabilization of platelet counts ($\geq 50 \times 10^9/L$) in the first year of life with a slower progression to aplastic anemia. These patients predominantly had missense mutations or altered splice sites, which were thought to correspond to a residual function of c-MPL receptor protein.

Bone marrow evaluation in CAMT patients initially shows normal cellularity with absent or severely reduced megakaryocytes, which are small and immature in appearance[84]; however, in rare cases, bone marrow findings have been reported normal at birth, with serial bone marrow aspirations being done to confirm the diagnosis.[90] In the systematic review by Ballmaier and Germeshausen,[88] the median age of onset of pancytopenia or bone marrow hypocellularity was 39 months, although 3 patients were described who had not developed pancytopenia at 10 years or more of age. Plasma TPO levels are uniformly elevated in patients with CAMT, often 10-fold or more above controls.[84] However this test is not routinely available in most coagulation laboratories. Molecular genetics should be used to confirm the diagnosis. Currently, the only definitive therapy for CAMT is hematopoietic stem cell transplantation (HSCT), with a matched sibling being the donor of choice.

Thrombocytopenia–Absent Radius Syndrome

Introduction

TAR syndrome was first described by Shaw and Oliver in 1959,[91] but it was Hall and colleagues[92] who reported the first major series of patients in 1969 and derived the current diagnostic criteria. TAR syndrome is an autosomal recessive syndrome complex characterized by absent radii with the presence of thumbs and congenital or early-onset thrombocytopenia, which is transient and improves with age.[93] The presence of thumbs distinguishes TAR syndrome from other disorders featuring radial aplasia, which are usually associated with absent thumbs.[94] In addition, patients may have skeletal, gastrointestinal, renal, and cardiac anomalies. TAR syndrome is rare, with an estimated prevalence of 1:500,000 to 1:1,000,000 and is thought to be more common in women.[94]

Molecular defect

TAR is inherited in an autosomal recessive manner secondary to compound-heterozygous mutations in the *RBM8A* gene.[95] In a study of 30 patients with TAR syndrome, all subjects were found to have a minimally deleted 200-kb region on chromosome 1q21.1. In 75% of the cases, this microdeletion was identified in 1 asymptomatic parent, whereas in the remaining 25%, it was thought to occur de novo.[96] This deletion involves multiple genes, including *RBM8A*. A subsequent study of 53 patients with TAR syndrome confirmed the 200-kb microdeletion in 51 patients. In addition, gene sequencing identified that the second *RBM8A* allele in all 51 patients had a hypomorphic mutation that was thought to diminish the transcript and protein level.[95,97] Two of the 53 patients who did not have the 200-kb microdeletion were found to have heterozygous mutations within *RBM8A*, of which 1 was an inactivating mutation (frameshift or nonsense), whereas the second was a known hypomorphic mutation.[95,97] *RBM8A* encodes 1 (Y14) of 4 subunits of the exon-junction complex that performs essential RNA processing tasks, such as nuclear export, subcellular localization, translational enhancement, and nonsense-mediated RNA decay, whereby reduced Y14 expression was noted in platelets (and presumably megakaryocytes) from individuals with TAR syndrome.[95] How reduced Y14 results in thrombocytopenia has yet to be determined.

Clinical presentation and laboratory evaluation

All cases of TAR syndrome have radial aplasia. Thumbs are present but are hypoplastic or proximally placed. In a review of 34 patients with TAR syndrome, Greenhalgh and colleagues[94] divided the upper limb anomalies into 3 categories. The first group (mild) had radial aplasia with hypoplasia of the ulna and humerus and a normal shoulder girdle (20/28 [71%]). The second group (moderate) had greater degree of limb shortening with underdevelopment of the shoulder girdle (5/28 [18%]), whereas the third consisted of severely affected patients who had severe shortening of the radius and humerus with phocomelia (3/28 [11%]). In addition to upper limb anomaly, 47% (13/28) of the cohort had lower limb anomalies, including hip dysplasia, small patella, and bowing of legs; 47% (14/30) had cow's milk intolerance; 23% (7/30) had renal anomalies; and 15% (5/33) had cardiac anomalies. Ninety five percent of the cohort had a height at or below the 50th percentile.[94]

Thrombocytopenia of TAR syndrome is usually present at birth or develops within the first few months of life, with platelet counts usually lower than 50×10^9/L.[93] In the series by Greenhalgh and colleagues,[94] platelet count was documented at birth for 17 cases and ranged from 7×10^9/L to 92×10^9/L. Platelet counts may fluctuate over time, although there is a general trend toward improvement, with counts approaching normal by school age.[93,97] Thrombocytopenia is often exacerbated by introduction of cow's milk. Platelet size and granularity are normal with bone marrow evaluation showing reduced and small megakaryocytes accompanied by elevated levels of plasma TPO. The most common clinical presentations of thrombocytopenia include gastrointestinal and intracranial hemorrhage.

Toriello[97] recommends performing deletion/duplication analysis in all children born with bilateral absence of radius and presence of thumbs to identify the deletion of 200-kb region at 1q21.1, with the presence of this deletion confirming the diagnosis. Patients with a high degree of clinical suspicion who lack of the typical deletion should undergo sequencing of the coding and noncoding regions of the *RBM8A* gene. Management includes a multidisciplinary approach with inputs from the hematology, orthopedics, and cardiology services. Platelet transfusions in infants should aim for a platelet count greater than or equal to 30×10^9/L to 50×10^9/L, given the risk in intracranial hemorrhage. Lower transfusion thresholds (platelet count $<10 \times 10^9$/L) have been suggested for older individuals to avoid the risk of alloimmunization.[97]

X-LINKED THROMBOCYTOPENIAS
Wiskott-Aldrich Syndrome and X-linked Thrombocytopenia

Introduction
In 1937, Alfred Wiskott, a Bavarian hematologist, described 3 brothers with a history of thrombocytopenia, bloody diarrhea, eczema, and recurrent skin infection who died early in life from intestinal bleeding and sepsis. Subsequently, in 1954, Robert Aldrich and colleagues[98] traced 6 generations of a family and described 16 male family members (but no female family members) who died of the syndrome described by Wiskott, suggesting a sex-linked recessive mode of inheritance. WAS is now recognized as an X-linked disorder characterized by microthrombocytopenia, eczema, combined immunodeficiency with an increased risk of lymphoid malignancies, and autoimmunity, which occurs secondary to mutations in the *WAS* gene located on Xp11.22-p11.23.[99] A milder allelic variant of the disease, which presents with intermittent thrombocytopenia and eczema, is known as X-linked thrombocytopenia (XLT).

Molecular defect
The *WAS* gene is composed of 12 exons and encodes a 502 amino acid protein (WASp). WASp is a key regulator of actin polymerization in hematopoietic cells where it is involved in signal transduction and cytoskeletal rearrangements.[56] In mouse models, deficiency of WASp is associated with premature proplatelet formation and altered megakaryocyte migration within sinusoids, severely compromising the efficiency of platelet production.[100] In addition, increased peripheral destruction of platelets may contribute to thrombocytopenia, specifically given that splenectomy and IVIG therapy result in improvement in platelet counts.[101]

More than 150 mutations in the *WAS* gene have been identified, with missense mutation in exons 1 to 3 being the most common, followed by nonsense and splice mutations (mostly in exons 6–11) and short deletions and insertions.[101] A genotype-phenotype correlation has been suggested. Missense mutations (usually in exons

1–3) accompanied by partial expression of WASp result in the milder XLT, whereas frameshift, nonsense mutations, and large deletions resulting in complete loss of WASp expression lead to the classical WAS phenotype.[102] X-linked neutropenia, an exceedingly rare phenotypic manifestation of WAS mutation, occurs secondary to gain-of-function missense mutations in the GTPase-binding domain of *WAS*, resulting in a constitutively active WASp. These patients present with profound neutropenia and risk of developing myelodysplasia, in the absence of thrombocytopenia or immunodeficiency.[103]

Clinical presentation and laboratory evaluation

A diagnosis of WAS/XLT should be suspected in any male patients presenting with microthrombocytopenia. Bleeding manifestations are present in more than 80% of patients and can range from mild symptoms, such as epistaxis, gingival bleeding, and petechiae in 78% of patients to life-threatening bleeds and intracranial hemorrhage in 30% of patients.[104] Eczema is seen in 80% of patients, although it is heterogeneous in severity and persistence.[104] Bacterial infections are common in classical WAS and include otitis media (78%), sinusitis (24%), and pneumonia (45%). Although less common, fungal, viral, and *Pneumocystis jiroveci* infections have also been reported.[104] Autoimmune complications and malignancies have been observed in 40% to 70% and 13% to 22% of patients, respectively.[102,104] WAS-associated tumors are typically lymphoreticular malignancies, with leukemia, myelodysplasia, and lymphoma (often Epstein-Barr virus positive) accounting for 90% of the cases.[103]

Based on the presence of these symptoms, a scoring system has been derived, which may help categorize patients into the 3 clinical phenotypes associated with *WAS* mutations, namely, classical WAS, XLT, and X-linked neutropenia, and predict outcome (see review by Albert and colleagues[101]). A score of 1 to 2 indicates a milder phenotype consistent with XLT whereas a score of 3 to 4 is thought consistent with classical WAS. A score of 5 is reserved for patients with either WAS or XLT who develop autoimmunity and/or malignancy. Given the evolution of disease phenotype with age, it is recommended that the score not be used to predict disease severity in infancy.

XLT is usually associated with a milder phenotype, although a recent, retrospective, multicenter study of 173 patients with XLT reported serious hemorrhage in 14%, life-threatening infections in 7%, autoimmunity in 12% and malignancy in 5% of the cohort.[105] Overall survival of the cohort at 60 years was excellent at 81% (95% CI, 66%–97%), although possibility of survival without having experienced a severe, disease-related adverse event at 60 years was only 27% (95% CI, 10%–44%).

The diagnostic hallmark of WAS are small platelets with an MPV of 3.5 fL to 5 fL accompanied by moderate to severe thrombocytopenia (5–50 × 10⁹/L).[10] Decreased T-cell subsets, decreased natural killer cell function, abnormal immunoglobulin levels, absent isohemagluttinin titers, and abnormal antibody production in response to vaccines support the diagnosis. Transmission electron microscopy reveals reduction in alpha and dense granules, and platelet aggregation studies demonstrate a decreased response to ADP, epinephrine, and collagen. Screening for WAS may be performed by flow cytometry of lymphocytes using anti-WASp antibodies, although sequencing of the *WAS* gene is recommended for confirmation.[106]

X-Linked Thrombocytopenia and Dyserythropoiesis (GATA1 Mutations)

Introduction

The zinc-finger transcription factor GATA1 plays a critical role in hematopoiesis, particularly in megakaryocyte and erythroid development. Several mutations have been described in the *GATA1* gene, located on Xp11.23, that result in dysregulation of hematopoietic function, manifesting primarily as macrothrombocytopenia and dyserythropoietic anemia.[107] XLT associated with *GATA1* mutations may be differentiated from WAS by the presence of normal-sized to large-sized platelets, absence of eczema, immunodeficiency, and lymphoma.[3]

Molecular defect
GATA1 is expressed on erythroid, megakaryocyte, eosinophil, and mast cells.[107] The only nonhematopoietic cells expressing GATA1 are the sertoli cells of the testis, although the exact role of GATA1 in these cells remains unclear. Mice studies have shown that GATA1 deficiency results in hyperproliferation of megakaryocytes, incomplete nuclear and cytoplasmic maturation, and macrothrombocytopenia.[108] Six germ-line mutations in *GATA1* have been described, which result in a phenotype of macrothrombocytopenia with mild to severe dyserythropoietic anemia (**Table 3**).[108–113] These mutations are clustered in the highly conserved N-zinc finger domain and result from single amino acid substitutions at 4 positions.[3] In 5 of these mutations, the substitutions interfere with the interaction of GATA1 with its transcription factor, friend of GATA1 (FOG-1). The sixth substitution (Arg216Gln) shows normal interaction of GATA1 with FOG-1 but decreased affinity to its palindromic DNA-binding site.[113] Recently, another mutation (p.Argt216Trp) was described at position 216, which manifests as congenital erythropoietic porphyria, mild thrombocytopenia, normal platelet size, β-thalassemia, and splenomegaly.[114]

Clinical presentation and laboratory evaluation
Patients typically present with a history of significant epistaxis, bruising, and hemorrhage after trauma or surgery that starts in the neonatal period. Thrombocytopenia is usually severe with peripheral smear showing large platelets. In addition, platelet

Table 3
Genotypic mutations and associated phenotypes of X-linked thrombocytopenia and dyserythropoietic anemia associated with *GATA1* mutations

Reference	Mutation	Laboratory Finding	Associated Clinical Findings
Nichols et al,[112] 2000	*p.Val205Met*	Macrothrombocytopenia, severe dyserythropoietic anemia	Cryptorchidism
Freson et al,[110] 2001	*p.Asp218Gly*	Macrothrombocytopenia, dyserythropoiesis but no anemia	None described
Freson et al,[111] 2002	*p.Asp218Tyr*	Macrothrombocytopenia, severe dyserythropoietic anemia	Early death in 6/7 affected subjects
Mehaffey et al,[108] 2001	*p.Gly208Ser*	Macrothrombocytopenia, no anemia	None described
Del Vecchio et al,[109] 2005	*p.Gly208Arg*	Macrothrombocytopenia, mild dyserythropoietic anemia	Cryptorchidism
Yu et al,[113] 2002	*p.Arg216Gln*	Macrothrombocytopenia, β-thalassemia	Splenomegaly
Phillips et al,[114] 2007	*p.Arg216Trp*	Thrombocytopenia, β-thalassemia	Congenital erythropoietic porphyria

aggregation studies suggest abnormal platelet function.[115] Platelet electron microscopy shows clusters composed of smooth endoplasmic reticulum and abnormal membrane complexes, with a paucity of alpha granules.[111] Bone marrow evaluation shows hypercellular marrow with dysplasia in the erythroid and megakaryocyte lineages, without evidence of progression to myelodysplasia, leukemia, or bone marrow failure. The degree of anemia, even for different substitutions at the same site, varies significantly and can range from life-threatening, requiring regular blood transfusions, to mild dyserythropoiesis in the bone marrow.[111]

XLT and dyserythropoiesis should be suspected in boys with congenital thrombocytopenia, anemia, and a hypercellular marrow.[3] GATA1 gene sequencing can be pursued to confirm the diagnosis. Management is largely supportive with platelet and red blood cell transfusion, although successful HSCT for severe cases has been reported.

VERY RARE THROMBOCYTOPENIAS

Very rare thrombocytopenias with few pedigrees reported in literature are included in **Table 1** but not discussed in this article. Readers are referred to a recent review by Balduini and Savoia[2] for further information on these cases.

MANAGEMENT OF PATIENTS WITH CONGENITAL THROMBOCYTOPENIAS

Given the rarity of congenital thrombocytopenias, it is important that patients be referred to a comprehensive bleeding disorders center with appropriate facilities for investigation, transfusion, and management. Education of patients and primary care providers about risk of bleeding and prevention of bleeding and related complications is important. Lifestyle modifications, including avoidance of contact and collision sports, routine dental care to reduce the risk of gingival bleeding, avoidance of platelet impairing medications (aspirin and nonsteroidal anti-inflammatory drugs), and use of medic alert bracelets, should be encouraged. In addition, identification cards bearing the name of underlying disorder and relevant contact information should be provided to all patients. Given the risk of exposure to blood products, patients should be vaccinated against hepatitis A and hepatitis B, and annual liver function tests should be performed on patients who require routine transfusions. Patients with evidence of iron deficiency should be treated with iron supplementation.

Most patients with mild-to-moderate bleeding episodes can be managed with local measures. Compression, use of gelatin sponge or gauze soaked in tranexamic acid may be used for superficial wounds. Epistaxis and oral mucosal bleeding may be managed by nasal packing and use of topical human thrombin. Moderate to major bleeding episodes require specific and nonspecific regimens, including antifibrinolytic medications (lysine analogs), desmopressin (1-deamino-8-D-arginine vasopressin [DDAVP]), and recombinant FVIIa (rFVIIa).[10] Life-threatening bleeds usually require platelet transfusions to compensate for dysfunctional platelets. Excellent reviews on management of patients with platelet disorders are available for further reading.

Antifibrinolytic Agents

Lysine analogs tranexamic acid and epsilon-aminocaproic acid (Amicar), may be used alone or in combination with other therapeutic modalities, such as DDAVP, rFVIIa, and platelet transfusion. They are particularly useful in patients with epistaxis, gingival bleeding, and menorrhagia. They may also be used for prevention of bleeding after minor surgical and dental procedures. Both agents can be used orally and intravenously. Tranexamic acid is preferred because it is cheaper and more potent (8-fold higher antifibrinolytic activity) on a weight-for-weight basis compared with epsilon-aminocaproic acid.[10] The dose of tranexamic acid is 15 mg/kg to 25 mg/kg orally, 3 to 4 times a day (or 10 mg/kg intravenously, 3 to 4 times a day). It is also available as a mouthwash (10 mL of a 5% solution 4 to 6 times a day), which, if swallowed, is equivalent to a dose of 500 mg.[1] Antifibrinolytics are contraindicated in hematuria, given the risk of clot formation in the renal collecting system.

Desmopressin

DDAVP, a synthetic analog of the antidiuretic hormone, vasopressin, is thought to exert its procoagulant effect by increasing the circulating levels of FVIII and VWF,[1,116] although its exact cellular mechanism of hemostatic effect in platelet disorders is still unknown. Since the initial description of the use of DDAVP in patients with platelet functional defects by Kobrinsky and colleagues[117] in 1984, several series have been reported.[118] DDAVP can be administered intravenously, subcutaneously, or intranasally. The standard dose of DDAVP is 0.3 µg/kg (not exceeding 20 µg) administered intravenously (or subcutaneously) or 300 µg administered intranasally (150 µg in children who weigh less than 50 kg). Peak VWF levels are reached within 30 to 60 minutes after intravenous injection and 90 to 120 minutes after intranasal and subcutaneous administration.[116] DDAVP causes fluid retention and hyponatremia and patients should be advised to limit their fluid intake for 24 hours after DDAVP administration. For the same reason, DDAVP should be avoided in children younger than 2 years of age.

Platelet Transfusions

Transfusion of platelets remains the cornerstone of therapy for congenital thrombocytopenia patients with life-threatening or organ-threatening bleeds and patients who are unresponsive to nonspecific hemostatic agents. Patients with severe congenital platelet defects, such as BSS, WAS, and Glanzmann thrombasthenia (GT), require a restrictive platelet transfusion policy given the risk of alloimmunization to either HLA antigens or the missing surface proteins (GPIb-IX-V in BSS or $\alpha IIb\beta_3$ in GT).[116] Development of such antibodies results in the rapid clearance of transfused platelets and consequent platelet refractoriness. Given the obvious therapeutic ramifications of the development of such alloantibodies, several recent reviews, including guidelines by the United Kingdom Hemophilia Center Doctor's Organization (UKHCDO), recommend the use of HLA-matched platelet transfusions to such patients.[1,116] However, getting HLA-matched platelets during a catastrophic bleed may not be practical and will not protect patients from developing antibodies to missing platelet surface proteins in BSS and GT.

Recombinant Factor VIIa

In 1996, Tengborn and Petruson[119] first described the use of rFVIIa (NovoSeven) to control epistaxis in a child with GT. Since then, several cohorts have reported on the successful use of rFVIIa in both children and adults with congenital platelet defects, specifically in patients with GT (and less commonly BSS).[120] rFVIIa is thought to enhance thrombin generation by both tissue factor–dependent and tissue factor–independent mechanisms. In Europe, rFVIIa is now approved for GT patients with platelet alloimmunization and a history of platelet refractoriness.[1] rFVIIa is typically given as an initial dose of 90 µg/kg, with repeat doses every 2 to 4 hours, depending on the clinical status of a patient. Thrombotic complications are a rare but serious side effect of rFVIIa.

Thrombopoietin Receptor Agonists

The recently reported TPO receptor agonists, romiplostim and eltrombopag, are now approved by the Food and Drug Administration as second-line treatment of chronic ITP. These drugs represent an appealing therapeutic modality for patients with certain congenital thrombocytopenias, such as MYH9-RD, specifically since in vitro studies have shown that the platelet aggregation is largely preserved in such patients. Therefore, increasing the platelet counts, at least theoretically, should reduce the bleeding tendency. Safety and efficacy data on eltrombopag, an oral nonpeptide TPO receptor agonist, was recently reported in 12 patients with MYH9-RD.[15] Subsequently, the same group reported the first major surgical procedure in a patient with MYH9-RD done under the cover of eltrombopag (50 mg/kg/d starting 20 days before the anticipated procedure with close monitoring of platelet counts).[121]

Renin-angiotensin System Blockage for Nephropathy Associated with MYH9-RD

Nephropathy associated with MYH9-RD tends to be progressive, eventually causing ESRD requiring dialysis or renal transplant. Pecci and colleagues[122] recently reported 4 patients with genetically confirmed MYH9-related nephropathy in whom the proteinuria significantly improved after treatment with angiotensin receptor blockers and/or angiotensin-converting enzyme inhibitors. Although these findings cannot be used to make clinical recommendations, blockage of the renin-angiotensin system as renoprotective treatment in patients remains an attractive hypothesis for testing in larger studies.

Hematopoietic Stem Cell Transplant

HSCT is an effective therapy for platelet disorders that are accompanied by other life-threatening conditions, where the risks of transplant outweigh the risks of supportive treatment modalities. These include diseases with severe long-term sequelae, such as progression to aplastic anemia (CAMT or amegakaryocytic thrombocytopenia with radioulnar synostosis) or risk of life-threatening infections (WAS).

Currently, the only definitive therapy for patients with CAMT is HSCT, with transplantation from a matched sibling donor, if available, being the treatment modality of choice.[84] In a retrospective, single-institution study by King and colleagues,[123] 15 of 20 patients with CAMT underwent HSCT at median age of 38 months (range 7–89 months). All 4 patients who received HSCT from a matched unrelated donor had a fatal outcome, whereas only 1 patient who received an HSCT from a related donor (HLA identical sibling/haploidentical parent) died. Similar findings were reported in a systematic review of literature by Ballmaier and Germeshausen,[88] where the HSCT-related mortality was 1 of 13 for matched related donors (7.7%) and 5 of 18 for unrelated donors (27.8%). However, more recent reports have documented that unrelated donor transplants may be a viable option in CAMT.[124]

Since the first description of successful HSCT for WAS in 1968,[125] HSCT has become the therapeutic modality of choice for boys with classic WAS. A retrospective analysis of 170 transplants reported to the International Bone Marrow Transplant Registry and/or National Marrow Donor Program reported a 5-year overall survival of 70% (95% CI, 63%–77%), with improved survival in HLA-identical sibling donors (84% [95% CI, 74%–93%]) compared with unrelated (71% [95% CI, 58%–80%]) and other related donors (53% [95% CI, 37%–65%]). Outcomes for MUD transplants, however, done in patients under 5 years of age were similar to those for HLA-identical sibling donors.[126] More recently, a study from Cincinnati Children's reported improved survival for transplants done from 2001 to 2009 (90.8% [95% CI, 66.7%–97.6%])

compared with transplants done during the years 1990 to 2000 (62.5% [95% CI, 34.9–81.1]). Extent of mismatch did not have an impact on the outcome in multivariate analysis.[127] Thus, stem cell transplant with the best available donor, done as early as possible, remains the therapeutic modality of choice for classic WAS. Successful HSCT has also been reported for patients with amegakaryocytic thrombocytopenia with radioulnar synostosis and BSS.[116]

Gene Therapy for WAS

Introduction of a normal *WAS* gene copy into CD34[+] stem cells isolated from WAS patients and the subsequent reinfusion of the manipulated cells into patients via a viral vector after administration of suboptimal doses of busulfan form the basis of gene therapy for WAS.[101] Recently, a gene therapy trial for WAS using a retroviral vector encoding the full WASp cDNA was initiated in Hanover, Germany. Preliminary results on 2 patients reported correction of thrombocytopenia and resolution of eczema and autoimmunity for more than 24 months after treatment, accompanied by sustained WASp expression in stem cells, lymphoid, and myeloid cells and platelets.[128] Other studies using lentiviral vectors, which are thought to be less genotoxic than retroviral vectors, are currently under way.

ACKNOWLEDGMENTS

The authors would like to thank Hilary Christensen for the platelet electron micrographs, William Brien for the BSS blood film, and Fred Pluthero for the NMMHC-IIA immunofluorescence images. Riten Kumar is a recipient of the Baxter Bioscience Pediatric Hemostasis and Thrombosis fellowship at the Hospital for Sick Children, Toronto (2011–2013).

REFERENCES

1. Bolton-Maggs PH, Chalmers EA, Collins PW, et al. A review of inherited platelet disorders with guidelines for their management on behalf of the UKHCDO. Br J Haematol 2006;135(5):603–33.
2. Balduini CL, Savoia A. Genetics of familial forms of thrombocytopenia. Hum Genet 2012;131(12):1821–32.
3. Drachman JG. Inherited thrombocytopenia: when a low platelet count does not mean ITP. Blood 2004;103(2):390–8.
4. Biss TT, Blanchette VS, Clark DS, et al. Quantitation of bleeding symptoms in children with von Willebrand disease: use of a standardized pediatric bleeding questionnaire. J Thromb Haemost 2010;8(5):950–6.
5. Rodeghiero F, Tosetto A, Abshire T, et al. ISTH/SSC bleeding assessment tool: a standardized questionnaire and a proposal for a new bleeding score for inherited bleeding disorders. J Thromb Haemost 2010;8(9):2063–5.
6. Balduini CL, Pecci A, Savoia A. Recent advances in the understanding and management of MYH9-related inherited thrombocytopenias. Br J Haematol 2011;154(2):161–74.
7. Hegglin R. [Not available]. Helv Med Acta 1945;12:439.
8. Kelley MJ, Jawien W, Ortel TL, et al. Mutation of MYH9, encoding non-muscle myosin heavy chain A, in May-Hegglin anomaly. Nat Genet 2000;26(1):106–8.
9. Seri M, Cusano R, Gangarossa S, et al. Mutations in MYH9 result in the May-Hegglin anomaly, and Fechtner and Sebastian syndromes. The May-Hegglin/Fechtner Syndrome Consortium. Nat Genet 2000;26(1):103–5.

10. Cox K, Price V, Kahr WH. Inherited platelet disorders: a clinical approach to diagnosis and management. Expert Rev Hematol 2011;4(4):455–72.

11. Chang Y, Aurade F, Larbret F, et al. Proplatelet formation is regulated by the Rho/ROCK pathway. Blood 2007;109(10):4229–36.

12. Chen Z, Naveiras O, Balduini A, et al. The May-Hegglin anomaly gene MYH9 is a negative regulator of platelet biogenesis modulated by the Rho-ROCK pathway. Blood 2007;110(1):171–9.

13. Pecci A, Malara A, Badalucco S, et al. Megakaryocytes of patients with MYH9-related thrombocytopenia present an altered proplatelet formation. Thromb Haemost 2009;102(1):90–6.

14. Leung TF, Tsoi WC, Li CK, et al. A Chinese adolescent girl with Fechtner-like syndrome. Acta Paediatr 1998;87(6):705–7.

15. Pecci A, Gresele P, Klersy C, et al. Eltrombopag for the treatment of the inherited thrombocytopenia deriving from MYH9 mutations. Blood 2010; 116(26):5832–7.

16. Pecci A, Panza E, Pujol-Moix N, et al. Position of nonmuscle myosin heavy chain IIA (NMMHC-IIA) mutations predicts the natural history of MYH9-related disease. Hum Mutat 2008;29(3):409–17.

17. Noris P, Klersy C, Zecca M, et al. Platelet size distinguishes between inherited macrothrombocytopenias and immune thrombocytopenia. J Thromb Haemost 2009;7(12):2131–6.

18. Pecci A, Panza E, De Rocco D, et al. MYH9 related disease: four novel mutations of the tail domain of myosin-9 correlating with a mild clinical phenotype. Eur J Haematol 2010;84(4):291–7.

19. Savoia A, De Rocco D, Panza E, et al. Heavy chain myosin 9-related disease (MYH9 -RD): neutrophil inclusions of myosin-9 as a pathognomonic sign of the disorder. Thromb Haemost 2010;103(4):826–32.

20. Breton-Gorius J, Favier R, Guichard J, et al. A new congenital dysmegakaryopoietic thrombocytopenia (Paris-Trousseau) associated with giant platelet alpha-granules and chromosome 11 deletion at 11q23. Blood 1995;85(7):1805–14.

21. Favier R, Douay L, Esteva B, et al. A novel genetic thrombocytopenia (Paris-Trousseau) associated with platelet inclusions, dysmegakaryopoiesis and chromosome deletion AT 11q23. C R Acad Sci III 1993;316(7):698–701.

22. Favier R, Jondeau K, Boutard P, et al. Paris-Trousseau syndrome: clinical, hematological, molecular data of ten new cases. Thromb Haemost 2003;90(5): 893–7.

23. Hart A, Melet F, Grossfeld P, et al. Fli-1 is required for murine vascular and megakaryocytic development and is hemizygously deleted in patients with thrombocytopenia. Immunity 2000;13(2):167–77.

24. Hashimoto Y, Ware J. Identification of essential GATA and Ets binding motifs within the promoter of the platelet glycoprotein Ib alpha gene. J Biol Chem 1995;270(41):24532–9.

25. Spyropoulos DD, Pharr PN, Lavenburg KR, et al. Hemorrhage, impaired hematopoiesis, and lethality in mouse embryos carrying a targeted disruption of the Fli1 transcription factor. Mol Cell Biol 2000;20(15):5643–52.

26. Raslova H, Komura E, Le Couedic JP, et al. FLI1 monoallelic expression combined with its hemizygous loss underlies Paris-Trousseau/Jacobsen thrombopenia. J Clin Invest 2004;114(1):77–84.

27. Noris P, Valli R, Pecci A, et al. Clonal chromosome anomalies affecting FLI1 mimic inherited thrombocytopenia of the Paris-Trousseau type. Eur J Haematol 2012;89(4):345–9.

28. Guerin A, Stavropoulos DJ, Diab Y, et al. Interstitial deletion of 11q-implicating the KIRREL3 gene in the neurocognitive delay associated with Jacobsen syndrome. Am J Med Genet A 2012;158(10):2551–6.

29. Weiss HJ, Meyer D, Rabinowitz R, et al. Pseudo-von Willebrand's disease. An intrinsic platelet defect with aggregation by unmodified human factor VIII/von Willebrand factor and enhanced adsorption of its high-molecular-weight multimers. N Engl J Med 1982;306(6):326–33.

30. Othman M. Platelet-type von Willebrand disease: a rare, often misdiagnosed and underdiagnosed bleeding disorder. Semin Thromb Hemost 2011;37(5):464–9.

31. Miller JL, Cunningham D, Lyle VA, et al. Mutation in the gene encoding the alpha chain of platelet glycoprotein Ib in platelet-type von Willebrand disease. Proc Natl Acad Sci U S A 1991;88(11):4761–5.

32. Russell SD, Roth GJ. Pseudo-von Willebrand disease: a mutation in the platelet glycoprotein Ib alpha gene associated with a hyperactive surface receptor. Blood 1993;81(7):1787–91.

33. Matsubara Y, Murata M, Sugita K, et al. Identification of a novel point mutation in platelet glycoprotein Ibalpha, Gly to Ser at residue 233, in a Japanese family with platelet-type von Willebrand disease. J Thromb Haemost 2003;1(10): 2198–205.

34. Said Enayat SR, Rassoulzadegan M, Jazebi M, et al. A novel D235Y mutation in the GP1BA gene enhances platelet interaction with VWF in an Iranian family with platelet type von Willebrand disease. Scientific and Standardization Committee of International Society of Thrombosis and Haemostasis. Liverpool (United Kingdom): 2012.

35. Othman M, Notley C, Lavender FL, et al. Identification and functional characterization of a novel 27-bp deletion in the macroglycopeptide-coding region of the GPIBA gene resulting in platelet-type von Willebrand disease. Blood 2005; 105(11):4330–6.

36. Othman M. Platelet-type Von Willebrand disease: three decades in the life of a rare bleeding disorder. Blood Rev 2011;25(4):147–53.

37. Suva LJ, Hartman E, Dilley JD, et al. Platelet dysfunction and a high bone mass phenotype in a murine model of platelet-type von Willebrand disease. Am J Pathol 2008;172(2):430–9.

38. Enayat MS, Guilliatt AM, Lester W, et al. Distinguishing between type 2B and pseudo-von Willebrand disease and its clinical importance. Br J Haematol 2006;133(6):664–6.

39. Favaloro EJ. Phenotypic identification of platelet-type von Willebrand disease and its discrimination from type 2B von Willebrand disease: a question of 2B or not 2B? A story of nonidentical twins? Or two sides of a multidenominational or multifaceted primary-hemostasis coin? Semin Thromb Hemost 2008;34(1): 113–27.

40. Giannini S, Cecchetti L, Mezzasoma AM, et al. Diagnosis of platelet-type von Willebrand disease by flow cytometry. Haematologica 2010;95(6):1021–4.

41. Thompson AA, Nguyen LT. Amegakaryocytic thrombocytopenia and radio-ulnar synostosis are associated with HOXA11 mutation. Nat Genet 2000;26(4):397–8.

42. Thompson AA, Woodruff K, Feig SA, et al. Congenital thrombocytopenia and radio-ulnar synostosis: a new familial syndrome. Br J Haematol 2001;113(4): 866–70.

43. Horvat-Switzer RD, Thompson AA. HOXA11 mutation in amegakaryocytic thrombocytopenia with radio-ulnar synostosis syndrome inhibits megakaryocytic differentiation in vitro. Blood Cells Mol Dis 2006;37(1):55–63.

44. Castillo-Caro P, Dhanraj S, Haut P, et al. Proximal radio-ulnar synostosis with bone marrow failure syndrome in an infant without a HOXA11 mutation. J Pediatr Hematol Oncol 2010;32(6):479–85.
45. Sola MC, Slayton WB, Rimsza LM, et al. A neonate with severe thrombocytopenia and radio-ulnar synostosis. J Perinatol 2004;24(8):528–30.
46. Dowton SB, Beardsley D, Jamison D, et al. Studies of a familial platelet disorder. Blood 1985;65(3):557–63.
47. Ho CY, Otterud B, Legare RD, et al. Linkage of a familial platelet disorder with a propensity to develop myeloid malignancies to human chromosome 21q22.1–22.2. Blood 1996;87(12):5218–24.
48. Song WJ, Sullivan MG, Legare RD, et al. Haploinsufficiency of CBFA2 causes familial thrombocytopenia with propensity to develop acute myelogenous leukaemia. Nat Genet 1999;23(2):166–75.
49. Liew E, Owen C. Familial myelodysplastic syndromes: a review of the literature. Haematologica 2011;96(10):1536–42.
50. Owen C, Barnett M, Fitzgibbon J. Familial myelodysplasia and acute myeloid leukaemia–a review. Br J Haematol 2008;140(2):123–32.
51. Levanon D, Glusman G, Bangsow T, et al. Architecture and anatomy of the genomic locus encoding the human leukemia-associated transcription factor RUNX1/AML1. Gene 2001;262(1–2):23–33.
52. Huang G, Shigesada K, Ito K, et al. Dimerization with PEBP2beta protects RUNX1/AML1 from ubiquitin-proteasome-mediated degradation. EMBO J 2001;20(4):723–33.
53. Ganly P, Walker LC, Morris CM. Familial mutations of the transcription factor RUNX1 (AML1, CBFA2) predispose to acute myeloid leukemia. Leuk Lymphoma 2004;45(1):1–10.
54. Bernard J, Soulier JP. [Not available]. Bull Mem Soc Med Hop Paris 1948;64(28–29):969–74.
55. Lanza F. Bernard-Soulier syndrome (hemorrhagiparous thrombocytic dystrophy). Orphanet J Rare Dis 2006;1:46.
56. Nurden A, Nurden P. Advances in our understanding of the molecular basis of disorders of platelet function. J Thromb Haemost 2011;9(Suppl 1):76–91.
57. Nurden AT, Caen JP. Specific roles for platelet surface glycoproteins in platelet function. Nature 1975;255(5511):720–2.
58. Wei AH, Schoenwaelder SM, Andrews RK, et al. New insights into the haemostatic function of platelets. Br J Haematol 2009;147(4):415–30.
59. Cranmer SL, Ashworth KJ, Yao Y, et al. High shear-dependent loss of membrane integrity and defective platelet adhesion following disruption of the GPIbalpha-filamin interaction. Blood 2011;117(9):2718–27.
60. Balduini A, Malara A, Pecci A, et al. Proplatelet formation in heterozygous Bernard-Soulier syndrome type Bolzano. J Thromb Haemost 2009;7(3):478–84.
61. Strassel C, Eckly A, Leon C, et al. Intrinsic impaired proplatelet formation and microtubule coil assembly of megakaryocytes in a mouse model of Bernard-Soulier syndrome. Haematologica 2009;94(6):800–10.
62. Savoia A, Pastore A, De Rocco D, et al. Clinical and genetic aspects of Bernard-Soulier syndrome: searching for genotype/phenotype correlations. Haematologica 2011;96(3):417–23.
63. Lopez JA, Andrews RK, Afshar-Kharghan V, et al. Bernard-Soulier syndrome. Blood 1998;91(12):4397–418.

64. Noris P, Pecci A, Di Bari F, et al. Application of a diagnostic algorithm for inherited thrombocytopenias to 46 consecutive patients. Haematologica 2004; 89(10):1219–25.
65. Hayward CP, Harrison P, Cattaneo M, et al. Platelet function analyzer (PFA)-100 closure time in the evaluation of platelet disorders and platelet function. J Thromb Haemost 2006;4(2):312–9.
66. Nurden P, Nurden AT. Congenital disorders associated with platelet dysfunctions. Thromb Haemost 2008;99(2):253–63.
67. Behrens WE. Mediterranean macrothrombocytopenia. Blood 1975;46(2):199–208.
68. Savoia A, Balduini CL, Savino M, et al. Autosomal dominant macrothrombocytopenia in Italy is most frequently a type of heterozygous Bernard-Soulier syndrome. Blood 2001;97(5):1330–5.
69. Noris P, Perrotta S, Bottega R, et al. Clinical and laboratory features of 103 patients from 42 Italian families with inherited thrombocytopenia derived from the monoallelic Ala156Val mutation of GPIbalpha (Bolzano mutation). Haematologica 2012;97(1):82–8.
70. Van Geet C, Devriendt K, Eyskens B, et al. Velocardiofacial syndrome patients with a heterozygous chromosome 22q11 deletion have giant platelets. Pediatr Res 1998;44(4):607–11.
71. Liang HP, Morel-Kopp MC, Curtin J, et al. Heterozygous loss of platelet glycoprotein (GP) Ib-V-IX variably affects platelet function in velocardiofacial syndrome (VCFS) patients. Thromb Haemost 2007;98(6):1298–308.
72. Budarf ML, Konkle BA, Ludlow LB, et al. Identification of a patient with Bernard-Soulier syndrome and a deletion in the DiGeorge/velo-cardio-facial chromosomal region in 22q11.2. Hum Mol Genet 1995;4(4):763–6.
73. Raccuglia G. Gray platelet syndrome. A variety of qualitative platelet disorder. Am J Med 1971;51(6):818–28.
74. Nurden AT, Nurden P. The gray platelet syndrome: clinical spectrum of the disease. Blood Rev 2007;21(1):21–36.
75. Maynard DM, Heijnen HF, Gahl WA, et al. The alpha-granule proteome: novel proteins in normal and ghost granules in gray platelet syndrome. J Thromb Haemost 2010;8(8):1786–96.
76. Gunay-Aygun M, Zivony-Elboum Y, Gumruk F, et al. Gray platelet syndrome: natural history of a large patient cohort and locus assignment to chromosome 3p. Blood 2010;116(23):4990–5001.
77. Tubman VN, Levine JE, Campagna DR, et al. X-linked gray platelet syndrome due to a GATA1 Arg216Gln mutation. Blood 2007;109(8):3297–9.
78. Fabbro S, Kahr WH, Hinckley J, et al. Homozygosity mapping with SNP arrays confirms 3p21 as a recessive locus for gray platelet syndrome and narrows the interval significantly. Blood 2011;117(12):3430–4.
79. Albers CA, Cvejic A, Favier R, et al. Exome sequencing identifies NBEAL2 as the causative gene for gray platelet syndrome. Nat Genet 2011;43(8):735–7.
80. Gunay-Aygun M, Falik-Zaccai TC, Vilboux T, et al. NBEAL2 is mutated in gray platelet syndrome and is required for biogenesis of platelet alpha-granules. Nat Genet 2011;43(8):732–4.
81. Kahr WH, Hinckley J, Li L, et al. Mutations in NBEAL2, encoding a BEACH protein, cause gray platelet syndrome. Nat Genet 2011;43(8):738–40.
82. Balduini CL, De Candia E, Savoia A. Why the disorder induced by GATA1 Arg216Gln mutation should be called "X-linked thrombocytopenia with thalassemia" rather than "X-linked gray platelet syndrome". Blood 2007;110(7): 2770–1 [author reply: 2771].

83. Ballmaier M, Germeshausen M. Advances in the understanding of congenital amegakaryocytic thrombocytopenia. Br J Haematol 2009;146(1):3–16.
84. Geddis AE. Congenital amegakaryocytic thrombocytopenia. Pediatr Blood Cancer 2011;57(2):199–203.
85. Ballmaier M, Germeshausen M, Schulze H, et al. c-mpl Mutations are the cause of congenital amegakaryocytic thrombocytopenia. Blood 2001;97(1):139–46.
86. Alexander WS, Roberts AW, Maurer AB, et al. Studies of the c-Mpl thrombopoietin receptor through gene disruption and activation. Stem Cells 1996;14(Suppl 1):124–32.
87. Ihara K, Ishii E, Eguchi M, et al. Identification of mutations in the c-mpl gene in congenital amegakaryocytic thrombocytopenia. Proc Natl Acad Sci U S A 1999;96(6):3132–6.
88. Ballmaier M, Germeshausen M. Congenital amegakaryocytic thrombocytopenia: clinical presentation, diagnosis, and treatment. Semin Thromb Hemost 2011;37(6):673–81.
89. Germeshausen M, Ballmaier M, Welte K. MPL mutations in 23 patients suffering from congenital amegakaryocytic thrombocytopenia: the type of mutation predicts the course of the disease. Hum Mutat 2006;27(3):296.
90. Rose MJ, Nicol KK, Skeens MA, et al. Congenital amegakaryocytic thrombocytopenia: the diagnostic importance of combining pathology with molecular genetics. Pediatr Blood Cancer 2008;50(6):1263–5.
91. Shaw S, Oliver RA. Congenital hypoplastic thrombocytopenia with skeletal deformaties in siblings. Blood 1959;14(4):374–7.
92. Hall JG, Levin J, Kuhn JP, et al. Thrombocytopenia with absent radius (TAR). Medicine (Baltimore) 1969;48(6):411–39.
93. Toriello HV. Thrombocytopenia-absent radius syndrome. Semin Thromb Hemost 2011;37(6):707–12.
94. Greenhalgh KL, Howell RT, Bottani A, et al. Thrombocytopenia-absent radius syndrome: a clinical genetic study. J Med Genet 2002;39(12):876–81.
95. Albers CA, Paul DS, Schulze H, et al. Compound inheritance of a low-frequency regulatory SNP and a rare null mutation in exon-junction complex subunit RBM8A causes TAR syndrome. Nat Genet 2012;44(4):435–9, S431–2.
96. Klopocki E, Schulze H, Strauss G, et al. Complex inheritance pattern resembling autosomal recessive inheritance involving a microdeletion in thrombocytopenia-absent radius syndrome. Am J Hum Genet 2007;80(2):232–40.
97. Toriello HV. Thrombocytopenia absent radius syndrome. In: Pagon RA, Bird TD, Dolan CR, et al, editors. GeneReviews. Seattle (WA): University of Washington; 1993.
98. Aldrich RA, Steinberg AG, Campbell DC. Pedigree demonstrating a sex-linked recessive condition characterized by draining ears, eczematoid dermatitis and bloody diarrhea. Pediatrics 1954;13(2):133–9.
99. Derry JM, Ochs HD, Francke U. Isolation of a novel gene mutated in Wiskott-Aldrich syndrome. Cell 1994;78(4):635–44.
100. Sabri S, Foudi A, Boukour S, et al. Deficiency in the Wiskott-Aldrich protein induces premature proplatelet formation and platelet production in the bone marrow compartment. Blood 2006;108(1):134–40.
101. Albert MH, Notarangelo LD, Ochs HD. Clinical spectrum, pathophysiology and treatment of the Wiskott-Aldrich syndrome. Curr Opin Hematol 2011;18:42–8.
102. Imai K, Morio T, Zhu Y, et al. Clinical course of patients with WASP gene mutations. Blood 2004;103(2):456–64.

103. Bosticardo M, Marangoni F, Aiuti A, et al. Recent advances in understanding the pathophysiology of Wiskott-Aldrich syndrome. Blood 2009;113(25):6288–95.

104. Sullivan KE, Mullen CA, Blaese RM, et al. A multiinstitutional survey of the Wiskott-Aldrich syndrome. J Pediatr 1994;125(6 Pt 1):876–85.

105. Albert MH, Bittner TC, Nonoyama S, et al. X-linked thrombocytopenia (XLT) due to WAS mutations: clinical characteristics, long-term outcome, and treatment options. Blood 2010;115(16):3231–8.

106. Ochs HD. The Wiskott-Aldrich syndrome. Clin Rev Allergy Immunol 2001;20(1): 61–86.

107. Millikan PD, Balamohan SM, Raskind WH, et al. Inherited thrombocytopenia due to GATA-1 mutations. Semin Thromb Hemost 2011;37(6):682–9.

108. Mehaffey MG, Newton AL, Gandhi MJ, et al. X-linked thrombocytopenia caused by a novel mutation of GATA-1. Blood 2001;98(9):2681–8.

109. Del Vecchio GC, Giordani L, De Santis A, et al. Dyserythropoietic anemia and thrombocytopenia due to a novel mutation in GATA-1. Acta Haematol 2005; 114(2):113–6.

110. Freson K, Devriendt K, Matthijs G, et al. Platelet characteristics in patients with X-linked macrothrombocytopenia because of a novel GATA1 mutation. Blood 2001;98(1):85–92.

111. Freson K, Matthijs G, Thys C, et al. Different substitutions at residue D218 of the X-linked transcription factor GATA1 lead to altered clinical severity of macro-thrombocytopenia and anemia and are associated with variable skewed X inactivation. Hum Mol Genet 2002;11(2):147–52.

112. Nichols KE, Crispino JD, Poncz M, et al. Familial dyserythropoietic anaemia and thrombocytopenia due to an inherited mutation in GATA1. Nat Genet 2000;24(3): 266–70.

113. Yu C, Niakan KK, Matsushita M, et al. X-linked thrombocytopenia with thalassemia from a mutation in the amino finger of GATA-1 affecting DNA binding rather than FOG-1 interaction. Blood 2002;100(6):2040–5.

114. Phillips JD, Steensma DP, Pulsipher MA, et al. Congenital erythropoietic porphyria due to a mutation in GATA1: the first trans-acting mutation causative for a human porphyria. Blood 2007;109(6):2618–21.

115. Kacena MA, Chou ST, Weiss MJ, et al. GATA1-Related X-Linked Cytopenia. In: Pagon RA, Bird TD, Dolan CR, et al, editors. GeneReviews. Seattle (WA): University of Washington; 1993.

116. Alamelu J, Liesner R. Modern management of severe platelet function disorders. Br J Haematol 2010;149(6):813–23.

117. Kobrinsky NL, Israels ED, Gerrard JM, et al. Shortening of bleeding time by 1-deamino-8-D-arginine vasopressin in various bleeding disorders. Lancet 1984;1(8387):1145–8.

118. Balduini CL, Noris P, Belletti S, et al. In vitro and in vivo effects of desmopressin on platelet function. Haematologica 1999;84(10):891–6.

119. Tengborn L, Petruson B. A patient with Glanzmann thrombasthenia and epistaxis successfully treated with recombinant factor VIIa. Thromb Haemost 1996;75(6): 981–2.

120. Almeida AM, Khair K, Hann I, et al. The use of recombinant factor VIIa in children with inherited platelet function disorders. Br J Haematol 2003;121(3): 477–81.

121. Pecci A, Barozzi S, d'Amico S, et al. Short-term eltrombopag for surgical preparation of a patient with inherited thrombocytopenia deriving from MYH9 mutation. Thromb Haemost 2012;107(6):1188–9.

122. Pecci A, Granata A, Fiore CE, et al. Renin-angiotensin system blockade is effective in reducing proteinuria of patients with progressive nephropathy caused by MYH9 mutations (Fechtner-Epstein syndrome). Nephrol Dial Transplant 2008; 23(8):2690–2.

123. King S, Germeshausen M, Strauss G, et al. Congenital amegakaryocytic thrombocytopenia: a retrospective clinical analysis of 20 patients. Br J Haematol 2005;131(5):636–44.

124. Frangoul H, Keates-Baleeiro J, Calder C, et al. Unrelated bone marrow transplant for congenital amegakaryocytic thrombocytopenia: report of two cases and review of the literature. Pediatr Transplant 2010;14(4):E42–5.

125. Bach FH, Albertini RJ, Joo P, et al. Bone-marrow transplantation in a patient with the Wiskott-Aldrich syndrome. Lancet 1968;2(7583):1364–6.

126. Filipovich AH, Stone JV, Tomany SC, et al. Impact of donor type on outcome of bone marrow transplantation for Wiskott-Aldrich syndrome: collaborative study of the International Bone Marrow Transplant Registry and the National Marrow Donor Program. Blood 2001;97(6):1598–603.

127. Shin CR, Kim MO, Li D, et al. Outcomes following hematopoietic cell transplantation for Wiskott-Aldrich syndrome. Bone Marrow Transplant 2012;47(11): 1428–35.

128. Boztug K, Schmidt M, Schwarzer A, et al. Stem-cell gene therapy for the Wiskott-Aldrich syndrome. N Engl J Med 2010;363(20):1918–27.

Immune Thrombocytopenia

Gaurav Kistangari, MD[a], Keith R. McCrae, MD[b],*

KEYWORDS

- Immune • Thrombocytopenia • ITP • Platelets • Thrombopoietin • Splenectomy

KEY POINTS

- Primary immune thrombocytopenia (ITP) presents as isolated thrombocytopenia (platelet count <100 × 10^9/L) in the absence of other causes or disorders that may be associated with thrombocytopenia, or as a secondary disorder, most commonly associated with autoimmune disease (such as systemic lupus erythematosus) or chronic infections (such as *Helicobacter pylori* or hepatitis C).
- Primary ITP in children is usually self-limited, with approximately 80% of cases resolving within 6 to 12 months. In contrast, ITP evolves into a chronic disorder in 80% of adults.
- Antiplatelet glycoprotein antibodies cause thrombocytopenia through 2 mechanisms: (1) reducing the survival of circulating platelets, and (2) inhibiting the production of new platelets by bone marrow megakaryocytes.
- The first line of therapy for ITP includes corticosteroids, sometimes in conjunction with intravenous immunoglobulin or anti–rhesus D. Although these are effective therapies, none reliably induce durable remission.
- Second-line therapy for ITP may include rituximab, splenectomy, or thrombopoietin receptor agonists. There is no consensus as to which is superior, and no controlled data to support the preferential use of one rather than the other. Splenectomy provides the greatest chance for long-term remission, but its use is declining.

DEFINITION AND HISTORY

Immune thrombocytopenia (ITP) is a common hematologic disorder that affects patient of all ages, genders, and races. Initially known as idiopathic thrombocytopenic purpura, an International Working Group (IWG) on ITP recently recommended that this disease be designated immune thrombocytopenia (retaining the abbreviation ITP); this terminology recognizes the immune pathogenesis of ITP and that patients with ITP may not uniformly exhibit purpura or bleeding manifestations.[1] The IWG also proposed terminology to allow standardized disease classification (**Table 1**). In

[a] Department of Hospital Medicine, Cleveland Clinic, 9500 Euclid Avenue, Cleveland, OH 44195, USA; [b] Taussig Cancer Institute, Department of Cellular and Molecular Medicine, Cleveland Clinic, R4-018, 9500 Euclid Avenue, Cleveland, OH 44195, USA
* Corresponding author.
E-mail address: mccraek@ccf.org

Hematol Oncol Clin N Am 27 (2013) 495–520
http://dx.doi.org/10.1016/j.hoc.2013.03.001
0889-8588/13/$ – see front matter © 2013 Elsevier Inc. All rights reserved.

hemonc.theclinics.com

Table 1 ITP IWG proposed definitions of disease	
Primary ITP	An autoimmune disorder characterized by isolated thrombocytopenia (platelet count <100 × 10⁹/L) in the absence of other causes and disorders that may be associated with thrombocytopenia. The diagnosis of primary ITP is one of exclusion, because no clinical or laboratory parameters are available to establish its diagnosis with accuracy. The main clinical problem in patients with primary ITP is an increased risk of bleeding, although bleeding symptoms are not always present
Secondary ITP	All forms of immune-mediated thrombocytopenia other than primary ITP. The acronym ITP should be followed by the name of the associated disease, (eg, secondary ITP–lupus associated, secondary ITP–drug induced)
Phases of the disease	Newly diagnosed ITP: within 3 mo of diagnosis Persistent ITP: 3–12 mo from diagnosis. Includes patients not reaching spontaneous remission or not maintaining complete response off therapy Chronic ITP: lasting for more than 12 mo Severe ITP: presence of bleeding symptoms at presentation sufficient to mandate treatment, or occurrence of new bleeding symptoms requiring additional therapeutic intervention with a different platelet-enhancing agent or an increased dose

Adapted from Rodeghiero F, Stasi R, Gernsheimer T, et al. Standardization of terminology, definitions and outcome criteria in immune thrombocytopenic purpura of adults and children: report from an international working group. Blood 2009;113:2386; with permission.

this scheme, primary ITP is defined as isolated thrombocytopenia (platelet count <100 × 10⁹/L) in the absence of other causes or disorders that may be associated with thrombocytopenia.[1] Secondary ITP is defined as any form of ITP other than primary; this might include thrombocytopenia secondary to systemic lupus erythematosus, hepatitis C infection, or lymphoproliferative disorders. The term acute ITP has been replaced by newly diagnosed ITP, which refers to ITP diagnosed within the preceding 3 months.[1] ITP of 3 to 12 months' duration is designated as persistent ITP, whereas chronic ITP is defined as disease of more than 12 months' duration. Severe ITP refers to the presence of bleeding symptoms at presentation, or the development of new bleeding symptoms while on therapy, requiring additional intervention. Refractory ITP designates cases of ITP that have not responded to splenectomy or have relapsed thereafter, and are sufficiently severe or pose sufficient risk of bleeding to require ongoing therapy. Definitions to standardize criteria for responses to ITP therapy have also been proposed.[1]

ITP has probably existed for centuries, and its history has recently been reviewed by Stasi and Newland.[2] Initial descriptions of purpura date to the Greco-Roman era and have been attributed to physicians such as Hippocrates and Galen. The most thorough early description of ITP was from Werhlof in 1735, who described a 16-year-old girl with postinfectious bleeding symptoms including epistaxis and hematemesis. In 1808, Willan described "purpura simplex," characterized by diffuse petechiae in the absence of systemic symptoms and occurring primarily in women and children. The recognition of platelets as a distinct entity in the blood with an important role in hemostasis is attributed to Bizzozero in 1882, and led to the correlation between purpura simplex and thrombocytopenia, reported by Brohm in 1883.[2] Kaznelson, a medical student, hypothesized that ITP resulted from destruction of platelets in the spleen; this led to the first splenectomy for ITP, performed by Kaznelson's mentor, Professor Doktor Schloffer, in 1916, inducing complete resolution of severe thrombocytopenia in a 36-year-old woman.[2]

CAUSES AND MECHANISMS OF PRIMARY AND SECONDARY ITP

The pathogenesis of ITP involves loss of tolerance to glycoproteins expressed on platelets and megakaryocytes.[3–10] ITP is not a single disorder, but a syndrome in which thrombocytopenia may be primary or occur secondary to underlying infectious or immune processes.[7,8]

Cines and colleagues[7] proposed that the immune tolerance defects in ITP can be divided into 3 categories that include (1) peripheral tolerance defects arising in the setting of immune stimulation, (2) differentiation blocks with skewed peripheral B-cell subsets, and (3) central tolerance defects arising during development or in the bone marrow. Underlying mechanisms associated with each of these may explain the clinical characteristics of individual cases of ITP. ITP resulting from loss of peripheral tolerance is proposed to be platelet specific, more amenable to therapy, and less likely to recur after treatment. In contrast, defects in central tolerance affect multiple cell types, and treated patients are more prone to relapse because of intrinsic autoreactivity.

Secondary ITP

Examples of secondary ITP related to loss of peripheral tolerance include ITP of childhood, which is preceded by a viral-like illness in two-thirds of affected children, and remits spontaneously in 80% of patients.[11,12] Loss of peripheral tolerance may also underlie the development of secondary ITP caused by vaccines or infectious exposures such as the mumps-measles-rubella (MMR) vaccine (incidence of 1 in 40,000 administrations), *Helicobacter pylori* infection, and infection with cytomegalovirus (CMV) or varicella-zoster virus (VZV).[13] Perhaps the most common infection associated with ITP is hepatitis C virus (HCV), which is present in up to 20% of ITP cases, with a higher incidence in certain geographic areas.[14] The pathogenesis of HCV-associated ITP may involve activation of B cells, as well as antibodies cross reactive with HCV and platelet glycoprotein (GP) IIIa.[15] Human immunodeficiency virus (HIV) is another well-described cause of ITP; thrombocytopenia results from decreased platelet production caused by infection of megakaryocytes as well as cross reactive antibodies that react with viral proteins and a linear epitope on GPIIIa (amino acids 44–66),[16] causing platelet lysis through generation of reactive oxygen species.[17] The incidence of thrombocytopenia in patients infected with HIV increases with disease progression, and decreases in response to highly active antiretroviral therapy (HAART).

Examples of ITP associated with blocks in differentiation with B-cell skewing include chronic lymphocytic leukemia (CLL), in which thrombocytopenia develops in 1% to 5% of cases[18] and may correlate with poor prognostic markers and decreased survival. Hodgkin disease, non-Hodgkin lymphomas, and large granulocytic leukemia (LGL) are associated with secondary ITP, although ITP develops in less than 1% of cases. ITP may develop in up to 10% of patients with common variable immunodeficiency. The pathogenesis of ITP or other immune disorders such as autoimmune hemolytic anemia that occur in these patients may involve defects in B-cell tolerance checkpoints and/or deficiencies of memory B-cell subsets.

Examples of defects in central tolerance associated with secondary ITP include the autoimmune lymphoproliferative syndrome (ALPS), a disorder linked to defective B-cell and T-cell apoptosis associated with mutations in genes encoding Fas, Fas-L, or other apoptosis mediators such as caspases.[19] Patients develop hepatosplenomegaly and lymphadenopathy, and 20% develop ITP, sometimes in association with autoimmune hemolytic anemia and/or neutropenia. Evans syndrome is characterized by ITP and autoimmune hemolytic anemia.[20] The antiphospholipid syndrome may be associated with ITP in up to one-third of patients, whereas up to 40% of patients with ITP may have antiphospholipid antibodies. The role of antiphospholipid versus antiplatelet glycoprotein antibodies in the development of thrombocytopenia is uncertain, because anti-GPIIIa antibodies have been described in thrombocytopenic patients with antiphospholipid antibodies.[21] ITP develops in up to one-third of patients with systemic lupus erythematosus, which is associated with a broad array of autoantibodies. The management of thrombocytopenia in patients with lupus is difficult, and corticosteroids and splenectomy are less effective than in primary ITP.[22] Defects in central tolerance also develop after transplantation; several mechanisms may be involved, including formation of alloantibodies against donor platelets in the setting of mixed chimerism.

Primary ITP

Like secondary ITP, diverse clinical features and responses to therapy in patients with primary ITP suggest that this apparently more defined disorder also derives from heterogeneous mechanisms. Most patients with primary ITP display a CD4+ Th0/Th1 cytokine profile[4,23] (associated with increased levels of interferon [IFN]-γ and interleukin [IL]-2) and decreased peripheral Th2+ and T regulatory (Treg) cells.[24] The increased Th1/Th2 ratio may correlate inversely with the platelet count. Alterations in levels of apoptosis regulatory factors in T cells from patients with ITP may influence T-cell subset expression and promote survival of autoreactive T-cell clones.[4] Reversions of Th1/Th2 ratios and normalization of T-cell Vβ spectratyping may follow therapy with rituximab or splenectomy.[10] Likewise, levels of regulatory T cells improve with responses to rituximab and other ITP therapies, including thrombopoietic agents, suggesting a more complex mechanism for rituximab than CD20+ B-cell depletion.[25,26] These findings are consistent with the hypothesis that autoantibodies in ITP develop as a consequence of T-cell–dependent antigen-driven clonal expansion and somatic mutation.[27] CD8+ Tc (cytotoxic) T cells may also contribute to the pathogenesis of primary ITP by causing platelet lysis through expression of granzymes A and B, Apo1/Fas, and perforin.[28] Cytotoxic T cells from patients with ITP also mediate toxicity toward megakaryocytes, and increased numbers of VLA4+CD3+CD8+ T cells expressing the homing receptor CX3Cr1+ have been observed in the bone marrow of patients with ITP.[29]

Antiplatelet antibodies

The observations of Kaznelson and Schloffer provided evidence for a central role of the spleen in the pathogenesis of ITP. Other studies showed that injection of an extract of splenic tissue from patients with ITP into rabbits produced a rapid decrease in the platelet count. The studies of Harrington and colleagues[30] in 1951 were the first to provide evidence of a circulating plasma component in the pathogenesis of human ITP. They arranged an exchange transfusion between Harrington and a woman with chronic ITP and a platelet count of 5×10^9/L. Afterward, he developed severe thrombocytopenia that resolved over the next 7 days. Subsequent studies with additional volunteers yielded similar results, although the response to ITP plasma was variable and severe thrombocytopenia developed in only 16 of 26 recipients. In 1965, Shulman and colleagues[31] reported that the thrombocytopenic factor in ITP plasma was a platelet-reactive immunoglobulin (Ig)G antibody. Studies performed in the 1970s showed increased levels of platelet-associated IgG in 90% of patients with ITP,[32] although subsequent work showed that much of this material bound to platelets nonspecifically or was contained within alpha granules. The development of antigen-specific antiplatelet antibody assays in the 1980s identified IgG reactive with platelet surface glycoproteins, primarily GPIIbIIIa (integrin αIIbβ3) and GPIb/IX, in 60% of patients with ITP.[6,33] Although antiplatelet antibodies may initially be directed toward a single platelet glycoprotein, following uptake of antibody-coated platelets and processing of antigenic peptides from originally nontargeted platelet glycoproteins, the production of antibodies against these new targets may ensue as a result of epitope spreading (**Fig. 1**).[34]

Antibody-dependent mechanisms of platelet destruction

Platelet survival is decreased in patients with ITP, with most platelets cleared in the spleen and liver.[35–38] Antibody-coated platelets are removed by splenic macrophages

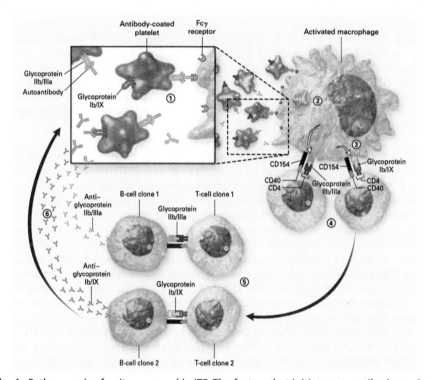

Fig. 1. Pathogenesis of epitope spread in ITP. The factors that initiate autoantibody production are unknown. Many patients have antibodies against several platelet surface glycoproteins at the time the disease becomes clinically evident. Here, GPIIb/IIIa is recognized by autoantibody (*orange, inset*), whereas antibodies that recognize the GPIb/IX complex have not been generated at this stage (1). Antibody-coated platelets bind to antigen-presenting cells (macrophages or dendritic cells) through Fcγ receptors and are then internalized and degraded (2). Antigen-presenting cells not only degrade GPIIb/IIIa (*light blue oval*), thereby amplifying the initial immune response, they also may generate cryptic epitopes from other platelet glycoproteins (*light blue cylinder*) (3). Activated antigen-presenting cells (4) express these novel peptides on the cell surface along with costimulatory help (represented in part by the interaction between CD154 and CD40) and the relevant cytokines that facilitate the proliferation of the initiating CD4-positive T-cell clones (T-cell clone 1) and those with additional specificities (T-cell clone 2) (5). B-cell immunoglobulin receptors that recognize additional platelet antigens (B-cell clone 2) are thereby also induced to proliferate and synthesize anti–GPIb/IX antibodies (*green*) in addition to amplifying the production of anti-GPIIb/IIIa antibodies (*orange*) by B-cell clone 1 (6). (*From* Cines DB, Blanchette VS. Immune thrombocytopenic purpura. N Engl J Med 2002;346(13):996; with permission.)

through Fcγ receptor–mediated phagocytosis.[9] Polymorphisms in the gene encoding FcγRIII (FcγRIIIA-581 V/V), a subtype of Fcγ receptor, are over-represented in adults and children with ITP; the V/V isoform of this receptor binds IgG1 and IgG3 with greater affinity than the F/F or F/V isoforms. An important role for FcγRIII in humans is also suggested by the ability of a monoclonal antibody to this receptor (mAb 3G8) to increase the platelet count in patients with refractory ITP.[39] Although one group has reported an essential role for FcγRIIa in the therapeutic effect of intravenous (IV) immunoglobulin (IVIg) in preclinical models, this finding has not been consistently reproduced.

Although uptake in the spleen is the primary mechanism by which antibody-coated platelets are cleared in patients with ITP, other mechanisms of platelet destruction exist. The failure of splenectomy in one-third of patients may reflect alternative mechanisms of platelet clearance and/or decreased platelet production.[10] Antiplatelet antibodies from more than half of a cohort of 240 patients with ITP were capable of fixing complement on platelets,[40] and some antiplatelet antibodies induce complement-dependent lysis of platelets in vitro. In patients with HIV, antibodies to platelet GPIIIa amino acids 49 to 66 cause platelet lysis in a complement-independent manner by generation of peroxides through the reduced nicotinamide adenine dinucleotide (NADH)/reduced nicotinamide adenine dinucleotide phosphate (NADPH) oxidase system.[17]

Evidence for decreased platelet production in patients with ITP
The concept of decreased platelet production as a cause of ITP was first suggested by Frank in 1915.[2] Like platelets, megakaryocytes express GPIIb/IIIa and GPIb/IX, which are targets for platelet-reactive autoantibodies. Increased numbers of histologically abnormal megakaryocytes, specifically younger and more immature forms, were noted more than 70 years ago in patients with ITP. Similar abnormalities were observed in the megakaryocytes of healthy individuals infused with ITP plasma, and marked inhibition of megakaryopoiesis was observed in rats treated with antiplatelet serum. Electron microscopic studies have confirmed ultrastructural abnormalities in megakaryocytes in patients with ITP consistent with apoptosis and para-apoptosis; these include cytoplasmic vacuolization, mitochondrial swelling, abnormal chromatin condensation, and increased staining for activated caspase-3.[41]

Chang and colleagues[42] showed that plasma from pediatric patients with ITP that contained anti-GPIb and/or anti-GPIIbIIIa antibodies inhibited the maturation of umbilical cord mononuclear cells into mature megakaryocytes in the presence of thrombopoietin. McMillan and colleagues[43] extended this work, showing that plasma from 12 of 18 adult patients with ITP decreased the production of megakaryocytes from CD34-positive cells: these effects were mediated by IgG, and prevented by adsorption of IgG fractions with immobilized GPIIb/IIIa.

Measurement of platelet turnover rates provides convincing evidence that platelet production is impaired in patients with ITP. Because platelet production is equal to platelet destruction at stable platelet concentrations, and because platelet destruction can be measured through the use of ^{111}In-labeled platelets, platelet production rates can be estimated. Early thrombokinetic studies suggested that platelet production rates were increased in ITP, although these studies relied on allogeneic platelets labeled with Cr[51,35,44] a less effective platelet label. However, later studies in which allogeneic and autologous platelet survival were studied in the same individuals showed significantly longer survival of autologous platelets,[36,45,46] particularly in patients in whom autologous platelet survival exceeded 1 day.[9] Platelet production rates estimated based on these later studies led to the conclusion that platelet production is normal or decreased in most patients with ITP.

Levels of plasma thrombopoietin are not increased in patients with ITP, reflecting that thrombopoietin production occurs in the liver and is largely constitutive.[47] Plasma thrombopoietin levels are regulated primarily via clearance, mediated through binding of thrombopoietin to the thrombopoietin receptor (c-Mpl) on circulating platelets and to bone marrow megakaryocytes. Accelerated clearance of platelets in ITP leads to enhanced metabolism of thrombopoietin, and thrombopoietin production rates do not increase proportionally.[48]

Role of cellular immunity in platelet destruction and impaired platelet production
The maturation of antiplatelet antibodies is T-cell–dependent and antigen-dependent.[27] However, antiplatelet antibodies are only detectable in 60% of patients,[33] and ITP may enter remission despite the continued presence of antiplatelet antibodies[10]; these observations suggest that antibody-independent mechanisms account for thrombocytopenia in some individuals. In one study, CD8[+] cytotoxic T cells from patients with active ITP but without detectable antiplatelet antibodies bound and lysed platelets in vitro, although CD8[+] T cells from patients with ITP in remission did not.[28] CD3[+] T cells from patients with ITP also showed increased expression of genes that mediate cell-dependent cytotoxicity, including perforin, tumor necrosis factor alpha, and granzymes A and B.[28] Li and colleagues[49] reported that CD8[+] T cells also prevented apoptosis of autologous megakaryocytes, which is involved in budding and release of proplatelets.

CLINICAL FEATURES OF ITP
Epidemiology

ITP affects patients of all genders, races, and ages.[50] Studies from Scandinavia suggest a prevalence of ITP ranging from 4.6 to 5.3 cases per 100,000 children.[51] In a study that analyzed data from the Maryland Health Care Commission, the prevalence of ITP was 9.5 per 100,000 children aged 1 to 5 years, 7.3 per 100,000 in children aged 6 to 10 years, and 4.1 per 100,000 in children of aged 11 to 14 years.[52] Analysis of the UK General Practice Research Database (GPRD) identified a higher incidence of ITP in boys between the ages of 2 and 5 years (9.7 cases vs 4.7 cases in girls per 100,000 patient years, respectively) compared with the incidence in teenagers between the ages of 13 and 17 years (2.4 cases per 100,000 patient years, with equal sex distribution).[53]

The overall prevalence of ITP in adults is comparable with that in children.[54] A prospective, population-based study of patients older than 16 years with newly diagnosed ITP showed an annual incidence of 1.6 cases per 100,000 patient years; the incidence was slightly higher in women between 45 and 49 years of age but otherwise no gender differences existed.[55] The highest age-specific incidence of ITP was in individuals more than 60 years old. A Scandinavian study identified an ITP incidence of between 2.25 and 2.68 per 100,000 individuals/y; the incidence was greater in women (female/male ratio 1.7) and the elderly.[56] Other studies have suggested a prevalence of ITP in adults ranging from 4.0 to 23.6/100,000 patient-years. A study based on queries of physicians' offices suggested a higher prevalence of ITP in women less than 70 years old, but a higher incidence in men more than 70 years old.[57]

Clinical Manifestations of ITP

Because ITP is often secondary, a patient with newly diagnosed thrombocytopenia should be evaluated for symptoms associated with disorders causing secondary ITP such as rashes, arthralgias, or serositis associated with systemic lupus; hepatomegaly and increased transaminase levels associated with hepatitis C; or fever and lymphadenopathy associated with infection or lymphoid malignancy. A history of prescription and nonprescription drug intake, including herbs and supplements, is of critical importance.

This section focuses on the manifestations of primary ITP, which may dominate even in cases of secondary ITP.

Bleeding

Bleeding is the most common clinical manifestation of ITP, presenting as mucocutaneous bleeding involving the skin, oral cavity, and gastrointestinal tract. Purpura, usually on the extremities (dry purpura), may often appear without an obvious precipitating event. Mucosal bleeding includes epistaxis, menorrhagia, and gingival and gastrointestinal bleeding.[55] Patients with severe thrombocytopenia may display oral hemorrhagic bullae (wet purpura), which may be a harbinger of more severe bleeding manifestations in the gastrointestinal tract or elsewhere. Bleeding from more distal sites in the gastrointestinal tract may develop at the site of unsuspected preexisting lesions.

Intracranial hemorrhage is the most feared complication of ITP. The incidence of intracranial hemorrhage in children has been estimated to be less than 0.2%, almost always occurring at platelet counts less than 10×10^9/L.[12,58] A recent report from the International Cooperative Study shows that this complication occurs more frequently in adults than in children, occurring in 10 of 1784 children and 6 of 340 adults with newly diagnosed ITP.[59] In a natural history study that enrolled 152 patients, 4 patients died of ITP-related causes in the first 2 years (1 because of hemorrhage, 3 because of infection), and 2 died of ITP-related causes during long-term follow-up (1 with postsplenectomy sepsis, 1 with refractory bleeding and a platelet count of 2×10^9/L).[60] Patients with ITP may be at increased risk of hematologic malignancy,[61] consistent with the demonstration of an increased frequency of CLL phenotype lymphocytes in patients with ITP.[62]

Several risk factors for bleeding in patients with ITP have been identified. Cohen and colleagues[63] identified 49 cases of fatal hemorrhage in 1718 patients from pooled ITP case series. The overall risk of fatal hemorrhage was between 0.0162 and 0.0389 cases per patient-year, with a risk of 0.004 in patients less than 40 years old increasing to 0.130 for patients more than 60 years of age. Cortelazzo and colleagues[64] observed an overall incidence of hemorrhagic events of 3.2% per patient-year in patients with ITP. Hemorrhagic events at similar platelet counts occurred in 10.4% of patients older than 60 years, compared with 0.4% in patients less than the age of 40 years. A previous history of hemorrhage also predicted bleeding (relative risk [RR] 27.5). Michel and colleagues[65] compared the incidence of bleeding and other outcomes in 55 patients with ITP older than 70 years (mean age 77.8 ± 6.1 years) with those of a younger cohort (mean age 40.3 ± 14.9 years). The median platelet count at diagnosis did not differ between the 2 groups, although bleeding symptoms were more frequent in the older (82%) versus the younger (62%) group.

In a prospective study of 245 patients older than 16 years with newly diagnosed ITP, 30 (12%) presented with frank bleeding, 28% were asymptomatic, and the remainder displayed purpura.[55] Bleeding was uncommon at platelet counts more than 30×10^9/L. However, in this and other studies, a direct correlation between the platelet count and severity of bleeding was not uniform, reflecting the observation that occasional individuals with very low platelet counts exhibit little bleeding, whereas others with platelet counts greater than 30×10^9/L bleed frequently. This conundrum might be explained by binding of some antiplatelet antibodies to highly restricted regions in the GPIIb beta-propeller domain[66] near the ligand (fibrinogen) binding site, potentially interfering with platelet aggregation.

Fatigue

Fatigue is an underappreciated symptom in patients with ITP, occurring in approximately 22% of children, and 22% to 39% of adults.[67] Significant improvements in fatigue and several health-related quality-of-life measurements have been observed in successfully treated patients.[68] In one study, univariate analyses showed that the presence of fatigue correlated with a platelet count less than 100×10^9/L, treatment with steroids, bleeding, and several other factors, but not with duration of ITP, age, or gender.[69] Fatigue in patients with ITP may reflect, in part, increased levels of inflammatory cytokines, including IL-2 and IFN-γ, associated with the Th1 profile.

Thrombosis

Recent studies suggest that patients with ITP have an increased risk of thrombosis. Aledort and colleagues[70] initially reported 18 thromboembolic events in 186 adults with chronic ITP. Sarpatwari and colleagues[71] observed that the adjusted hazard ratio for venous, arterial, or combined thromboembolic events in patients with ITP mined from the UK GPRD were 1.58 (95% confidence interval [CI], 1.01–2.48), 1.37 (95% CI, 0.94–2.00), and 1.41 (95% CI, 1.04–1.91), respectively. The severity of thrombocytopenia correlated with the development of thrombosis. A study using a matched ITP cohort from the Danish National Patient Registry observed an incidence rate ratio for venous thromboembolism in patients with ITP of 2.04 (95% CI, 1.45–2.87).[72]

The mechanisms underlying the paradoxic development of thrombosis in patients with ITP are uncertain. The incidence of antiphospholipid antibodies (APLA) is increased in patients with ITP, and patients with ITP with APLA may develop thrombosis more frequently.[73] Although current guidelines do not recommend routine screening of patients with ITP for APLA,[74,75] this should be considered in patients who develop thrombosis. Other factors that may contribute to the development of thrombosis include increased levels of prothrombotic, platelet-derived microparticles and complement activation on antibody-coated platelets.[76]

The management of thrombosis in thrombocytopenic patients with ITP is not addressed by current guidelines. Many experts consider anticoagulation to be justified at platelet counts more than approximately 40×10^9 L, although this should be individualized depending on the severity of the thrombotic event and characteristics of the patient. Aggressive treatment of ITP is warranted during anticoagulation therapy.

LABORATORY STUDIES

ITP is characterized by isolated thrombocytopenia without abnormalities in erythrocyte or leukocyte number or morphology. Platelet size may be normal or increased, although not usually to the degree observed in inherited causes of thrombocytopenia such as MYH9-related macrothrombocytopenias.[77] A careful examination of the peripheral blood smear is essential to exclude other causes of thrombocytopenia such as microangiopathic processes, platelet satellitism, or pseudothrombocytopenia. Myelodysplastic syndromes or acute and chronic leukemias occasionally present with isolated thrombocytopenia, although in many cases review of the peripheral blood reveals characteristic changes in other hematopoietic lineages. A recent report showed decreases in the absolute immature platelet fraction (A-IPF) in patients with ITP. Treatment with eltrombopag increased the A-IPF.[78]

Normal or increased numbers of megakaryocytes are present in the bone marrow of patients with ITP, sometimes with an increase in immature megakaryocytes. Ultrastructural examination may show evidence of megakaryocyte apoptosis.[41]

The sensitivity of measurements of platelet-associated IgG for the diagnosis of ITP is 91%, although the specificity is only 27%; thus, the positive predictive value is only

48% and the diagnostic usefulness of such assays is poor. Measurement of specific platelet glycoprotein antibodies offers greater specificity (78%–92%), although their diagnostic value is limited by low sensitivity (49%–66%) leading to a positive predictive value of only 80% to 83%.[6,34]

Several other laboratory parameters in the diagnostic evaluation of ITP have been recommended by the ITP IWG[75]; those considered to comprise the basic evaluation or to be potentially useful are listed in **Table 2**. A reticulocyte count and direct antiglobulin (Coombs) test are recommended to exclude concurrent autoimmune hemolytic anemia. Blood type may be useful in determining the usefulness of therapy with anti-Rhesus D [anti-Rh(D)], whereas quantitative immunoglobulin levels may lead to the diagnosis of common variable immunodeficiency. Screening for HIV, HCV, and H pylori is recommended regardless of geographic location, although the importance of H pylori in the development of ITP in North America is not well established.

DIFFERENTIAL DIAGNOSIS

The diagnosis of primary ITP is one of exclusion. Both nonimmune causes of thrombocytopenia and secondary ITP must be considered (**Table 3**). Nonimmune causes of thrombocytopenia include exposure to drugs or toxins that suppress platelet production (alcohol, chemotherapeutic agents), splenic sequestration of platelets, primary bone marrow disorders, prior radiation exposure (therapeutic or incidental), and inherited thrombocytopenias.

Inherited thrombocytopenias may be misdiagnosed as ITP.[79] The diagnosis should be suspected in a patient with a family history of thrombocytopenia and in patients who do not respond appropriately to standard ITP therapy. In some cases, characteristic

Table 2
Diagnostic recommendations (laboratory) of the ITP IWG

Basic Evaluation	Potential Usefulness	Uncertain or Unproven Benefit
Complete blood count and reticulocyte count	Glycoprotein-specific antiplatelet antibody	Thrombopoietin level
Peripheral blood film	Antiphospholipid antibodies	Reticulated platelets
Quantitative immunoglobulin level (consider in children, recommend in children with persistent or chronic ITP)	Thyroid function and antithyroid antibodies	Platelet-associated IgG
Bone marrow examination (may be informative in patients >60 y old, with systemic symptoms, or before splenectomy)	Pregnancy test (women of childbearing potential)	Platelet survival study
Blood group (Rh)	Antinuclear antibodies	Bleeding time
Direct antiglobulin test	PCR for parvovirus and CMV	Serum complement
H pylori	—	—
HCV	—	—
HIV	—	—

Abbreviation: PCR, polymerase chain reaction.
Data from Provan D, Stasi R, Newland AC, et al. International consensus report on the investigation and management of primary immune thrombocytopenia. Blood 2010;115:168.

Table 3 Differential diagnosis of primary ITP	
Nonimmunologic	**Immunologic (Secondary ITP)**
Decreased platelet production	Autoimmune disorders
Acute or chronic leukemia	Systemic lupus erythematosus
Myelodysplasia	Evans syndrome
Aplastic anemia	Antiphospholipid antibodies
Congenital or acquired amegakaryocytic thrombocytopenia	Drug-induced thrombocytopenia
Toxic exposure (radiation, chemotherapy, alcohol)	Antibiotics (eg, Bactrim, vancomycin)
Nutritional deficiency (B_{12}, folate)	Quinine
Myelofibrosis	Valproic acid
Myelophthistic processes	Heparin
Viral infection of hematopoietic precursors	Others (oxaliplatin, alemtuzumab, purine analogs)
Enhanced platelet destruction	Infection
Splenic sequestration	H pylori
Disseminated intravascular coagulation	HIV
Thrombotic thrombocytopenic purpura (no direct immune response to platelets)	HCV
Cardiopulmonary bypass	Lymphoproliferative disorders
Infection/sepsis	Immunodeficiency (ALPS, CVID)
Inherited thrombocytopenia	Posttransfusion purpura
	Vaccinations

Abbreviation: CVID, common variable immunodeficiency.

findings such as absent radii (thrombocytopenia with absent radii [TAR] syndrome), right heart defects (DiGeorge syndrome), or specific laboratory features such as large platelets and Döhle bodies in neutrophils (MYH9-related disorders) support the diagnosis of familial thrombocytopenia.[80]

The Bernard-Soulier syndrome is an autosomal recessive familial thrombocytopenic disorder characterized by the absence of the platelet GPIb-IX complex and associated with large platelets, lack of platelet aggregation by high-dose ristocetin, and bleeding.[81] Wiskott-Aldrich syndrome is an X-linked disorder characterized by severe immunodeficiency and small platelets. Congenital amegakaryocytic thrombocytopenia (CAMT) is an autosomal recessive disorder characterized by severe thrombocytopenia and absence of megakaryocytes, resulting from mutations in c-Mpl. Inherited thrombocytopenias also occur in association with mutations in transcription factors that regulate megakaryocyte development, including GATA1 (sex-linked inheritance) and RUNX1 (autosomal dominant). Laboratories in Europe and the United States provide genetic testing for these disorders (see www.genetests.org).

THERAPEUTIC OPTIONS AND PROGNOSIS
Management of ITP in Children

Spontaneous recovery from ITP occurs in approximately 80% of children with ITP, usually within 6 months, but occasionally taking a year or more.[11,12] Severe hemorrhage occurs in 1 in 200 children with newly diagnosed ITP, and intracerebral hemorrhage occurs in less than 1 in 500, most often in the first month after diagnosis.[82] For those requiring treatment, a short course of corticosteroids, IVIg, or anti-D (in Rh-positive individuals) usually results in rapid improvement.

Several therapeutic approaches exist for the 20% of children who develop persistent thrombocytopenia. Rituximab has similar efficacy in children as in adults and is associated with a long-term remission rate of 22% in retrospective analyses.[83] Romiplostim induces platelet responses in 83% to 88% of children with chronic ITP,[84] although long-term safety in children is not established. Splenectomy is reserved for severe persistent thrombocytopenia and bleeding and results in complete remission in approximately 75% of children.[11] The risk of postsplenectomy sepsis is greater in children than in adults, and splenectomy is usually deferred until at least 5 years of age.[85] Vaccination against *Streptococcus pneumoniae*, *Neisseria meningitidis*, and *Haemophilus influenzae* type b should be administered before splenectomy in children and adults, and penicillin prophylaxis is recommended until adulthood.

Management of ITP in Adults

Adult patients with ITP have increased morbidity and mortality (RR 2.3; 95% CI, 1.8–3.0) compared with the general population, particularly those unable to maintain a hemostatic platelet count greater than 30 × 10^9/L despite therapy.[60,61] Bleeding and infection contribute equally to mortality.[60]

The management of ITP in adults is more complex than in children because most cases evolve into chronic disease, and the risk of bleeding is increased.[55,61,64] The goal of therapy is to achieve a hemostatic platelet count, generally considered to be at least 20 × 10^9/L to 30 × 10^9/L,[60] while causing the least toxicity. Treatment is rarely required beyond a platelet count of 50 × 10^9/L,[75] and must be individualized to account for age, lifestyle, individual bleeding risk, and patient preference.

There are no controlled studies showing the superiority of any specific treatment algorithm in ITP, and hence no well-delineated standard of care. The ITP IWG has divided therapies into first-line treatments consisting of corticosteroids, IVIg, and IV anti-D, and second-line therapies consisting of splenectomy and all other medical approaches (**Table 4**).[75]

First-line therapy

Corticosteroids remain the most commonly used first-line therapy for ITP. At least 80% of patients with ITP initially respond to corticosteroids, although most of these individuals relapse when steroids are tapered.[75,86] Several studies have examined whether more intensive dosing of steroids in newly diagnosed ITP leads to more durable remissions. Cheng and colleagues[87] reported that treatment with a single course of dexamethasone (40 mg/d for 4 days) led to sustained responses (platelet count >50 × 10^9/L at 6 months) in 50% of responders. Mazzucconi and colleagues[86] observed that treatment of newly diagnosed ITP with 4 to 6 cycles of dexamethasone given at 2-week intervals led to relapse-free survival of 80% to 90% at 15 months. However, in a small, randomized study, a single course of high-dose dexamethasone did not induce a greater percentage of sustained responses than standard doses of prednisolone.[88] Zaja and colleagues[89] compared a combination of dexamethasone and rituximab with dexamethasone alone in the initial treatment of ITP, showing a higher sustained response rate at 6 months in patients who received the combination (63% vs 36%; n = 52; P<.004; 95% CI, 0.079–0.455); however, these differences were lost on longer follow-up.

IVIg is often used in conjunction with corticosteroids, particularly when a rapid increase in the platelet count is desired. IVIg is also used to support the platelet count until more definitive therapy can be delivered to patients whose platelets decrease on

Table 4
Treatment options for ITP

First Line	Second Line	Third Line[a]
Corticosteroids	Rituximab	Combination chemotherapy
Prednis(ol)one	Thrombopoietin receptor agonists	Combination of first-line and second-line therapies
Dexamethasone	Romiplostim	Campath 1H (currently withdrawn from market)
Methylprednisolone	Eltrombopag	Hematopoietic stem cell transplantation
IVIg	Splenectomy	
Anti-Rh(D)	Azathioprine[b]	
	Cyclophosphamide	
	Danazol	
	Dapsone	
	Cyclosporine	
	Mycophenylate mofetil	

[a] Considered to be treatment options supported by minimal data with the potential for inducing significant toxicity.
[b] Agents that are italicized are used less commonly in the current era of ITP therapy and might be considered third line by some clinicians.
   Data from Provan D, Stasi R, Newland AC, et al. International consensus report on the investigation and management of primary immune thrombocytopenia. Blood 2010;115:168.

tapering of corticosteroids. IVIg increases the platelet count in 60% to 80% of treated patients, often within days, and is effective in both nonsplenectomized and splenectomized patients, although responses are usually of short duration (1–3 weeks). Several IVIg regimens are used, but many clinicians prefer the convenience of a 1-gm/kg/d infusion for 1 or 2 days.[10] The activity of IVIg is mediated through several mechanisms, including modulation of Fcγ receptor expression and activity, inhibition of cytotoxic T-cell activation, complement neutralization, cytokine modulation, and inhibition of megakaryocyte apoptosis.[90,91] Toxicities include aseptic meningitis, fluid overload, nephrotoxicity, thrombosis, and rarely, severe hemolytic anemia.

Anti-Rh(D) binds to the Rh(D) antigen on erythrocytes leading to clearance of antibody-coated cells and inhibiting the clearance of opsonized platelets by the reticuloendothelial system[91]; other mechanisms including reduction in antigen-specific B-cell priming and modulation of Fcγ receptor and inflammatory cytokine levels may contribute. Anti-D is effective only in Rh(D) positive individuals with an intact spleen. Anti-D causes a hemolytic response that results in a decrease in hemoglobin of 0.5 to 2 gm/dL, although more severe hemolysis may occur in approximately 1 in 1000 patients, rarely accompanied by disseminated intravascular coagulation, renal failure, and death.[92] Many of these toxicities can be avoided by appropriate patient selection.[93] At the approved dose of 50 μg/kg, anti-D increases platelet counts in 70% of treated patients, although higher doses (75 μg/kg) increase response rates. In a single-arm study, repeated dosing of patients with ITP with IVIg for recurring thrombocytopenia led to durable responses in 43% of patients.[94]

Second-line therapy
Several second-line therapies exist for treatment of ITP resistant to corticosteroids, IVIg, or anti-D. The use of older second-line agents has decreased significantly

because of the emergence of rituximab and thrombopoietin receptor agonists (TRAs), which offer greater efficacy with lower toxicity (see **Table 4**). The use of newer agents in ITP is discussed later; excellent reviews on the safety and efficacy of older agents are available.[95,96]

Rituximab is a chimeric anti-CD20 antibody approved for treatment of lymphoma that is often used for ITP in patients who fail first-line therapy. Whether it is best positioned before or after splenectomy or TRAs is not established. In a systematic review of 313 patients with ITP, half of whom were not splenectomized, 62.5% (95% CI, 52.6%–72.5%) of patients treated with rituximab achieved a platelet count response (platelet increment of 50×10^9/L), with a median time to response of 5.5 weeks (range, 2–18 weeks) and a median duration of response of 10.5 months.[97] In another systematic review that included 364 nonsplenectomized patients, the complete response rate was 41.5% with a mean time to response of 6.34 weeks and a median duration of response of 49 weeks.[98] In a single-arm prospective study of 60 nonsplenectomized patients with ITP, 40% achieved a platelet count at or more than 50×10^9/L with at least a doubling from baseline at 1 year, and 33.3% of these responses were sustained at 2 years.[99] However, a pilot, randomized, placebo-controlled trial that assessed a composite end point showed only a nonsignificant trend toward superior responses to rituximab within 6 months of therapy initiation.[100] An appealing aspect of rituximab therapy is its ability to induce durable responses in approximately 21% of adults.[83] Rituximab is usually administered at a dose of 375 mg/m^2 weekly for 4 weeks, although a lower dose regimen of 100 mg/m^2 may have similar efficacy.[101] Despite targeting CD20 on B cells, the mechanism of rituximab may involve more complex immunologic modulation. Successful therapy correlated in one report with normalization of T-cell subset distribution,[102] and in another with reappearance of normal numbers and function of regulatory T cells.[26]

Adverse effects of rituximab include infusion reactions, serum sickness, and cardiac arrhythmias. Fatal reactivation of hepatitis B infection has occurred; thus, rituximab is contraindicated in patients infected with hepatitis B. Reactivation of latent JC virus leading to progressive multifocal leukoencephalopathy occurred in several patients treated with rituximab, one of whom had ITP, although most were heavily pretreated with other immunosuppressive agents.[103]

Splenectomy was the first successful treatment of ITP, and is still considered by some to be the gold standard because it provides the greatest opportunity for a durable remission.[104] Splenectomy may be offered to patients who fail to achieve sustained responses after steroid therapy, or may be used before or after a trial of rituximab or TRAs. In a systematic review of 135 case series between 1966 and 2004, complete responses to splenectomy were observed in 66% of patients, with a median duration of follow-up of 28 months (range 1–153 months).[105] In another systematic review of 1223 patients with ITP undergoing laparoscopic splenectomy, a 5-year success rate of 72% was reported[106]; most relapses occurred within the first 2 years after splenectomy. The use of splenectomy, especially in the United States and some European countries, has decreased from between 50% and 60% to between 20% and 25% in recent years.[107] Laparoscopic splenectomy carries a mortality risk and complication rate of 0.2% and 9.6%, respectively (compared with 1.0% and 12.9% with open laparotomy).[105] Splenectomy has been associated with an increased risk of infection and postsplenectomy sepsis, with an estimated mortality of 0.73 per 1000 patient-years determined from a historical cohort undergoing splenectomy for hereditary spherocytosis.[108] However, whether patients with ITP experience an increased risk of postsplenectomy infection compared with other patients with ITP who have not undergone splenectomy has not been established. In a large

Danish study, infection in patients splenectomized for ITP relative to infection in non-splenectomized individuals with a matched indication (ITP) was observed only within the first 90 days following splenectomy (RR, 2.6; 95% CI, 1.3–5.1). No significantly increased risk was seen thereafter, with an RR of 1.0 between 91 and 365 days, and 1.4 (95% CI, 1.0–2.0) beyond the first year.[109] Early infections result primarily from enteric pathogens.[109] Nevertheless, immunization against encapsulated organisms and aggressive treatment of febrile illness may reduce long-term infection-related morbidity and mortality postsplenectomy.

Current guidelines differ on the relative place of splenectomy in the management of ITP. Although both the IWG[75] and revised American Society of Hematology (ASH) guidelines[74] consider splenectomy an acceptable second-line option, the former group weights splenectomy similarly to several other options, whereas the ASH guidelines recommend splenectomy (grade 1B evidence) for patients who fail corticosteroids, and only suggest rituximab or thrombopoietic agents (grade 2C evidence). Given the lack of comparative data between splenectomy, rituximab, or TRA therapy, treatment decisions should be individualized and encompass both physician and patient preferences.[110]

The position of TRAs in ITP therapy continues to evolve. Although some clinicians reserve these agents for patients with refractory ITP, others suggest their use in newly diagnosed ITP with the goal of sustaining the platelet count for the first year after diagnosis in hopes of spontaneous remission.[111] Neither of the two approved TRAs, romiplostim and eltrombopag, have direct sequence homology with thrombopoietin (**Fig. 2**). Both enhance platelet production following binding to the thrombopoietin receptor, c-Mpl, on megakaryocytes, stimulating megakaryocyte proliferation and differentiation.[112]

Romiplostim (Nplate) is a fusion protein comprising 4 thrombopoietin peptidomimetic regions linked to an IgG Fc domain that provides in vivo stability.[113] It is administered as a weekly subcutaneous injection, dosed according to the platelet count. After initial phase I dose-finding trials, the efficacy of romiplostim over a 6 month period was assessed in 2 placebo-controlled, phase III trials that that enrolled 63 splenectomized and 62 nonsplenectomized patients, respectively, with severe, chronic ITP.[114] A durable platelet response, defined as a platelet count greater than $50 \times 10^9/L$ during 6 of the final 8 weeks of treatment, was achieved in 38% of splenectomized patients (vs 0% in placebo) and 61% of nonsplenectomized patients (vs 5% in placebo) who received romiplostim. Romiplostim-treated patients were more likely to reduce or discontinue concomitant treatment (usually corticosteroids) and less likely to require rescue medications.[114] Romiplostim was also compared with standard of care in a randomized study involving 234 adult patients with ITP who had not undergone splenectomy. Over a 12-month period, romiplostim-treated patients showed a 2.3-fold higher incidence of platelet responses, a decreased incidence of treatment failure (11% vs 30%), a lower incidence of splenectomy (9% vs 36%), less bleeding, and a better quality of life.[111] The efficacy and safety of romiplostim over a longer treatment period has also been assessed in a single-arm extension trial of 407 patients.[115] This trial revealed that 90% of patients achieved the platelet response definitions (doubling of the platelet count and platelet count $>50 \times 10^9/L$, or platelets $>20 \times 10^9$ from baseline) at a mean romiplostim dose of 3.62 µg/kg.

Eltrombopag (Promacta) is an oral, small-molecule TRA with a similar mechanism to romiplostim, although eltrombopag binds to the transmembrane portion of c-Mpl rather than the ligand (thrombopoietin) binding site (see **Fig. 2**).[116] Following phase I dose-finding trials, the drug was tested in patients with severe, chronic ITP in 6-week and 6-month[117] (RAISE [Randomized Placebo-Controlled Idiopathic Thrombocytopenic

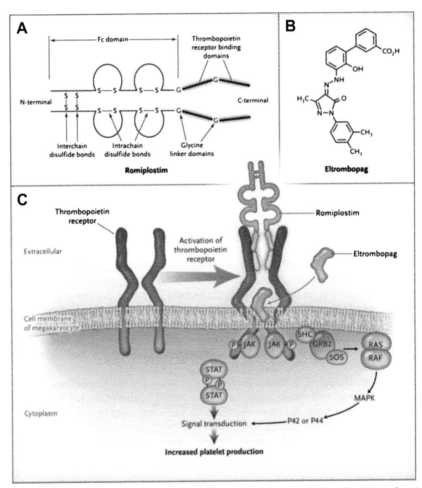

Fig. 2. Structure of romiplostim and eltrombopag and the cellular mechanisms of action. (A) The chemical structure of romiplostim, which is composed of the Fc portion of IgG1, to which 2 thrombopoietin peptides consisting of 14 amino acids are coupled through glycine bridges at the C-terminal of each gamma heavy chain. (B) The chemical structure of eltrombopag. (C) The cellular mechanisms of action of romiplostim, which binds to the thrombopoietin receptor, and of eltrombopag, which binds to the thrombopoietin receptor's transmembrane domain, thereby activating signaling that leads to increased platelet production. GRB2, growth factor receptor-binding protein 2; JAK, Janus kinase; MAPK, mitogen-activated protein kinase; P, phosphorylation; RAF, rapidly accelerated fibrosarcoma kinase; RAS, rat sarcoma GTPase; SHC, Src homology collagen protein; STAT, signal transducer and activator of transcription. (*From* Imbach P, Crowther M. Thrombopoietin-receptor agonists for primary immune thrombocytopenia. N Engl J Med 2011;365(8):736; with permission.)

Purpura (ITP) Study With Eltrombopag]), randomized, placebo-controlled trials. Platelet responses were seen in 59% to 79% of patients, compared with 16% to 28% of placebo-treated patients. Splenectomized and nonsplenectomized patients responded similarly, and treated patients experienced less bleeding, with many able to reduce concomitant ITP medications. The long-term safety and efficacy of eltrombopag has been studied in the EXTEND (Eltrombopag Extended Dosing) study, which enrolled 301 patients, with 84 and 28 patients treated for at least 3 and 4 years.[118] Overall, 88% of patients achieved a platelet count greater than 50×10^9/L at least once during the study; the pretreatment platelet count, history of splenectomy, or previous use of ITP medication did not predict response. Clinically significant bleeding decreased from 16% at baseline to 0% at week 156. A unique toxicity of eltrombopag is the development of hepatobiliary abnormalities, which occurred in 34 (11%) of patients.

Both romiplostim and eltrombopag are well tolerated, although several class-specific toxicities have been identified.[119] Rebound thrombocytopenia occurs in 8% to 10% of patients following discontinuation of TRAs and can lead to increased bleeding.[119,120] Platelet counts should be monitored closely for the first 2 weeks after discontinuation, and tapering of the medication may be considered. Arterial and venous thrombosis is a concern with increased platelet counts in response to TRAs, but must be considered against the background of a potentially increased thrombosis risk in ITP.[71] In randomized phase III studies, the incidence of thrombosis was not increased in patients treated with TRAs. Of 407 patients reported in the romiplostim extension study, cerebrovascular accident, deep venous thrombosis, and pulmonary embolism each occurred in 2 patients (0.5%),[115] whereas in 301 patients in the eltrombopag extension study, 25 thromboembolic events developed in 19 patients for an incidence rate of 3.02/100 patient-years.[118] In neither study did the development of thrombosis correlate with the platelet count. Increased bone marrow reticulin has been observed in approximately 5% of patients treated with TRAs.[119] In most cases, this process has been limited to reticulin, and not associated with clinical signs of bone marrow dysfunction.[121] Both the platelet count and peripheral blood film should be regularly monitored in patients on TRAs, and myelophthisic changes or loss of response to therapy should prompt consideration of discontinuation and bone marrow examination.

Special Situations

Emergency treatment of ITP
Patients with severe thrombocytopenia, particularly those with newly diagnosed ITP, should be hospitalized. Therapy is directed at increasing the platelet count as quickly as possible through the use of corticosteroids and IVIg. Platelet transfusion provides transient increases in the platelet count in emergent situations, and concurrent infusion of IVIg may prolong survival of transfused platelets in some patients.[122] Splenectomy offers the potential for increasing the platelet count most quickly, and has been used to treat ITP in patients with acute intracranial hemorrhage. Recombinant factor VIIa has been used in anecdotal reports.

Pregnancy
ITP affects 0.1 to 1.0 of every 1000 pregnancies, and accounts for 3% to 5% of cases of pregnancy-associated thrombocytopenia; it is 50-fold to 100-fold less common than incidental thrombocytopenia of pregnancy. However, because incidental thrombocytopenia usually does not develop until the second or third trimester, ITP is the most common cause of isolated thrombocytopenia in the first trimester.[123,124] In the first and second trimesters, patients with no bleeding and a platelet count more than 20×10^9/L to 30×10^9/L do not require treatment.[74,75] As term approaches, a more aggressive approach is indicated to raise the platelet count to greater than 50×10^9/L to 70×10^9/L, a level generally considered safe for epidural anesthesia and delivery.[124] Corticosteroids are effective in pregnant patients, but their association with toxicities such as pregnancy-induced hypertension have led some to suggest that IVIg (2 gm/kg) should be considered as initial therapy.[123] Refractory patients may

undergo splenectomy, which is optimally performed during the second trimester. Teratogenic agents such as danazol, cyclophosphamide, or vinca alkaloids should be avoided[74,75]; azathioprine has been used in pregnant patients without teratogenicity, and rituximab has also been used effectively, although it may delay neonatal B-cell maturation.

Antiplatelet antibodies may cross the placenta and induce neonatal thrombocytopenia; approximately 10% of the offspring of mothers with ITP are born with a platelet count less than 50×10^9/L, and 1% to 5% have platelet counts less than 20×10^9/L. There is no effective means to predict neonatal thrombocytopenia, although it is more common in neonates with a sibling who was born thrombocytopenic. Although up to 50% of severely thrombocytopenic neonates experience bleeding during delivery, intracranial hemorrhage is rare (<1.0%).[125] There is no evidence that the risk of fetal intracranial hemorrhage is reduced by cesarean section, thus the use of cesarean section should be dictated by maternal indications only.[74,75] In some offspring of patients

Table 5
Treatment options for refractory ITP

Medication	Approximate Response Rate	Major Toxicities
Azathioprine 1–2 mg/kg (maximum 150 mg/d)	Up to two-thirds, 40% in anecdotal reports	Infrequent and mild: weakness, sweating, transaminitis, severe neutropenia, pancreatitis
Cyclosporine A 5 mg/kg/d for 6 d then 2.5–3.0 mg/kg/d (titrate to blood levels of 100–200 ng/mL)	Dose dependent, up to 50%–80% in small series	Moderate but transient in most patients: increased creatinine, hypertension, fatigue, paresthesias, myalgia, gingival hyperplasia, dyspepsia, hypertrichosis, tremor
Danazol 200 mg 2–4 times daily	67% CR or PR, 40% in anecdotal reports	Frequent: transaminitis, acne, hirsutism, increased cholesterol, amenorrhea
Cyclophosphamide 1–2 mg/kg orally daily for at least 16 wk, or IV 0.3–1 gm/m² for 1–3 doses every 2–4 wk	24%–85%	Usually mild to moderate: neutropenia, DVT, nausea
Dapsone 75–100 mg	Up to 50%	Infrequent and reversible: anorexia, nausea, abdominal distention, methemoglobinuria, hemolytic anemia in G6PD deficiency Severe: skin rash, requires discontinuation
Vinca alkaloids: Vincristine: 1–2 mg weekly- total 6 mg Vinblastine: 10 mg weekly, total 30 mg	Highly variable, 10%–75%	Neuropathy, particularly in elderly, Neutropenia, fever Thrombophlebitis at infusion site

Abbreviations: CR, complete remission; PR, partial remission.
Data from Provan D, Stasi R, Newland AC, et al. International consensus report on the investigation and management of primary immune thrombocytopenia. Blood 2010;115:168.

with ITP, thrombocytopenia may develop several days after delivery, thus careful monitoring of the neonate is indicated during this critical period.

Refractory ITP is often managed with several immunosuppressant and chemotherapeutic agents, such as azathioprine, cyclophosphamide, vinca alkaloids, danazol, cyclosporine, and mycophenylate mofitil.[96] The efficacy of many of these agents has not been prospectively studied and estimates are derived from small series (**Table 5**).[95] The ITP IWG categorizes these agents as second line,[75] although most patients with refractory ITP are currently managed with TRAs or rituximab, with the approaches listed in **Table 5** used less frequently.[126] However, recent reports suggest that the use of such approaches in combination with other agents listed in **Table 4** may induce responses in patients with refractory ITP, and emerging data suggest that these agents may also be effective in combination with more contemporary treatment schemes.

SUMMARY

- Primary ITP presents as isolated thrombocytopenia (platelet count $<100 \times 10^9/L$) in the absence of other causes or disorders that may be associated with thrombocytopenia, or as a secondary disorder, most commonly associated with autoimmune disease, lymphoproliferative disorders, or chronic infections.
- Primary ITP in children is usually self-limited, with approximately 80% of cases resolving within 6 to 12 months. In contrast, ITP evolves into a chronic disorder in 80% of adults.
- Bleeding is the most common clinical manifestation of ITP, occurring most commonly in the elderly, in whom the incidence of ITP is highest.
- The pathogenesis of ITP involves loss of tolerance to glycoproteins expressed on platelets and megakaryocytes. Epitope spreading may explain why many patients have antibodies against more than 1 glycoprotein.
- Antiplatelet glycoprotein antibodies cause thrombocytopenia through 2 mechanisms: (1) reducing the survival of circulating platelets, and (2) inhibiting the production of new platelets by bone marrow megakaryocytes.
- Cellular immunity contributes significantly to the pathogenesis of ITP. Alterations in T-cell subsets and decreased numbers and activity of regulatory T cells are common. Cytotoxic T cells may also mediate toxicity against platelets and megakaryocytes.
- The first line of therapy for ITP includes corticosteroids, sometimes in conjunction with IVIg or anti-Rh(D). Although both of these are effective therapies, neither reliably induces durable remission.
- The second-line therapy for ITP may include rituximab, splenectomy, or TRAs. There is no consensus as to which is superior, and no controlled data to support the preferential use of one rather than the other. Splenectomy provides the greatest chance for long-term remission.

REFERENCES

1. Rodeghiero F, Stasi R, Gernsheimer T, et al. Standardization of terminology, definitions and outcome criteria in immune thrombocytopenic purpura of adults and children: report from an international working group. Blood 2009;113:2386–93.
2. Stasi R, Newland AC. ITP: a historical perspective. Br J Haematol 2011;153(4): 437–50.
3. Cuker A, Cines DB. Immune thrombocytopenia. Hematology Am Soc Hematol Educ Program 2010;2010:377–84.

4. Toltl LJ, Nazi I, Jafari R, et al. Piecing together the humoral and cellular mechanisms of immune thrombocytopenia. Semin Thromb Hemost 2011;37(6):631–9.

5. Semple JW, Provan D, Garvey MB, et al. Recent progress in understanding the pathogenesis of immune thrombocytopenia. Curr Opin Hematol 2010;17(6):590–5.

6. McMillan R. Antiplatelet antibodies in chronic immune thrombocytopenia and their role in platelet destruction and defective platelet production. Hematol Oncol Clin North Am 2009;23(6):1163–75.

7. Cines DB, Bussel JB, Liebman HA, et al. The ITP syndrome: pathogenic and clinical diversity. Blood 2009;113:6511–21.

8. Cines DB, Liebman H, Stasi R. Pathobiology of secondary immune thrombocytopenia. Semin Hematol 2009;46:S2–14.

9. Nugent D, McMillan R, Nichol JL, et al. Pathogenesis of chronic immune thrombocytopenia: increased platelet destruction and/or decreased platelet production. Br J Haematol 2009;146(6):585–96.

10. Stasi R. Immune thrombocytopenia: pathophysiologic and clinical update. Semin Thromb Hemost 2012;38(5):454–62.

11. Blanchette V, Bolton-Maggs P. Childhood immune thrombocytopenic purpura: diagnosis and management. Hematol Oncol Clin North Am 2010;24(1):249–73.

12. Breakey VR, Blanchette VS. Childhood immune thrombocytopenia: a changing therapeutic landscape. Semin Thromb Hemost 2011;37(7):745–55.

13. Liebman HA. Viral-associated immune thrombocytopenic purpura. Hematology Am Soc Hematol Educ Program 2008;212–8.

14. Rajan SK, Espina BM, Liebman HA. Hepatitis C virus-related thrombocytopenia: clinical and laboratory characteristics compared with chronic immune thrombocytopenic purpura. Br J Haematol 2005;129(6):818–24.

15. Zhang W, Nardi MA, Borkowsky W, et al. Role of molecular mimicry of hepatitis C virus protein with platelet GPIIIa in hepatitis C-related immunologic thrombocytopenia. Blood 2009;113(17):4086–93.

16. Li Z, Nardi MA, Karpatkin S. Role of molecular mimicry to HIV-1 peptides in HIV-1 related immunologic thrombocytopenia. Blood 2005;106:572–6.

17. Nardi M, Tomlinson S, Greco MA, et al. Complement-independent, peroxide-induced antibody lysis of platelets in HIV-1-related immune thrombocytopenia. Cell 2001;106:551–61.

18. Liebman HA. Recognizing and treating secondary immune thrombocytopenic purpura associated with lymphoproliferative disorders. Semin Hematol 2009;46(1 Suppl 2):S33–6.

19. Teachey DT. New advances in the diagnosis and treatment of autoimmune lymphoproliferative syndrome. Curr Opin Pediatr 2012;24(1):1–8.

20. Michel M, Chanet V, Dechartres A, et al. The spectrum of Evans syndrome in adults: new insight into the disease based on the analysis of 68 cases. Blood 2009;114(15):3167–72.

21. Lipp E, von Felten A, Sax H, et al. Antibodies against platelet glycoproteins and antiphospholipid antibodies in autoimmune thrombocytopenia. Eur J Haematol 1998;60:282–8.

22. Arnal C, Piette JC, Leone J, et al. Treatment of severe immune thrombocytopenia associated with systemic lupus erythematosus: 59 cases. J Rheumatol 2002;29(1):75–83.

23. Panitsas FP, Theodoropoulou M, Kouraklis A, et al. Adult chronic idiopathic thrombocytopenic purpura (ITP) is the manifestation of a type-1 polarized immune response. Blood 2004;103(7):2645–7.

24. Sakakura M, Wada H, Tawara I, et al. Reduced Cd4+Cd25+ T cells in patients with idiopathic thrombocytopenic purpura. Thromb Res 2007;120(2):187–93.
25. Bao W, Bussel JB, Heck S, et al. Improved regulatory T-cell activity in patients with chronic immune thrombocytopenia treated with thrombopoietic agents. Blood 2010;116(22):4639–45.
26. Stasi R, Cooper N, Del PG, et al. Analysis of regulatory T-cell changes in patients with idiopathic thrombocytopenic purpura receiving B cell-depleting therapy with rituximab. Blood 2008;112(4):1147–50.
27. Roark JH, Bussel JB, Cines DB, et al. Genetic analysis of autoantibodies in idiopathic thrombocytopenic purpura reveals evidence of clonal expansion and somatic mutation. Blood 2002;100:1388–98.
28. Olsson B, Andersson PO, Jernas M, et al. T-cell-mediated cytotoxicity toward platelets in chronic idiopathic thrombocytopenic purpura. Nat Med 2003;9(9): 1123–4.
29. Olsson B, Ridell B, Carlsson L, et al. Recruitment of T cells into bone marrow of ITP patients possibly due to elevated expression of VLA-4 and CX3CR1. Blood 2008;112(4):1078–84.
30. Harrington WJ, Minnich V, Hollingsworth JW, et al. Demonstration of a thrombocytopenic factor in the blood of patients with thrombocytopenic purpura. J Lab Clin Med 1951;38:1–8.
31. Shulman NR, Marder VJ, Weinrach RS. Similarities between known antiplatelet antibodies and the factor responsible for thrombocytopenia in idiopathic purpura. Physiologic, serologic and isotopic studies. Ann N Y Acad Sci 1965; 124(2):499–542.
32. Dixon RH, Rosse WF. Platelet antibody in autoimmune thrombocytopenia. Br J Haematol 1975;31(2):129–34.
33. McMillan R. Antiplatelet antibodies in chronic adult immune thrombocytopenic purpura: Assays and epitopes. J Pediatr Hematol Oncol 2003;25:S57–61.
34. Cines DB, Blanchette VS. Immune thrombocytopenic purpura. N Engl J Med 2002;346(13):995–1008.
35. Branehog I, Kutti J, Weinfeld A. Platelet survival and platelet production in idiopathic thrombocytopenic purpura (ITP). Br J Haematol 1974;27(1):127–43.
36. Ballem PJ, Segal GM, Stratton JR, et al. Mechanisms of thrombocytopenia in chronic autoimmune thrombocytopenic purpura. Evidence of both impaired platelet production and increased platelet clearance. J Clin Invest 1987;80(1): 33–40.
37. Najean Y, Rain JD, Billotey C. The site of destruction of autologous 111In-labelled platelets and the efficiency of splenectomy in children and adults with idiopathic thrombocytopenic purpura: a study of 578 patients with 268 splenectomies. Br J Haematol 1997;97(3):547–50.
38. Stratton JR, Ballem PJ, Gernsheimer T, et al. Platelet destruction in autoimmune thrombocytopenic purpura: kinetics and clearance of indium-111-labeled autologous platelets. J Nucl Med 1989;30(5):629–37.
39. Clarkson SB, Bussel JB, Kimberly RP, et al. Treatment of refractory immune thrombocytopenic purpura with an anti-Fc gamma-receptor antibody. N Engl J Med 1986;314(19):1236–9.
40. Najaoui A, Bakchoul T, Stoy J, et al. Autoantibody-mediated complement activation on platelets is a common finding in patients with immune thrombocytopenic purpura (ITP). Eur J Haematol 2012;88(2):167–74.
41. Houwerzijl EJ, Blom NR, van der Want JJ, et al. Ultrastructural study shows morphologic features of apoptosis and para-apoptosis in megakaryocytes

from patients with idiopathic thrombocytopenic purpura. Blood 2004;103(2): 500–6.

42. Chang M, Nakagawa PA, Williams SA, et al. Immune thrombocytopenic purpura (ITP) plasma and purified ITP monoclonal autoantibodies inhibit megakaryocytopoiesis in vitro. Blood 2003;102:887–95.

43. McMillan R, Wang L, Tomer A, et al. Suppression of in vitro megakaryocyte production by antiplatelet autoantibodies from adult patients with chronic ITP. Blood 2004;103:1364–9.

44. Harker LA. Thrombokinetics in idiopathic thrombocytopenic purpura. Br J Haematol 1970;19(1):95–104.

45. Branehog I, Weinfeld A. Platelet survival and platelet production in idiopathic thrombocytopenic purpura (ITP) before and during treatment with corticosteroids. Scand J Haematol 1974;12(1):69–79.

46. Heyns AP, Badenhorst PN, Lotter MG, et al. Platelet turnover and kinetics in immune thrombocytopenic purpura: results with autologous 111In-labeled platelets and homologous 51Cr-labeled platelets differ. Blood 1986;67(1): 86–92.

47. Kaushansky K. Thrombopoietin. N Engl J Med 1998;339(11):746–54.

48. Nichol JL. Endogenous TPO (eTPO) levels in health and disease: possible clues for therapeutic intervention. Stem Cells 1998;16(Suppl 2):165–75.

49. Li S, Wang L, Zhao C, et al. CD8+ T cells suppress autologous megakaryocyte apoptosis in idiopathic thrombocytopenic purpura. Br J Haematol 2007;139(4): 605–11.

50. Fogarty PF, Segal JB. The epidemiology of immune thrombocytopenic purpura. Curr Opin Hematol 2007;14(5):515–9.

51. Zeller B, Rajantie J, Hedlund-Treutiger I, et al. Childhood idiopathic thrombocytopenic purpura in the Nordic countries: epidemiology and predictors of chronic disease. Acta Paediatr 2005;94(2):178–84.

52. Segal JB, Powe NR. Prevalence of immune thrombocytopenia: analyses of administrative data. J Thromb Haemost 2006;4(11):2377–83.

53. Yong M, Schoonen WM, Li L, et al. Epidemiology of paediatric immune thrombocytopenia in the General Practice Research Database. Br J Haematol 2010; 149(6):855–64.

54. Terrell DR, Beebe LA, Vesely SK, et al. The incidence of immune thrombocytopenic purpura in children and adults: A critical review of published reports. Am J Hematol 2010;85(3):174–80.

55. Neylon AJ, Saunders PW, Howard MR, et al, Northern Region Haematology Group. Clinically significant newly presenting autoimmune thrombocytopenic purpura in adults: a prospective study of a population-based cohort of 245 patients. Br J Haematol 2003;122:966–74.

56. Frederiksen H, Schmidt K. The incidence of idiopathic thrombocytopenic purpura in adults increases with age. Blood 1999;94(3):909–13.

57. Terrell DR, Beebe LA, Neas BR, et al. Prevalence of primary immune thrombocytopenia in Oklahoma. Am J Hematol 2012;87(9):848–52.

58. Psaila B, Petrovic A, Page LK, et al. Intracranial hemorrhage (ICH) in children with immune thrombocytopenia (ITP): study of 40 cases. Blood 2009;114(23): 4777–83.

59. Kuhne T, Berchtold W, Michaels LA, et al. Newly diagnosed immune thrombocytopenia in children and adults: a comparative prospective observational registry of the Intercontinental Cooperative Immune Thrombocytopenia Study Group. Haematologica 2011;96(12):1831–7.

60. Porteilje JE, Westendorp RG, Kluin-Nelemans HC, et al. Morbidity and mortality in adults with idiopathic thrombocytopenic purpura. Blood 2001;97:2549–54.
61. Norgaard M, Jensen AO, Engebjerg MC, et al. Long-term clinical outcomes of patients with primary chronic immune thrombocytopenia: a Danish population-based cohort study. Blood 2011;117(13):3514–20.
62. Mittal S, Blaylock MG, Culligan DJ, et al. A high rate of CLL phenotype lymphocytes in autoimmune hemolytic anemia and immune thrombocytopenic purpura. Haematologica 2008;93(1):151–2.
63. Cohen YC, Djulbegovic B, Shamai-Lubovitz O, et al. The bleeding risk and natural history of idiopathic thrombocytopenic purpura in patients with persistent low platelet counts. Arch Intern Med 2000;160(11):1630–8.
64. Cortelazzo S, Finazzi G, Buelli M, et al. High risk of severe bleeding in aged patients with chronic idiopathic thrombocytopenic purpura. Blood 1991;77(1):31–3.
65. Michel M, Rauzy OB, Thoraval FR, et al. Characteristics and outcome of immune thrombocytopenia in elderly: results from a single center case-controlled study. Am J Hematol 2011;86(12):980–4.
66. Kiyomizu K, Kashiwagi H, Nakazawa T, et al. Recognition of highly restricted regions in the β-propeller domain of αllb by platelet-associated anti-αllbβ3 autoantibodies in primary immune thrombocytopenia. Blood 2012;120(7):1499–509.
67. Newton JL, Reese JA, Watson SI, et al. Fatigue in adult patients with primary immune thrombocytopenia. Eur J Haematol 2011;86(5):420–9.
68. Kuter DJ, Mathias SD, Rummel M, et al. Health-related quality of life in nonsplenectomized immune thrombocytopenia patients receiving romiplostim or medical standard of care. Am J Hematol 2012;87(5):558–61.
69. Mathias SD, Bussel JB, George JN, et al. A disease-specific measure of health-related quality of life for use in adults with immune thrombocytopenic purpura: its development and validation. Health Qual Life Outcomes 2007;5:11.
70. Aledort LM, Hayward CP, Chen MG, et al. Prospective screening of 205 patients with ITP, including diagnosis, serological markers, and the relationship between platelet counts, endogenous thrombopoietin, and circulating antithrombopoietin antibodies. Am J Hematol 2004;76(3):205–13.
71. Sarpatwari A, Bennett D, Logie JW, et al. Thromboembolic events among adult patients with primary immune thrombocytopenia in the United Kingdom General Practice Research Database. Haematologica 2010;95:1167–75.
72. Severinsen MT, Engebjerg MC, Farkas DK, et al. Risk of venous thromboembolism in patients with primary chronic immune thrombocytopenia: a Danish population-based cohort study. Br J Haematol 2011;152(3):360–2.
73. Diz-Kucukkaya R, Hacehanefioglu A, Yenerel M, et al. Antiphospholipid antibodies and antiphospholipid syndrome in patients presenting with immune thrombocytopenic purpura: a prospective cohort study. Blood 2001;98:1760–4.
74. Neunert C, Lim W, Crowther M, et al. The American Society of Hematology 2011 evidence-based practice guideline for immune thrombocytopenia. Blood 2011;117(16):4190–207.
75. Provan D, Stasi R, Newland AC, et al. International consensus report on the investigation and management of primary immune thrombocytopenia. Blood 2010;115:168–86.
76. Peerschke EI, Yin W, Ghebrehiwet B. Complement activation on platelets: implications for vascular inflammation and thrombosis. Mol Immunol 2010;47(13):2170–5.

77. Noris P, Klersy C, Zecca M, et al. Platelet size distinguishes between inherited macrothrombocytopenias and immune thrombocytopenia. J Thromb Haemost 2009;7(12):2131–6.

78. Barsam SJ, Psaila B, Forestier M, et al. Platelet production and platelet destruction: assessing mechanisms of treatment effect in immune thrombocytopenia. Blood 2011;117(21):5723–32.

79. Nurden AT, Freson K, Seligsohn U. Inherited platelet disorders. Haemophilia 2012;18(Suppl 4):154–60. http://dx.doi.org/10.1111/j.1365-2516.2012.02856.x.

80. Balduini CL, Pecci A, Savoia A. Recent advances in the understanding and management of MYH9-related inherited thrombocytopenias. Br J Haematol 2011;154(2):161–74.

81. Berndt MC, Andrews RK. Bernard-Soulier syndrome. Haematologica 2011;96(3):355–9.

82. Kuhne T, Imbach P, Bolton-Maggs PH, et al. Newly diagnosed idiopathic thrombocytopenic purpura in childhood: an observational study. Lancet 2001;358(9299):2122–5.

83. Patel VL, Mahevas M, Lee SY, et al. Outcomes 5 years after response to rituximab therapy in children and adults with immune thrombocytopenia. Blood 2012;119(25):5989–95.

84. Bussel JB, Buchanan GR, Nugent DJ, et al. A randomized, double-blind study of romiplostim to determine its safety and efficacy in children with immune thrombocytopenia. Blood 2011;118(1):28–36.

85. Kuhne T, Blanchette V, Buchanan GR, et al. Splenectomy in children with idiopathic thrombocytopenic purpura: a prospective study of 134 children from the Intercontinental Childhood ITP Study Group. Pediatr Blood Cancer 2007;49(6):829–34.

86. Mazzucconi MG, Fazi P, Bernasconi S, et al. Therapy with high-dose dexamethasone (HD-DXM) in previously untreated patients affected by idiopathic thrombocytopenic purpura: a GIMEMA experience. Blood 2007;109:1401–7.

87. Cheng Y, Wong RS, Soo YO, et al. Initial treatment of immune thrombocytopenic purpura with high-dose dexamethasone. N Engl J Med 2003;349:831–6.

88. Bae SH, Ryoo H, Lee WS, et al. High dose dexamethasone vs conventional dose prednisolone for adults with immune thrombocytopenia: a prospective multicenter phase III trial [abstract]. Blood 2010;116.

89. Zaja F, Baccarani M, Mazza P, et al. Dexamethasone plus rituximab yields higher sustained response rates than dexamethasone monotherapy in adults with primary immune thrombocytopenia. Blood 2010;115(14):2755–62.

90. Leontyev D, Katsman Y, Branch DR. Mouse background and IVIG dosage are critical in establishing the role of inhibitory Fcγ receptor for the amelioration of experimental ITP. Blood 2012;119(22):5261–4.

91. Cooper N. Intravenous immunoglobulin and anti-RhD therapy in the management of immune thrombocytopenia. Hematol Oncol Clin North Am 2009;23(6):1317–27.

92. Gaines AR. Disseminated intravascular coagulation associated with acute hemoglobinemia or hemoglobinuria following Rh(0)(D) immune globulin intravenous administration for immune thrombocytopenic purpura. Blood 2005;106(5):1532–7.

93. Despotovic JM, Lambert MP, Herman JH, et al. RhIG for the treatment of immune thrombocytopenia: consensus and controversy (CME). Transfusion 2012;52(5):1126–36.

94. Cooper N, Wolowski BM, Fodero EM, et al. Does treatment with intermittent infusion of intravenous anti-D allow a proportion of adults with recently diagnosed

immune thrombocytopenic purpura to avoid splenectomy. Blood 2002;99: 1922–7.

95. George JN, Kojouri K, Perdue JJ, et al. Management of patients with chronic, refractory idiopathic thrombocytopenic purpura. Semin Hematol 2000;37:290–8.

96. Psaila B, Bussel JB. Refractory immune thrombocytopenic purpura: current strategies for investigation and management. Br J Haematol 2008;143(1):16–26.

97. Arnold DM, Dentali F, Crowther MA, et al. Systematic review: efficacy and safety of rituximab for adults with idiopathic thrombocytopenic purpura. Ann Intern Med 2007;146(1):25–33.

98. Auger S, Duny Y, Rossi JF, et al. Rituximab before splenectomy in adults with primary idiopathic thrombocytopenic purpura: a meta-analysis. Br J Haematol 2012;158(3):386–98.

99. Godeau B, Porcher R, Fain O, et al. Rituximab efficacy and safety in adult splenectomy candidates with chronic immune thrombocytopenic purpura: results of a prospective multicenter phase 2 study. Blood 2008;112(4):999–1004.

100. Arnold DM, Heddle NM, Carruthers J, et al. A pilot randomized trial of adjuvant rituximab or placebo for nonsplenectomized patients with immune thrombocytopenia. Blood 2012;119(6):1356–62.

101. Provan D, Butler T, Evangelista ML, et al. Activity and safety profile of low-dose rituximab for the treatment of autoimmune cytopenias in adults. Haematologica 2007;92(12):1695–8.

102. Stasi R, Del Poeta G, Evangelista ML, et al. Response to B-cell depleting therapy with rituximab reverts the abnormalities of T-cell subsets in patients with idiopathic thrombocytopenic purpura. Blood 2007;110:2924–30.

103. Carson KR, Focosi D, Major EO, et al. Monoclonal antibody-associated progressive multifocal leucoencephalopathy in patients treated with rituximab, natalizumab, and efalizumab: a review from the Research on Adverse Drug Events and Reports (RADAR) Project. Lancet Oncol 2009;10(8):816–24.

104. Rodeghiero F. First-line therapies for immune thrombocytopenic purpura: re-evaluating the need to treat. Eur J Haematol Suppl 2008;(69):19–26.

105. Kojouri K, Vesely SK, Terrell DR, et al. Splenectomy for adult patients with idiopathic thrombocytopenic purpura: a systematic review to assess long-term platelet responses, prediction of response, and surgical complications. Blood 2004;104: 2623–34.

106. Mikhael J, Northridge K, Lindquist K, et al. Short-term and long-term failure of laparoscopic splenectomy in adult immune thrombocytopenic purpura patients: a systematic review. Am J Hematol 2009;84(11):743–8.

107. Rodeghiero F, Ruggeri M. Is splenectomy still the gold standard for the treatment of chronic ITP? Am J Hematol 2008;83(2):91.

108. Schilling RF. Estimating the risk for sepsis after splenectomy in hereditary spherocytosis. Ann Intern Med 1995;122:187–8.

109. Thomsen RW, Schoonen WM, Farkas DK, et al. Risk for hospital contact with infection in patients with splenectomy: a population-based cohort study. Ann Intern Med 2009;151(8):546–55.

110. Ghanima W, Godeau B, Cines DB, et al. How I treat immune thrombocytopenia: the choice between splenectomy or a medical therapy as a second-line treatment. Blood 2012;120(5):960–9.

111. Kuter DJ, Rummel M, Boccia R, et al. Romiplostim or standard of care in patients with immune thrombocytopenia. N Engl J Med 2010;363(20):1889–99.

112. Stasi R, Bosworth J, Rhodes E, et al. Thrombopoietic agents. Blood Rev 2010; 24(4–5):179–90.

113. Kuter DJ. Romiplostim. Cancer Treat Res 2011;157:267–88.
114. Kuter DJ, Bussel JB, Lyons RM, et al. Efficacy of romiplostim in patients with chronic immune thrombocytopenic purpura: a double-blind randomised controlled trial. Lancet 2008;371(9610):395–403.
115. Janssens A, Tarantino MD, Bird R, et al. Final results from a multicenter, international, single arm study evaluating the efficacy and safety of romiplostim in adults with primary immune thrombocytopenia [abstract]. Blood 2011;118.
116. Bussel JB, Pinheiro MP. Eltrombopag. Cancer Treat Res 2011;157:289–303.
117. Cheng G, Saleh MN, Marcher C, et al. Eltrombopag for management of chronic immune thrombocytopenia (RAISE): a 6-month, randomised, phase 3 study. Lancet 2011;377(9763):393–402.
118. Saleh MN, Cheng G, Bussel JB, et al. Safety and efficacy of extended treatment with eltrombopag in adults with chronic immune thrombocytopenia from June 2006 to February 2011 [abstract]. Blood 2011;118.
119. Cuker A, Chiang EY, Cines DB. Safety of the thrombopoiesis-stimulating agents for the treatment of immune thrombocytopenia. Curr Drug Saf 2010;5(2):171–81.
120. Imbach P, Crowther M. Thrombopoietin-receptor agonists for primary immune thrombocytopenia. N Engl J Med 2011;365(8):734–41.
121. Brynes RK, Orazi A, Verma S, et al. Evaluation of bone marrow reticulin in patients with chronic immune thrombocytopenic purpura (ITP) treated with eltrombopag-data from the EXTEND study [abstract]. Blood 2011;118.
122. Spahr JE, Rodgers GM. Treatment of immune-mediated thrombocytopenia purpura with concurrent intravenous immunoglobulin and platelet transfusion: a retrospective review of 40 patients. Am J Hematol 2008;83(2):122–5.
123. Gill KK, Kelton JG. Management of idiopathic thrombocytopenic purpura in pregnancy. Semin Hematol 2000;37:275–83.
124. McCrae KR. Thrombocytopenia in pregnancy. Hematology Am Soc Hematol Educ Program 2010;2010:397–402.
125. Burrows RF, Kelton JG. Fetal thrombocytopenia and its relation to maternal thrombocytopenia. N Engl J Med 1993;329:1463–6.
126. Lakshmanan S, Cuker A. Contemporary management of primary immune thrombocytopenia in adults. J Thromb Haemost 2012;10(10):1988–98.

Drug-induced Immune Thrombocytopenia

Beng H. Chong, PhD, MBBS, FRACP, FRCPA, FRCP (Glasgow)[a,b,]*,
Philip Young-Ill Choi, MBBS[b,c], Levon Khachigian, PhD[c],
Jose Perdomo, PhD[b,c]

KEYWORDS

- Drugs • Thrombocytopenia • Immune • Antibodies

KEY POINTS

- Thrombocytopenia is caused by immune reactions elicited by diverse drugs in clinical practice.
- The activity of the drug-dependent antibodies produces a marked decrease in blood platelets and a high risk of serious bleeding.
- Understanding of the cellular mechanisms that drive drug-induced thrombocytopenia has advanced recently but there is still a need for improved laboratory tests and treatment options.
- This article includes an overview of the different types of drug-induced thrombocytopenia, discusses potential pathologic mechanisms, and considers diagnostic methods and treatment options.

HISTORY, DEFINITION, AND CLASSIFICATION

Purpura in association with pestilential fevers was described by Hippocrates, but it was not until the sixteenth century that purpura in the absence of fever was observed by Lusitanus. It took another 3 centuries for Krauss (1883) and Denys (1887) to recognize that purpura hemorrhagica was caused by a decrease in blood platelets.[1] The association of drug and purpura was first reported by Vipan[2] in 1865 before the role of platelets in hemostasis was known. Later, Rosenthal in 1928 provided evidence that

[a] Haematology Department, Level 4, Clinical Services Building, Gray Street, St George Hospital, Kogarah, NSW 2217, Australia; [b] Department of Medicine, St George Clinical School, University of New South Wales, Level 2, Pitney Building, St George Hospital, Gray Street, Kogarah, NSW 2217, Australia; [c] Centre of Vascular Research, Lowy Building, University of New South Wales, Kensington, Sydney, NSW 2033, Australia
* Corresponding author. St George Hospital, Level 4, Clinical Services Building, Gray Street, Kogarah, New South Wales 2217, Australia.
E-mail address: beng.chong@unsw.edu.au

Hematol Oncol Clin N Am 27 (2013) 521–540
http://dx.doi.org/10.1016/j.hoc.2013.02.003
0889-8588/13/$ – see front matter © 2013 Elsevier Inc. All rights reserved.

drug ingestion caused thrombocytopenia by rechallenging a patient with quinine-induced thrombocytopenia with the drug and showing a prompt decrease in platelet count.[1]

Drug-induced thrombocytopenia (DIT) can be divided into 2 categories according to the mechanism responsible for the thrombocytopenia, namely (1) suppression of platelet production and (2) increase in peripheral platelet destruction or clearance. The former, which usually occurs as pancytopenia, is caused mostly by myelosuppressive agents (mainly chemotherapeutic drugs) and their suppressive effect is dose dependent. The latter can be further divided into 3 subtypes:

1. Nonimmune DIT (caused by a direct toxic effect of the drug on platelets; eg, ristocetin, an antibiotic that is no longer used in clinical practice)
2. Immune DIT (mediated by a drug-dependent antibody)
3. Autoimmune DIT (mediated by a drug-independent antibody that binds and prematurely clears platelets even in the absence of the drug such as alpha-methyldopa)

Most drugs are thought to cause thrombocytopenia by a drug-dependent immune mechanism (ie, the second mechanism); this is the focus of this article and other types of DIT are not discussed.

Drug-induced immune thrombocytopenia (DITP) is a common problem in clinical practice, particularly in hospital inpatients. Patients usually develop extensive petechiae or purpura, with markedly low blood platelet levels (frequently $<10 \times 10^9/L$), about 1 to 2 weeks after commencing a new medication.[3–5] Serious bleeding including intracranial hemorrhage can occur,[6,7] presenting a challenging diagnostic and management problem. Diagnosis of DITP is usually made clinically but can be difficult when there are comorbid conditions (eg, infection) and concomitant drugs that can also cause thrombocytopenia. Despite significant advances in this area of hematology, there is still a need for more research to increase understanding of the mechanisms of DITP, and to improve diagnostic tests and patient management. This article discusses the pathogenesis, diagnosis, and management of DITP, focusing on recent advances.

CAUSATIVE DRUGS

More than 200 drugs (including some herbal medicines) have been reported to cause DITP.[3,4] Aster and Bougie[3] identified 85 drugs that they considered as definite or probable causes of thrombocytopenia. Among these are drugs commonly used in clinical practice: heparin, quinine, antibiotics (eg, penicillin, cephalosporin, rifampicin, vancomycin, sulfonamides), antiplatelet agents, glycoprotein IIb/IIIa (GPIIb/IIIa) inhibitors (tirofiban, eptifibatide, abciximab), antirheumatic agents (gold, D-penicillamine), antiepileptics (sodium valproate, phenytoin), cardiac agents (amrinone), and the new biologic agents infliximab and rituximab.[3,8] Heparin causes an immune thrombocytopenia that leads to severe thrombosis rather than bleeding,[9] through a mechanism different from other DITPs.

INCIDENCE

DITP incidence is not well defined and is reported to be low, ranging from 0.6 to 1.6 per 100,000.[10–16] These studies used national surveillance programs and hospital records, and probably underestimate the frequency of DITP.[8] However, the incidence of thrombocytopenia induced by GPIIb/IIIa inhibitors (tirofiban, eptifibatide, and abciximab) and heparin is higher. DITP-associated GPIIb/IIIa inhibitors have an incidence of 0.1% to 2% on first drug exposure and about 5% to 10% on subsequent exposures.[3,4]

This incidence suggests that thousands of patients globally must develop this drug complication every year because millions of cardiac patients receive these drugs for prevention of coronary artery thrombosis following coronary angioplasty, stent insertion, and acute coronary syndrome. Despite the variable frequencies, DITP represents a significant clinical problem because of the large number of drugs involved and the large number of patients who can be affected.

PATHOPHYSIOLOGY

DITP is usually mediated by a drug-dependent antibody that binds to platelets or megakaryocytes (Mks) only in the presence of the sensitizing drug.[17] Over the years, several hypotheses have been proposed for the antibody-platelet interactions.[3–5] These hypotheses are discussed later (**Tables 1** and **2**).

HAPTEN-INDUCED ANTIBODY OR HAPTEN MECHANISM

Early immunologic studies in the 1900s suggested that small molecules like drugs are not antigenic and can only trigger an immune response when linked covalently to a macromolecule (a protein) acting as a hapten.[3–5,18] The resulting antibodies recognize the carrier molecule only where the hapten is attached covalently. In the 1950s and 1960s, Shulman[19,20] proposed the innocent-bystander or immune-complex mechanism that replaced the hapten mechanism as the dogma, and it remained accepted until the 1980s.[5] According to the immune-complex mechanism, drug-antibody complexes bind to platelets via platelet Fc receptors. Platelets are targeted for destruction as innocent bystanders as the antibody recognizes the drug but not the platelet.[5] It is now well recognized that the hapten and the immune-complex mechanisms are relevant for only a few drugs: high-dose penicillins cause immune hemolysis by haptens[21,22] and heparin causes thrombocytopenia via immune-complex binding.[23] These mechanisms are not discussed further in this article. Heparin-induced thrombocytopenia (HIT) represents a unique clinical-pathologic entity with strong platelet activation and frequent thrombosis. HIT merits a separate discussion with a full article to itself.

QUININE-TYPE IMMUNE THROMBOCYTOPENIA

As stated earlier, thrombocytopenia caused by quinine or its isomer, quinidine, is the prototype of most DITPs. This mechanism or a variation thereof mediates immune

Table 1
Mechanisms of drug-induced immune thrombocytopenia

Major Mechanisms	Hypotheses
Increase in peripheral platelet destruction or clearance	Increased platelet clearance by splenic and hepatic macrophages Platelet lysis by complements in circulation Platelet lysis by free oxygen radicals in circulation
Suppression of platelet production	Suppression by megakaryocyte proliferation and differentiation Increase in megakaryocyte apoptosis Inhibition of proplatelet production Suppression of megakaryocyte GPIb-IX expression

Table 2
Hypotheses of platelet-antibody-drug interactions

Hypotheses	Descriptions
Quinine-type DITP	Drug binds to a hyperflexible domain of a platelet glycoprotein (GPIX or GPIIIa) and the antibody recognizes an epitope on the GP. There are 2 proposed models: • Model 1: antibody binds to a neoantigen that emerges after glycoprotein conformational change following drug binding. Antibody binding fixes the glycoprotein in a new configuration trapping the drug in a pocket; drug removal becomes more difficult (see **Fig. 1**A) • Model 2: the antibody binds to a drug-platelet glycoprotein complex with the drug sandwiched in between, making drug removal difficult (see **Fig. 1**B)
Fiban-induced DITP	Fiban drug binds to GPIIb or GPIIIa near the RGD binding site, inducing a conformational change and formation of a neo-epitope (MIBS; see text) to which the antibody binds (see **Fig. 3**A)
Abciximab-induced DITP	The patient's antibodies recognize and bind to a mouse sequence of abciximab chimeric Fab (see **Fig. 3**B)
Immune-complex mechanism	The antibody binds to a plasma protein-drug complex (with drug acting as a hapten) and immune complex binds to platelet via its Fc receptor and the platelet is destroyed/activated as an innocent bystander (see **Fig. 3**C)

Abbreviations: MIBS, mimetic-induced binding sites; RGD, recognition sequence arginine-glycine-aspartic acid.

thrombocytopenia caused by most drugs (see **Table 2**).[3,4] In 1983, we showed for the first time that, using staphylococcal protein A, we could immunoprecipitate the drug-platelet antigen (glycoprotein Ib-IX [GPIb-IX]) complex with the antibody of a patient with quinidine-induced thrombocytopenia.[24] This radical finding contradicted the immune-complex mechanism dogma at that time, because this finding suggests that the antibody binds to platelets by its Fab but not its Fc domain. This finding was confirmed by subsequent studies from our and other laboratories.[25–29] It became clear that the immune-complex mechanism does not contribute to thrombocytopenia caused by quinine, quinidine, or most other drugs, except heparin.

Current evidence suggests that the drug binds to platelet GPIb-IX (von Willebrand factor receptor complex)[25–27] and/or GPIIb/IIIa (fibrinogen receptor complex).[25,27,30]

One hypothesis (model 1, **Fig. 1**A) is that drug binding induces a conformational change of the platelet surface protein, resulting in the emergence of a cryptic epitope or neoantigen previously unseen by the immune system.[5] The resultant antibody recognizes and binds this epitope only in the presence of the drug. In the absence of the drug, this epitope or neoantigen is buried in the glycoprotein folds or does not exist. Aster and colleagues[3,4] recently proposed a new model (model 2, see **Fig. 1**B) that is slightly different from the model discussed earlier. The essential difference is that, unlike model 1 in which the drug and the antibody bind the glycoprotein at different sites, in model 2 the drug and the antibody bind the target platelet glycoprotein at the same site (the drug is considered an essential component of the antibody binding site). Model 2 is supported by observations that quinine bound to platelets is more resistant to removal in the presence of the drug-dependent antibody, suggesting that the drug may be part of the binding pocket and is, therefore, entrapped by the

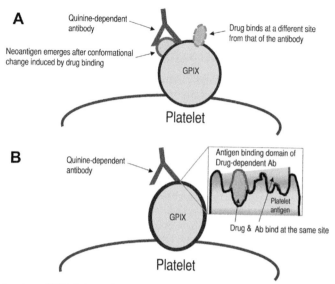

Fig. 1. Quinine-type DITP. (*A*) Model 1. Drug binding induces a conformational change on the glycoprotein, resulting in the emergence of a cryptic epitope or neoantigen. The drug and the antibody bind at different sites. (*B*) Model 2. The drug and the antibody bind the target platelet glycoprotein at the same site. GPIX, glycoprotein IX.

bound antibody. Nevertheless, there is no conclusive or direct experimental evidence to support this model.

WHY DO THE DRUG-DEPENDENT ANTIBODIES TARGET SPECIFIC PLATELET GLYCOPROTEINS SUCH AS GPIB-IX?

We have consistently found that all patients with quinine-induced and quinidine-induced thrombocytopenia had antibodies that reacted drug dependently with GPIb-IX[24–27]; almost all of these antibodies recognized GPIX[25,27] and only an occasional antibody had specificity for GPIbα.[27] In addition, a minority of patients (<30%) had drug-dependent antibodies reactive with GPIIb-IIIa.[25,27] In contrast, other investigators found a higher proportion of anti–GPIIb-IIIa antibodies.[30,31] Furthermore, we have mapped the binding site of the GPIX-specific quinine-dependent antibodies to a restricted site in the membrane-proximal ectodomain of platelet GPIX (R110–Q115)[25] and the GPIbα-specific antibody to the N-terminal domain of GPIbα (residues 283–293).[26]

Peterson and colleagues[30] located the binding sites of the quinine-dependent antibodies to a 29-kDa region of GPIIIa comprising the hybrid and the plextrin-semaphorinintegrin (PSI) domains, and residues A50 and D66 played a critical role in the formation of the antibody binding sites. Patients with rifampicin-induced and ranitidine-induced thrombocytopenia also have antibodies that react with GPIX.[32,33] An anti-GPIX monoclonal antibody (mAb) SZ1 cross-blocked the binding of quinine-dependent, quinidine-dependent, rifampicin-dependent, and ranitidine-dependent antibodies to GPIX,[25,27] suggesting that these four antibodies bind to a site that coincides with or is close to the epitope of SZ1. It is possible that, when other less well-characterized drug-induced antibodies (eg, vancomycin-induced antibody) are studied, they may also bind to this restricted GPIX site. These data also suggest that this region must have unique characteristics that render it unusually antigenic on drug binding.

FLEXIBLE DOMAINS AND IMMUNOGENICITY

Protein structure studies have recently provided additional information to refine the current hypothesis. The crystal structure of GPIIIa showed that the PSI domain (which is targeted by quinine-dependent antibodies)[30] could not be completely resolved,[34] indicating that it possesses a degree of mobility (hyperflexibility), adopting several transient state conformations.[34] The membrane-proximal part of the ectodomain of GPIX is also highly flexible[35] and is likely to adopt a range of non-native or denatured states (model in **Fig. 2**).[36,37] We have mapped the binding sites of anti-GPIX quinine-dependent antibodies to this hyperflexible GPIX region as described earlier.[25]

The presence of these unstructured protein domains may allow the binding of drugs of diverse chemical structures as the protein changes from one non-native conformation to another (see **Fig. 2**). Non-native conformations are characterized by an increase in their hydrophobic surface,[38] which may facilitate interaction by drugs containing hydrophobic pockets, such as quinine and quinidine, and it could also explain why drugs of different chemical structure, such as quinine, rifampicin, and ranitidine, interact with GPIX or GPIIIa. It is likely that each drug binds to distinct non-native structures, which then adopt a particular conformation. Under some

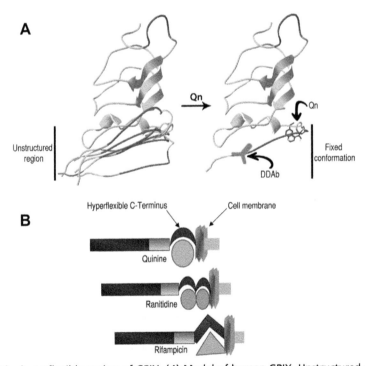

Fig. 2. The hyperflexible region of GPIX. (A) Model of human GPIX. Unstructured domains (in this case, the membrane-proximal domain of GPIX) may allow the binding of drugs of diverse chemical structures. Binding of the drug fixes a particular conformation (right panel) that, in some circumstances, is deemed foreign by the immune system. An antibody is then generated that binds to the glycoprotein in the presence of the drug (DDAb). (B) Hyperflexible region of GPIX binding drugs of different chemical structures.

conditions, this fixed configuration may elicit an immune response resulting in the generation of drug-dependent antibodies (see **Fig. 2**).[39]

THROMBOCYTOPENIA INDUCED BY GPIIB/IIIA INHIBITORS (FIBAN)

GPIIb/IIIa inhibitors, tirofiban and eptifibatide (fiban), are synthetic small molecules that bind tightly to the arginine-glycine-aspartic acid (recognition sequence arginine-glycine-aspartic acid [RGD]) recognition site on GPIIb/IIIa, inhibit fibrinogen binding, block platelet aggregation, and prevent platelet thrombus formation.[40] These drugs are widely used in clinical medicine to reduce cardiac complications following percutaneous transluminal coronary angioplasty (PTCA) and to treat acute coronary syndrome.[41,42] Clinical trials and subsequent clinical experience with the fibans showed that about 0.2% and 2% of patients receiving these compounds developed an acute, frequently severe, thrombocytopenia (platelet $<10 \times 10^9$/L) within a few hours of first drug exposure.[3,4,43–45] Previous studies have shown that naturally occurring antibodies against GPIIb/IIIa cause the thrombocytopenia, thus explaining the occurrence of thrombocytopenia on first drug exposure.[43,44] These antibodies are found not only in patients with fiban-induced thrombocytopenia (FIT) but also in normal volunteers never exposed to the drug.[46] It is still uncertain whether healthy individuals with these naturally occurring antibodies will develop severe thrombocytopenia if they receive a fiban.[46,47] If so, detection of the antibody before drug administration may prevent this serious complication.

Integrin research has revealed that RGD peptide and RGD mimetic compounds induce conformational changes in GPIIb/IIIa, resulting in the emergence of cryptic integrin domains that could be recognized by monoclonal antibodies specific for these ligand-induced binding sites (LIBSs).[48–55] It has been suggested that antibodies from patients with FIT probably have specificity for these LIBSs. Until recently, it was uncertain whether the ligand-induced GPIIb/IIIa determinants that resulted from fibrinogen/RGD peptide binding (ie, LIBSs) are the same as those induced by fiban drugs. Bougie and colleagues[56] showed that LIBSs are different from mimetic-induced binding sites (MIBSs), a term they used for determinants induced by fiban, but not fibrinogen, binding to GPIIb/IIIa. They also found that FIT antibodies did not recognize LIBS determinants as previously expected but instead recognized conformational changes in GPIIb/IIIa induced by the fiban drugs (MIBSs). In most patients with eptifibatide-induced and tirofiban-induced thrombocytopenia, antibody binding was drug specific and occurred only when the integrin complexed with the sensitizing drug. However, antibody cross-reactivity occurred only in a minority of patients.[56,57] These investigators also reported that the MIBSs resided in the head region of GPIIb/IIIa, near the RGD recognition site, probably on the β-propeller domain of GPIIb or the βA domain of GPIIIa (**Fig. 3A**). More precise epitope mapping, particularly identification of GPIIb or GPIIIa sequences that mediate antibody binding, may have to await further studies.

ABCIXIMAB-INDUCED THROMBOCYTOPENIA

Abciximab is a chimeric (mouse/human) monoclonal antibody (Fab fragment) that has specificity for the βA domain of GPIIIa. Because abciximab binds close to the RGD recognition site of GPIIIa, it blocks fibrinogen binding to activated GPIIb/IIIa and hence inhibits platelet thrombus formation. About 1% to 2% of patients given the drug develop acute, often severe, thrombocytopenia on first drug exposure,[58] and 10% to 12% on the second and subsequent exposure.[59] Like FIT, naturally occurring abciximab-dependent antibodies were detected in patients receiving the drug and in healthy volunteers never previously exposed to abciximab.[60,61] There is a subgroup

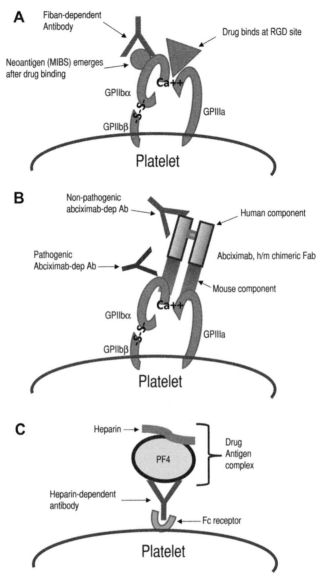

Fig. 3. Thrombocytopenia induced by GPIIb/IIIa inhibitors. (*A*) Fiban-induced DITP. A neoantigen emerges after drug binding. This is recognized by the antibody. (*B*) Abciximab-induced DITP. Naturally occurring nonpathogenic antibodies recognize the papain cleavage site at the C terminus of abciximab. Pathogenic antibodies may recognize the murine portion of the molecule. (*C*) Immune-complex or innocent-bystander mechanism. The immune complex binds to platelets via the Fc receptor and the platelet is destroyed/activated as an innocent bystander.

of patients who developed acute thrombocytopenia about a week after infusion of the drug.[60,61] These patients presumably did not have naturally occurring antibodies and acquired the antibody on drug sensitization. The antibody reached a level that could react with the abciximab that remained on platelets approximately 7 days later.[62]

Unlike other DITPs, both abciximab-dependent antibodies recognize the drug (abciximab) when bound to platelets. However, the patient antibody recognizes a mouse domain in the chimeric Fab.[58] In contrast, the antibody in healthy individuals is specific for the papain cleavage site introduced during the manufacturing process and, consequently, binding can be inhibited by Fab fragments prepared from normal immunoglobulin (Ig) G (see **Fig. 3**B).[60,61]

HOW MAY DRUG-DEPENDENT ANTIBODIES CAUSE THROMBOCYTOPENIA?
Platelet Destruction or Clearance

Thrombocytopenia occurs when there is an increase in platelet clearance/destruction or a decrease in platelet production in the bone marrow. The most widely held view is that in DITP, like other immune thrombocytopenias, antibody-coated platelets are cleared in the spleen and/or liver by macrophage phagocytosis.[63] However, there is little or no direct evidence for this. We and Bougie and colleagues[64] recently provided in vivo evidence using a nonobese diabetic/severe combined immunodeficiency (NOD/SCID) mouse model.[65] We were able to show that human platelets injected immediately after administration of DITP serum or purified IgG resulted in rapid platelet clearance. This rapid and marked platelet clearance was uniformly seen across 7 patients with quinine-induced thrombocytopenia, consistent with the clinical picture of severe thrombocytopenia of abrupt onset in this condition.[65] In comparison, platelet clearance using this in vivo model by antibodies from patients with primary immune thrombocytopenia (ITP) is gradual and variable in rate and extent, in keeping with the heterogenous clinical picture in ITP. Additional mechanisms have been proposed for the thrombocytopenia in DITP; these include platelet destruction in circulation by complement-mediated or radical oxygen species (ROS)–mediated lysis,[9] but there is no direct evidence for these hypotheses.

Early studies in the 1950s showed in vitro complement deposition on platelets following DITP antibody-platelet interaction.[19,20] Platelet lysis caused by oxidative stress has been shown in immune thrombocytopenia associated with human immunodeficiency virus (HIV) infection.[66–68] Platelet lysis by cytotoxic T cells has also been implicated in platelet number decline in ITP.[69] There is no convincing or direct evidence of complement-mediated, ROS-mediated, or T-cell–mediated platelet destruction in DITP.

Suppression of Platelet Production

Despite evidence that antibodies of patients with DITP can directly destroy platelets in vivo,[64,65] there is considerable support for additional platelet-independent processes that may contribute to the thrombocytopenia in DITP. One of these is antibody-mediated megakaryocytic damage. Most experimental data in this aspect come from studies in patients with ITP or using antiplatelet monoclonal antibodies. However, there is also recent evidence indicating that this is also applicable to DITP.[17]

In the 1970s, McMillan and colleagues[70] observed that antiplatelet antibodies produced by patients with ITP could recognize Mks. Subsequent experiments suggested a possible role of Mks in the pathogenesis of ITP.[71] These ideas were strengthened by Chang and colleagues[72] who showed that anti-GPIb/IX ITP antibodies affected Mk differentiation, and by McMillan and colleagues[73] who showed a reduction in Mk production after in vitro culture of Mks in the presence of antiplatelet antibodies. These investigations implied that megakaryocytic damage by antiplatelet antibodies may result in a decrease in platelet production and consequently thrombocytopenia.

DITP antibodies causing Mk damage have been shown in vitro using serum from a patient with eptifibatide-induced thrombocytopenia.[74] Furthermore, inhibition of Mk differentiation and proliferation together with decreased platelet production capacity were recently shown in a more in-depth study using IgG/sera from patients with quinine-induced thrombocytopenia antibodies.[17] Therefore, DITP antibodies may also contribute to thrombocytopenia by suppressing platelet production.

WHAT MECHANISMS MAY ACCOUNT FOR ANTIBODY-MEDIATED MK DAMAGE?

That the association of drug-dependent antibodies with Mks causes cellular injury seems puzzling. Nonetheless, potential explanations have been proposed: induction of apoptosis and a decrease in GPIb/IX expression.[17,75] Induction of apoptosis on antibody binding is an appealing proposition that has some experimental support in studies with both Mks[17] and platelets.[76] In this model, binding of drug-dependent antibodies, especially anti-GPIb/IX antibodies, to Mks triggers an apoptotic signaling cascade (reviewed in Ref.[75]). As apoptosis plays an essential role in Mk differentiation,[77] interfering with this process hinders platelet production.[75]

The physical association of antibodies with the GPIb/IX complex may also affect platelet production. It is known that GPIb/IX expression is required for platelet formation[78] and we have found that binding of quinine-dependent antibodies to Mks causes a reduction in the number of GPIb/IX receptors expressed on the cell surface.[17] This finding suggests that the decline in platelet production capacity in antibody-treated Mks may also be a consequence of lower GPIb/IX expression. This idea is substantiated by previous observations of impaired platelet production after incubation of Mks with anti-GPIbα monoclonal antibodies.[79] The experimental evidence suggests that platelet production is affected by DITP antibodies, and this is most likely caused by both induction of Mk apoptosis and reduction of GPIb/IX complex expression.

DIAGNOSIS OF DITP

All patients with an unexpected severe thrombocytopenia with an abrupt onset should be suspected to have DITP. A careful, detailed history is a key element of the patient evaluation.[8] The patient should be asked specifically about taking drugs that can cause thrombocytopenia, including herbal medicine, tonics, certain foods, and health supplements even if they are taken intermittently. Patients often do not report drugs or remedies that they take themselves because they assume that doctors are only interested in prescription drugs. Quinine, a drug that commonly causes DITP,[3–5] is present in quinine-containing beverages such as tonic water and Schweppes Bitter Lemon and may be missed if this is not explicitly questioned. The quantity of quinine present in these beverages, even though small, is enough to trigger the development of QITP.[8] Attention should also be given to herbal remedies such as traditional Chinese herbal medicine, jui, and food items such as tahini (pulped sesame seeds), the principal ingredient of the traditional Middle Eastern food hummus,[80] because ingestion of these herbs and foods have been reported to cause DITP.

CLINICAL PICTURE

The clinical picture of the patient should also be assessed. The clinical picture of patients with DITP varies with the causative drug and the patient's platelet count. For most drugs such as quinine, the thrombocytopenia is severe and platelet count decreases frequently to less than $10 \times 10^9/L$ and even to $0 \times 10^9/L$. The patient classically presents with extensive petechiae, bruising, mucosal bleeding, and occasionally overt hemorrhage. Serious bleeding can occur[6] but fatal intracranial bleed is uncommon.[7] The thrombocytopenia characteristically has an acute onset, occurring usually 5 to 14 days after drug commencement, but it can occur earlier if there is a recent exposure to the drug in question. However, in patients with thrombocytopenia caused by GPIIb/IIIa inhibitors, the platelet count usually decreases sharply to very low levels as early as a few hours after first exposure to the drug.[43–45]

In general, the clinician has to consider 2 sets of data when making a diagnosis of DITP (**Table 3**), namely:

1. Patient-specific data
2. Information regarding the capability of a suspected drug to cause DITP

For patient-specific data, the clinician needs to consider the temporal relationship between the commencement of the suspect drug and the onset of thrombocytopenia and then decide whether the time interval between the two events is consistent with the drug causing DITP in the patient.[5] Other causes of thrombocytopenia such as other drugs or comorbid conditions should be carefully considered and excluded.[4,8] In some patients, exclusion of other causes may be difficult or impossible clinically. In this situation, the suspect drugs may have to be stopped one at a time; this may be impractical, because it may take too long. As an alternative, the patient may be rechallenged with the suspect drug after its withdrawal with platelet recovery but this is seldom performed nowadays because it incurs too great a risk to the patient, unless it is deemed necessary for patient management. Furthermore, it is now possible to identify the sensitizing drug by a laboratory assay (discussed later). For a clinical diagnosis of DITP, diagnostic criteria as listed in **Table 1** could be helpful.

DRUG CAPACITY TO CAUSE DITP

The clinician should seek evidence from previous published studies or specific Web sites about the potential of the suspect drug to cause DITP, in particular the frequency and the strength of evidence for the drug causing DITP.[81] One helpful Web site[8] is

Table 3
Clinical diagnostic criteria

Criteria	Description
1	Administration of the suspected drug was commenced before the onset of thrombocytopenia and platelet count returned to normal or baseline levels after drug withdrawal
2	The suspected drug was the only drug administered before the onset of thrombocytopenia or other drugs were continued or reintroduced after withdrawal of the suspected drug and the platelet counts remained normal
3	Other causes of thrombocytopenia were excluded
4	Rechallenge with the suspected drug resulted in prompt recurrence of thrombocytopenia or the offending drug can be identified by a laboratory test
	Level of evidence • Definite: criteria 1, 2, 3, and 4 met • Probable: criteria 1, 2, and 3 met • Possible: Criteria 1 met • Unlikely: criteria 1 not met

Data from George JN, Chong BH, Li X. Drug-induced Thrombocytopenia. In: Colman RW, Marder VJ, Clowes AW, editors. Hemostasis and thrombosis: basic principles and clinical practice. 5th edition. Philadelphia: Lippincott Williams & Wilkins; 2006. p. 1095–102.

http://w3.ouhsc.edu/platelets. This site provides comprehensive and current information on all case reports of DITP and objective assessment of the level of evidence supporting a given drug as the cause of DITP.

LABORATORY DIAGNOSIS

The clinical diagnosis of DITP should be confirmed if possible by the detection of the specific drug-dependent antibody by a laboratory assay (**Table 4**). The assay can be:

- A direct test or
- An indirect test

A direct test measures antibodies or immunoglobulins attached to the patient's platelets, and is a method used in ITP in which the autoantibody is located predominantly on patients' platelets and not in the serum.[82] An indirect test measures antibodies or immunoglobulins in the patient's serum that bind to normal platelets when the serum and platelets are incubated together.[82] Unlike in ITP, the indirect test is the assay of choice in DITP because, after drug withdrawal and in the absence of

| Table 4 | | |
| Types of laboratory assays for detection of DITP antibodies (Abs)[a] | | |
Types of Assays	**Descriptions**	**Reliability**
Functional assays	Patient Abs and drug bind to platelets inducing an activation change such as platelet aggregation or serotonin release (used mainly to detect HIT Abs)	Not sensitive or specific because DITP Abs do not usually activate platelets
PA-IgG assays	Patient Ab binds to normal platelets only in the presence of the drug but not in its absence. Second negative control is also used, comprising normal serum, normal platelets, and drugs. Ab binding can be assessed using flow cytometry or ELISA (see **Fig. 4**A)	Highly sensitive and specific for detection of DITP Abs (eg, quinine, fiban, abciximab, vancomycin Abs)
Antigen-capture assays	Platelet antigen (GPIb-IX or GPIIb/IIIa) is captured onto microtiter wells by GP-specific monoclonal Abs. Captured antigen is incubated with patient serum and drug. Detection of the Ab is made with an ELISA. Two commonly used methods are MACE and MAIPA (see **Fig. 4**B, C)	Highly sensitive and specific for detection of DITP Abs (eg, quinine, fiban, abciximab, vancomycin Abs)
Other assays (old)	These include complement fixation,[19] platelet lysis,[84] and induction of platelet procoagulant activity[85]	Sensitivity and specificity uncertain

Abbreviations: MACE, modified antigen-capture enzyme-linked immunoadsorbent assay; MAIPA, monoclonal antibody-specific immobilization of platelet antigen.
[a] In these assays indirect testing is used, comprising patient serum, normal platelets, and drug.

the offending drug in the patient's blood, the drug-dependent antibody no longer binds to platelets but is present in the patient's plasma/serum in high titer. The patient's serum can be tested in the laboratory with each of the suspected drugs that the patient was taking. The finding of a drug-dependent antibody binding to platelets allows the causative drug to be identified.[8] This is often termed in vitro drug rechallenge.

Types of DITP Antibody Assays

Platelet activation or functional assays

These are indirect tests that measure antibody-induced platelet activation changes such as platelet aggregation and serotonin release when the patient's serum is incubated with normal platelets in the presence of therapeutic concentration of the drug.[82] Tests such as the ^{14}C-serotonin release assay and heparin-induced platelet aggregation tests are widely used for diagnosing HIT[9] but are seldom used to detect drug-dependent antibody in other DITPs such as quinine-induced thrombocytopenia, because antibodies in non-HIT DITP seldom cause platelet activation and thus these assays are of no practical use.

Platelet-associated IgG

These assays measure IgG associated with or bound to platelets (**Fig. 4**A). The test can be designed to measure IgG, IgA, and IgM separately or together. There are 3 different approaches to measure platelet-associated IgG (PA-IgG): (1) 2-stage assays such as competitive inhibition assays, (2) direct binding, and (3) total PA-IgG assays.[83] These assays are unreliable for measurement of platelet autoantibodies in ITP because of their low specificity caused by the presence of nonimmune IgG on platelets in both ITP and nonimmune thrombocytopenias.[83] In contrast, these assays are useful for detection of the drug-dependent antibodies in DITP.[5,82] We have found that they are both highly sensitive and specific for the detection of drug-induced antibodies, particularly quinine-dependent, quinidine-dependent, rifampicin-dependent, vancomycin-dependent, fiban-dependent, and abciximab-dependent antibodies. The commonly used PA-IgG assays for drug-dependent antibodies are enzyme-linked immunosorbent assay and flow cytometry. The latter involves common technology that is available in many clinical laboratories.

Platelet glycoprotein–specific antibody assays

These assays include the:

- Modified antigen-capture enzyme-linked immunoadsorbent assay (MACE)
- Monoclonal antibody-specific immobilization of platelet antigen (MAIPA) assay.

In MACE (see **Fig. 4**B), a glycoprotein-specific monoclonal antibody (eg, anti-GPIb-IX, FMC25) is used to capture the target platelet antigen in the wells of a microtiter plate from added platelet lysate.[82,83] Following incubation of captured glycoprotein with patient serum, the serum antibody binds drug dependently to the target antigen and is then detected using an enzyme-linked secondary antibody (antihuman IgG). In MAIPA (see **Fig. 4**C), an antimouse IgG coated on the microtiter well captures a trimolecular complex consisting of a mouse glycoprotein–specific antibody (eg, anti-GPIb-IX, FMC25), the platelet antigen (eg, GPIb-IX), and the patient drug-dependent antibody. The trimolecular complex is preformed in a test tube before its transfer to the microtiter wells so that patient serum is not added to the microtiter wells, to prevent high background readings.[25–27] The drug-dependent antibody is then detected by an enzyme-linked secondary antibody as in MACE.

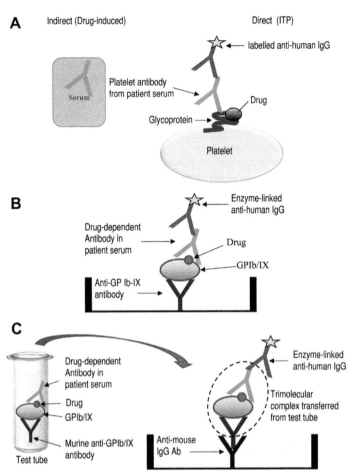

Fig. 4. Antiplatelet antibody assays. (*A*) Platelet associated IgG (PA-IgG): direct and indirect binding assay. (*B*) Modified antigen-capture enzyme-linked immunoadsorbent assay. (*C*) Monoclonal antibody-specific immobilization of platelet antigen assay.

Other Methods

Other methods used for drug-dependent antibody detection include complement fixation,[19] platelet lysis,[84] and induction of platelet procoagulant activity.[85] These methods were commonly used from the 1950s to the 1970s and their sensitivity is uncertain.

INTERPRETATION OF TEST RESULTS

With each of the tests discussed earlier, a positive result is seen when antibody binding occurs with patient serum and normal platelets in the presence of the suspected drug. Normal donor platelets are commonly used because of the patient's marked thrombocytopenia. After platelet recovery, the patient's platelets can be used. Two negative controls are required: (1) platelets and patient serum in the absence of the drug, and (2) platelets and normal serum in the presence of the drug; both controls should show negative results. The first control shows drug-dependent antibody binding and the second excludes the possibility of a false-positive result caused by drug autofluorescence.

COMPARISON OF ASSAYS

In our experience, the MAIPA assay is slightly more sensitive than flow cytometry in detecting drug-dependent antibodies.[25,82] However, there are some caveats. First, it is technically more difficult than flow cytometry. Second, prior knowledge of the antigen of the drug-dependent antibody is required so that an appropriate antibody can be used to capture the platelet antigen.[25,82] This is usually not a problem because the epitopes of drug-dependent antibodies are known to be located on platelet GPIb-IX and/or GPIIb-IIIa, and occasionally other glycoproteins such as PECAM-1.

In summary, unlike ITP, laboratory tests are often helpful in the diagnosis of DITP, in particular the drug-related thrombocytopenias discussed earlier. A technique like flow cytometry is widely available but assays such as MACE and MAIPA are not. At present, there are still challenges in the laboratory testing for drug-dependent antibodies. These include:

1. Knowing the optimum drug concentration for the test (often corresponds with the therapeutic plasma concentrations of the drug)[25,82]
2. Obtaining soluble drug for testing, because some drugs are difficult to dissolve[4]
3. The availability of drug metabolites, because some antibodies react only with the drug metabolite and do not react with the parent drug (examples are nonsteroidal antiinflammatory drugs and acetaminophen)[4]
4. The titer and/or avidity of some DITP antibodies may be too low to be detectable by current assays

MANAGEMENT

In most patients, the most appropriate treatment is withdrawal of the specific drug, herbal medicine, tonic, or food.[8] After drug removal, the drug-dependent antibody no longer binds to the platelets and Mks even though the antibody may persist for months in the patient's circulation. If the patient has severe thrombocytopenia with bleeding or high risk of bleeding, treatment with high-dose corticosteroid (1–2 mg/kg/d) and high-dose pooled human immunoglobulin (intravenous immunoglobulin [IVIG]) (2 g/kg over 2–5 days) is nearly always given.[5,8] because the platelet count of patients invariably returns to normal in 1 to 2 weeks, it is difficult to know whether these treatments are efficacious. In a recent study, we provided in vivo evidence in a mouse model of DITP that IVIG is partially effective in preventing the rapid platelet clearance by the drug-dependent antibody.[65] However, at present, if the patient has critical bleeding such as cerebral hemorrhage during the first few days after drug withdrawal when the patient is still markedly thrombocytopenic, there is no effective treatment to promptly increase the patient's platelet count. If major bleeding occurs during the acute phase of DITP, the patient should be given platelet transfusions, preferably following IVIG infusions, which may provide Fc receptor blockage to prevent premature platelet clearance by macrophages in the liver and spleen. Antifibrinolytic therapy such as tranexamic acid may also be helpful because the fibrinolytic pathway is activated in patients with active bleeding. If the bleeding is persistent and serious, measures such as plasma exchange to remove the drug should be considered, particularly when the drug has a long plasma half-life and/or when significant renal failure is present.

In DITP, unlike ITP, corticosteroids should be stopped abruptly when the platelet count recovers 1 to 2 weeks after drug withdrawal. In contrast, adult patients with ITP characteristically require a prolonged course of corticosteroids for continuing immunosuppression.[8]

In conclusion, recent work has provided considerable new knowledge concerning the pathogenesis of DITP, particularly thrombocytopenia caused by quinine (the prototype drug) and DITP caused by GPIIb/IIIa inhibitors. The antibody binding sites in DITP caused by quinine and possibly rifampicin and ranitidine have been mapped to a hyperflexible region in the membrane-proximal domain of GPIX and the PSI domain of GPIIIa. It is now understood that the drug-dependent antibodies not only coat platelets and induce their premature clearance by the reticuloendothelial system, they also bind Mks, inhibit their proliferation and maturation, and suppress proplatelet and platelet production. Diagnosis of DITP is made clinically based on diagnostic criteria that define the causal relationship between the suspected drug and thrombocytopenia. The diagnosis of DITP is further confirmed by the detection of the drug-dependent antibody using laboratory tests. The most important treatment is withdrawal of the offending drug, following which the platelet count invariably returns to normal. Nevertheless, corticosteroid and high-dose IVIG are usually given to most patients because of the severe thrombocytopenia and high risk of bleeding.

REFERENCES

1. Jones H, Tocantins L. The history of purpura haemorrhagica. Ann Med Hist 1933; 5:349–59.
2. Vipan WH. Quinine as a cause of purpura. Lancet 1865;2:37.
3. Aster RH, Bougie DW. Drug-induced immune thrombocytopenia. N Engl J Med 2007;357:580–7.
4. Aster RH, Curtis BR, McFarland JG, et al. Drug-induced immune thrombocytopenia: pathogenesis, diagnosis, and management. J Thromb Haemost 2009;7: 911–8.
5. Chong BH. Drug-induced immune thrombocytopenia. Platelets 1991;2:173–81.
6. Fireman Z, Yust I, Abramov AL. Lethal occult pulmonary hemorrhage in drug-induced thrombocytopenia. Chest 1981;79:358–9.
7. Freiman JP. Fatal quinine-induced thrombocytopenia. Ann Intern Med 1990;112: 308–9.
8. George JN, Chong BH, Li X. Drug-induced thrombocytopenia. In: Colman RW, Marder VJ, Clowes AW, et al, editors. Hemostasis and thrombosis: basic principles and clinical practice. 5th edition. Philadelphia: Lippincott Williams & Wilkins; 2006. p. 1095–102.
9. Chong BH, Isaacs A. Heparin-induced thrombocytopenia: what clinicians need to know. Thromb Haemost 2009;101:279–83.
10. Bottiger LE, Bottiger B. Incidence and cause of aplastic anemia, hemolytic anemia, agranulocytosis and thrombocytopenia. Acta Med Scand 1981;210:475–9.
11. Bottiger LE, Westerholm B. Thrombocytopenia. II. Drug-induced thrombocytopenia. Acta Med Scand 1972;191:541–8.
12. Danielson DA, Douglas SW, Herzog P, et al. Drug-induced blood disorders. JAMA 1984;252:3257–60.
13. Kaufman DW, Kelly JP, Johannes CB, et al. Acute thrombocytopenic purpura in relation to the use of drugs. Blood 1993;82:2714–8.
14. Pedersen-Bjergaard U, Andersen M, Hansen PB. Thrombocytopenia induced by noncytotoxic drugs in Denmark 1968-91. J Intern Med 1996;239:509–15.

15. Pedersen-Bjergaard U, Andersen M, Hansen PB. Drug-induced thrombocyto-penia: clinical data on 309 cases and the effect of corticosteroid therapy. Eur J Clin Pharmacol 1997;52:183–9.
16. Pedersen-Bjergaard U, Andersen M, Hansen PB. Drug-specific characteristics of thrombocytopenia caused by non-cytotoxic drugs. Eur J Clin Pharmacol 1998;54: 701–6.
17. Perdomo J, Yan F, Ahmadi Z, et al. Quinine-induced thrombocytopenia: drug-dependent GPIb/IX antibodies inhibit megakaryocyte and proplatelet production in vitro. Blood 2011;117:5975–86.
18. Ackroyd JF. Allergic purpura, including purpura due to foods, drugs and infec-tions. Am J Med 1953;14:605–32.
19. Shulman NR. Immunoreactions involving platelets. A steric and kinetic model for formation of a complex from a human antibody, quinidine as a haptene, and plate-lets; and for fixation of complement by the complex. J Exp Med 1958;107:665–90.
20. Shulman NR. A mechanism of cell destruction in individuals sensitized to foreign antigens and its implications in auto-immunity. Ann Intern Med 1964;60:506–21.
21. Garratty G. Immune cytopenia associated with antibiotics. Transfus Med Rev 1993;7:255–67.
22. Murphy MF, Riordan T, Minchinton RM, et al. Demonstration of an immune-mediated mechanism of penicillin-induced neutropenia and thrombocytopenia. Br J Haematol 1983;55:155–60.
23. Shantsila E, Lip GY, Chong BH. Heparin-induced thrombocytopenia. A contem-porary clinical approach to diagnosis and management. Chest 2009;135: 1651–64.
24. Chong BH, Berndt MC, Koutts J, et al. Quinidine-induced thrombocytopenia and leukopenia: demonstration and characterization of distinct antiplatelet and anti-leukocyte antibodies. Blood 1983;62:1218–23.
25. Asvadi P, Ahmadi Z, Chong BH. Drug-induced thrombocytopenia: localization of the binding site of GPIX-specific quinine-dependent antibodies. Blood 2003;102: 1670–7.
26. Burgess JK, Lopez JA, Berndt MC, et al. Quinine-dependent antibodies bind a restricted set of epitopes on the glycoprotein Ib-IX complex: characterization of the epitopes. Blood 1998;92:2366–73.
27. Chong BH, Du XP, Berndt MC, et al. Characterization of the binding domains on platelet glycoproteins Ib-IX and IIb/IIIa complexes for the quinine/quinidine-dependent antibodies. Blood 1991;77:2190–9.
28. Christie DJ, Mullen PC, Aster RH. Fab-mediated binding of drug-dependent an-tibodies to platelets in quinidine- and quinine-induced thrombocytopenia. J Clin Invest 1985;75:310–4.
29. Smith ME, Reid DM, Jones CE, et al. Binding of quinine- and quinidine-dependent drug antibodies to platelets is mediated by the Fab domain of the immunoglobulin G and is not Fc dependent. J Clin Invest 1987;79:912–7.
30. Peterson JA, Nelson TN, Kanack AJ, et al. Fine specificity of drug-dependent an-tibodies reactive with a restrictive domain of platelet GPIIIa. Blood 2008;111: 1234–9.
31. Bougie DW, Wilker PR, Aster RH. Patients with quinine-induced immune thrombo-cytopenia have both "drug-dependent" and "drug-specific" antibodies. Blood 2006;108:922–7.
32. Burgess JK, Lopez JA, Gaudry LE, et al. Rifampicin-dependent antibodies bind a similar or identical epitope to glycoprotein IX-specific quinine-dependent anti-bodies. Blood 2000;95:1988–92.

33. Gentilini G, Curtis BR, Aster RH. An antibody from a patient with ranitidine-induced thrombocytopenia recognizes a site on glycoprotein IX that is a favored target for drug-induced antibodies. Blood 1998;92:2359–65.
34. Xiong JP, Stehle T, Diefenbach B, et al. Crystal structure of the extracellular segment of integrin alphaV/beta3. Science 2001;294:339–45.
35. Mo X, Nguyen NX, McEwan PA, et al. Binding of platelet glycoprotein Ibbeta through the convex surface of leucine-rich repeats domain of glycoprotein IX. J Thromb Haemost 2009;7:1533–40.
36. Jürgen K, Schwede T. The SWISS-MODEL Repository of annotated three-dimensional protein structure homology models. Nucleic Acids Res 2004;32: D230–4.
37. Kiefer F, Arnold K, Künzli M, et al. The SWISS-MODEL Repository and associated resources. Nucleic Acids Res 2009;37:D387–92.
38. Dill KA. Denatured states of proteins. Annu Rev Biochem 1991;60:795–825.
39. Li R. A hypothesis that explains the heterogeneity of drug-induced immune thrombocytopenia. Blood 2010;115:914.
40. Topol EJ, Byzova TV, Plow EF. Platelet GPIIb-IIIa blockers. Lancet 1999;353: 227–31.
41. The RESTORE Investigators. Effects of platelet glycoprotein IIb/IIIa blockade with tirofiban on adverse cardiac events in patients with unstable angina or acute myocardial infarction undergoing coronary angioplasty. Circulation 1997;96:1445–53.
42. The PURSUIT Trial Investigators. Inhibition of platelet glycoprotein IIb/IIIa with eptifibatide in patients with acute coronary syndromes. N Engl J Med 1998;339: 436–43.
43. Coons JC, Barcelona RA, Freedy T, et al. Eptifibatide-associated acute, profound thrombocytopenia. Ann Pharmacother 2005;39:368–72.
44. Patel S, Patel M, Din I, et al. Profound thrombocytopenia associated with tirofiban: case report and review of literature. Angiology 2005;56:351–5.
45. Rezkalla SH, Hayes JJ, Curtis BR, et al. Eptifibatide-induced acute profound thrombocytopenia presenting as refractory hypotension. Catheter Cardiovasc Interv 2003;58:76–9.
46. Bougie DW, Wilker PR, Wuitschick ED, et al. Acute thrombocytopenia after treatment with tirofiban or eptifibatide is associated with antibodies specific for ligand-occupied GPIIb/IIIa. Blood 2002;100:2071–6.
47. Billheimer JT, Dicker IB, Wynn R, et al. Evidence that thrombocytopenia observed in humans treated with orally bioavailable glycoprotein IIb/IIIa antagonists is immune mediated. Blood 2002;99:3540–6.
48. Artoni A, Li J, Mitchell B, et al. Integrin beta3 regions controlling binding of murine mAb 7E3: implications for the mechanism of integrin alphaIIbbeta3 activation. Proc Natl Acad Sci U S A 2004;101:13114–20.
49. Du X, Gu M, Weisel JW, et al. Long range propagation of conformational changes in integrin alpha IIb beta 3. J Biol Chem 1993;268:23087–92.
50. Frelinger AL, Du XP, Plow EF, et al. Monoclonal antibodies to ligand-occupied conformers of integrin alpha IIb beta 3 (glycoprotein IIb-IIIa) alter receptor affinity, specificity, and function. J Biol Chem 1991;266:17106–11.
51. Honda S, Tomiyama Y, Pelletier AJ, et al. Topography of ligand-induced binding sites, including a novel cation-sensitive epitope (AP5) at the amino terminus, of the human integrin beta 3 subunit. J Biol Chem 1995;270:11947–54.
52. Jennings LK, Haga JH, Slack SM. Differential expression of a ligand induced binding site (LIBS) by GPIIb-IIIa ligand recognition peptides and parenteral antagonists. Thromb Haemost 2000;84:1095–102.

53. Kouns WC, Newman PJ, Puckett KJ, et al. Further characterization of the loop structure of platelet glycoprotein IIIa: partial mapping of functionally significant glycoprotein IIIa epitopes. Blood 1991;78:3215–23.

54. Kouns WC, Wall CD, White MM, et al. A conformation-dependent epitope of human platelet glycoprotein IIIa. J Biol Chem 1990;265:20594–601.

55. Loftus JC, Plow EF, Frelinger AL, et al. Molecular cloning and chemical synthesis of a region of platelet glycoprotein IIb involved in adhesive function. Proc Natl Acad Sci U S A 1987;84:7114–8.

56. Bougie DW, Rasmussen M, Zhu J, et al. Antibodies causing thrombocytopenia in patients treated with RGD-mimetic platelet inhibitors recognize ligand-specific conformers of alphaIIb/beta3 integrin. Blood 2012;119:6317–25.

57. Chong BH. Drug-induced thrombocytopenia: MIBS trumps LIBS. Blood 2012; 119:6177–8.

58. Jubelirer SJ, Koenig BA, Bates MC. Acute profound thrombocytopenia following C7E3 Fab (Abciximab) therapy: case reports, review of the literature and implications for therapy. Am J Hematol 1999;61:205–8.

59. Dery JP, Braden GA, Lincoff AM, et al. Final results of the ReoPro readministration registry. Am J Cardiol 2004;93:979–84.

60. Curtis BR, Divgi A, Garritty M, et al. Delayed thrombocytopenia after treatment with abciximab: a distinct clinical entity associated with the immune response to the drug. J Thromb Haemost 2004;2:985–92.

61. Curtis BR, Swyers J, Divgi A, et al. Thrombocytopenia after second exposure to abciximab is caused by antibodies that recognize abciximab-coated platelets. Blood 2002;99:2054–9.

62. Mascelli MA, Lance ET, Damaraju L, et al. Pharmacodynamic profile of short-term abciximab treatment demonstrates prolonged platelet inhibition with gradual recovery from GP IIb/IIIa receptor blockade. Circulation 1998;97:1680–8.

63. Newland AC, Macey MG. Immune thrombocytopenia and Fc receptor-mediated phagocyte function. Ann Hematol 1994;69:61–7.

64. Bougie DW, Nayak D, Boylan B, et al. Drug-dependent clearance of human platelets in the NOD/scid mouse by antibodies from patients with drug-induced immune thrombocytopenia. Blood 2010;116:3033–8.

65. Liang SX, Pinkevych M, Khachigian LM, et al. Drug-induced thrombocytopenia: development of a novel NOD/SCID mouse model to evaluate clearance of circulating platelets by drug-dependent antibodies and the efficacy of IVIG. Blood 2010;116:1958–60.

66. Li Z, Nardi MA, Karpatkin S. Role of molecular mimicry to HIV-1 peptides in HIV-1-related immunologic thrombocytopenia. Blood 2005;106:572–6.

67. Nardi M, Feinmark SJ, Hu L, et al. Complement-independent Ab-induced peroxide lysis of platelets requires 12-lipoxygenase and a platelet NADPH oxidase pathway. J Clin Invest 2004;113:973–80.

68. Nardi M, Tomlinson S, Greco MA, et al. Complement-independent, peroxide-induced antibody lysis of platelets in HIV-1-related immune thrombocytopenia. Cell 2001;106:551–61.

69. Olsson B, Andersson PO, Jernås M, et al. T-cell-mediated cytotoxicity toward platelets in chronic idiopathic thrombocytopenic purpura. Nat Med 2003;9:1123–4.

70. McMillan R, Luiken GA, Levy R. Antibody against megakaryocytes in idiopathic thrombocytopenic purpura. JAMA 1978;239:2460–2.

71. Hoffman R, Zaknoen S, Yang HH. An antibody cytotoxic to megakaryocyte progenitor cells in a patient with immune thrombocytopenic purpura. N Engl J Med 1985;312:1170–4.

72. Chang M, Nakagawa PA, Williams SA, et al. Immune thrombocytopenic purpura (ITP) plasma and purified ITP monoclonal autoantibodies inhibit megakaryocytopoiesis in vitro. Blood 2003;102:887–95.

73. McMillan R, Wang L, Tomer A, et al. Suppression of in vitro megakaryocyte production by antiplatelet autoantibodies from adult patients with chronic ITP. Blood 2004;103:1364–9.

74. Greinacher A, Fuerll B, Zinke H, et al. Megakaryocyte impairment by eptifibatide-induced antibodies causes prolonged thrombocytopenia. Blood 2009;114: 1250–3.

75. Perdomo J, Yan F, Chong BH. A megakaryocyte with no platelets: anti-platelet antibodies, apoptosis, and platelet production. Platelets 2013;24(2):98–106.

76. Piguet PF, Vesin C. Modulation of platelet caspases and life-span by anti-platelet antibodies in mice. Eur J Haematol 2002;68:253–61.

77. Li J, Kuter DJ. The end is just the beginning: megakaryocyte apoptosis and platelet release. Int J Hematol 2001;74:365–74.

78. Poujol C, Ware J, Nieswandt B, et al. Absence of GPIbalpha is responsible for aberrant membrane development during megakaryocyte maturation: ultrastructural study using a transgenic model. Exp Hematol 2002;30:352–60.

79. Takahashi R, Sekine N, Nakatake T. Influence of monoclonal antiplatelet glycoprotein antibodies on in vitro human megakaryocyte colony formation and proplatelet formation. Blood 1999;93:1951–8.

80. Arnold J, Ouwehand WH, Smith GA, et al. A young woman with petechiae. Lancet 1998;352:618.

81. George JN, Raskob GE, Shah SR, et al. Drug-induced thrombocytopenia: a systematic review of published case reports. Ann Intern Med 1998;129:886–90.

82. Chong BH. Diagnosis of drug-induced thrombocytopenia. Int J Lab Hematol 2008;30:10–11.

83. Chong BH, Keng TB. Advances in the diagnosis of idiopathic thrombocytopenic purpura. Semin Hematol 2000;37:249–60.

84. Cimo PL, Pisciotta AV, Desai RG, et al. Detection of drug-dependent antibodies by the 51Cr platelet lysis test: documentation of immune thrombocytopenia induced by diphenylhydantoin, diazepam, and sulfisoxazole. Am J Hematol 1977;2:65–72.

85. Karpatkin M, Siskind GW, Karpatkin S. The platelet factor 3 immunoinjury technique re-evaluated. Development of a rapid test for antiplatelet antibody. Detection in various clinical disorders, including immunologic drug-induced and neonatal thrombocytopenias. J Lab Clin Med 1977;89:400–8.

Diagnosis and Management of Heparin-Induced Thrombocytopenia

Grace M. Lee, MD[a], Gowthami M. Arepally, MD[b],*

KEYWORDS

• Platelet factor 4 • PF4 • Heparin • PF4/H complexes • HIT

KEY POINTS

• Heparin-induced thrombocytopenia (HIT) is a prothrombotic disorder caused by antibodies to platelet factor 4/heparin complexes. It classically presents with declining platelet counts 5 to 14 days after heparin administration and results in a predisposition to arterial and venous thrombosis.
• Establishing the diagnosis of HIT can be extremely challenging, especially in patients with multiple medical comorbidities.
• Once HIT is recognized, an alternative anticoagulant (direct thrombin inhibitor or fondaparinux) should be initiated to prevent further complications.

DEFINITION AND HISTORY

Unfractionated heparin (UFH) and its derivatives, the low-molecular weight heparins (LMWHs; henceforth, collectively referred to as *heparin*), remain the most commonly prescribed anticoagulants for the prophylaxis and treatment of venous thromboembolism (VTE) in hospitalized patients.[1] In a subset of treated patients (<5%), heparin elicits a life-threatening immune complication, heparin-induced thrombocytopenia (HIT). HIT is a self-limited hypercoagulable disorder occurring predominantly in hospitalized patients. The cardinal manifestations of HIT are declining platelet counts within 5 to 14 days after heparin exposure and a predilection for arterial and venous thrombosis.[2]

In the 1950s, Weismann and Tobin[3] first described the clinical syndrome of HIT. Subsequent studies revealed the immune origins of this syndrome[4] with the

Supported by the National Institutes of Health HL110860, HL109825, AI101992 (G.M. Lee), and 2T32HL007057-36 (G.M. Arepally).
[a] Division of Hematology, Department of Medicine, Duke University Medical Center, DUMC Box 3841, Room 304 Sands Building, Durham, NC 27710, USA; [b] Division of Hematology, Department of Medicine, Duke University Medical Center, DUMC Box 3486, Room 301 Sands Building, Durham, NC 27710, USA
* Corresponding author.
E-mail address: arepa001@mc.duke.edu

Hematol Oncol Clin N Am 27 (2013) 541–563
http://dx.doi.org/10.1016/j.hoc.2013.02.001
0889-8588/13/$ – see front matter © 2013 Elsevier Inc. All rights reserved.

identification of antibodies directed to antigenic complexes of platelet factor 4 (PF4) and heparin.[5] With the advent of immunoassays for the detection of PF4/heparin (PF4/H) antibodies, it is now recognized that an asymptomatic immune response to PF4/H occurs far more commonly than clinical complications of the disease (thrombocytopenia and/or thrombosis). This article reviews our current understanding of the pathogenesis, clinical features, laboratory testing, and therapeutic options for patients with HIT.

CAUSE AND PATHOGENESIS
PF4/H Complexes and the Immune Response in HIT

The primary physiologic role of PF4 is to neutralize the antithrombotic effect of heparin and heparin-like molecules (heparan sulfate, chondroitin sulfate) on cell surfaces. On platelet activation, PF4, a positively charged protein residing in platelet α-granules, is released in large amounts, binds to endothelial heparin sulfate, and displaces antithrombin from the cell surface. When patients are administered pharmacologic doses of heparin for thromboprophylaxis or for treatment, cell-bound PF4 dissociates from endothelial sites to form ultralarge complexes with circulating heparin. Recent murine studies have shown that these circulating and/or cell-bound PF4/H complexes are highly immunogenic in vivo.[6] Once antibodies are formed, immune complexes containing immunoglobulin G (IgG) antibody and antigen are capable of engaging cellular Fc receptors on platelets,[7] monocytes,[8,9] and neutrophils[10] to promote cellular activation and thrombin generation.[11]

Epidemiology of HIT

In recent prospective investigations using UFH and/or LMWH, the overall incidence of HIT is estimated at 0.5% to 0.8% of the treated patients.[12,13] Drug and host characteristics contribute to the risk of developing HIT. Of the various drug-dependent characteristics influencing immunogenicity, chain-length (UFH > LMWH ≥ fondaparinux), animal source of heparin (bovine > porcine),[14] and route (intravenous > subcutaneous),[15] heparin chain length seems to be the most clinically significant. The incidence of HIT is approximately tenfold higher with UFH ($\sim$3%) as compared with LMWH (0.2%)[16] in patients receiving thromboprophylactic doses. These differences in UFH and LMWH subside, however, when treatment doses are administered. In a meta-analysis involving 13 studies and more than 5000 patients, the rates of HIT were comparable in patients receiving UFH or LMWH (LMWH 1.2% vs UFH 1.5%).[13] Despite the increased utilization of LMWHs in recent years for the prevention of hospital-acquired VTE, there has been, surprisingly, no increase in the HIT incidence.[17,18] Although rates of seroconversion are similar for fondaparinux and LMWH,[19] the occurrence of HIT seems to be infrequent with fondaparinux.[20]

Host risk factors include clinical context of heparin exposure and patient characteristics (age, gender, and race). Patients on the general medical, cardiology, and surgical services (orthopedic and trauma) are at higher risk than patients on obstetric, pediatric, or renal (chronic hemodialysis) services.[2,21] The reasons for this variable risk are presently unknown but are thought to arise from differences in basal levels of platelet activation and circulating PF4 levels. Consistent with observations of a low incidence of HIT in pediatric and obstetric patients, a recent large analysis of hospital discharges of approximately 270 000 inpatient records showed that HIT was exceedingly rare in patients less than 40 years of age.[13] In this same study, among patients with VTE, the incidence of secondary thrombocytopenia, presumably caused by HIT, was higher among blacks (relative risk [RR] 1.3) as compared with whites.

Although one recent study showed a higher incidence of HIT among women (odds ratio of 2.4[22]), other studies have found a slightly higher risk among men (RR 1.1).[13] Several genetic polymorphisms, including homozygosity of the FcγRIIIa-158V allele,[23] the protein tyrosine phosphatase CD148,[24] and the interleukin-10 promoter,[25] have been described in single-center studies of patients with and without HIT. The clinical significance of these findings remains to be established in larger studies.

CLINICAL ELEMENTS OF DIAGNOSIS

Because of the high incidence of asymptomatic PF4/H conversion (see the "Laboratory Elements of Diagnosis" section) in patients exposed to heparin, it is essential to understand the clinical features associated with disease presentation. Three diagnostic elements should comprise the clinical evaluation of patients suspected of HIT: (1) documenting the presence of thrombocytopenia and/or thrombosis, (2) establishing the temporal course of thrombocytopenia relative to heparin exposure, and (3) excluding other causes of thrombocytopenia. A detailed discussion of these clinical diagnostic elements and commonly used diagnostic algorithms is provided subsequently in the section Clinical Algorithms in Assessing Likelihood of HIT. **Table 1** summarizes the clinical features commonly or infrequently seen in HIT.

Documenting the Presence of Thrombocytopenia and/or Thrombosis

Thrombocytopenia in HIT

Thrombocytopenia is an essential diagnostic feature of HIT and is reported to occur in approximately 95% of patients with HIT during the course of illness.[26–28] Patients who develop skin necrosis are a notable exception to this diagnostic rule because thrombocytopenia frequently does not accompany this atypical manifestation.[29,30]

Table 1
Clinical features consistent/not consistent with HIT

Consider HIT	HIT Unlikely
Following clinical symptoms within 4–14 d of new heparin therapy *or* within 24 h of heparin reexposure[a]	• Pancytopenia or chronic thrombocytopenia
• Absolute thrombocytopenia (<150 K/μL)	• Petechiae or hemorrhage in the absence of DIC
• Relative thrombocytopenia (30%–50% decrease from baseline platelet count)	• Thrombocytopenia
• New or progressive arterial or venous thrombosis on heparin therapy	◦ Within 24–72 h in patients without prior heparin exposure
• New thrombocytopenia and/or thrombosis presenting 14–30 d after recent hospitalization and heparin exposure	◦ In association with intra-aortic balloon pump, ventricular assist device, or extracorporeal membrane oxygenation
• Thrombosis at catheter sites	◦ In patients with documented severe bacterial, fungal, or viral infection
• Thrombosis at unusual sites (venous limb gangrene, skin necrosis, spinal ischemia, cerebral venous thrombosis)	◦ After recent chemotherapy or pelvic radiation
• Bilateral adrenal hemorrhage (secondary to adrenal thrombosis)	◦ With microangiopathic changes on blood film in absence of DIC
• Skin necrosis at subcutaneous injection sites	◦ Within 72–96 h of cardiopulmonary bypass
• Severe thrombocytopenia (<20 K/μL) in association with DIC or extensive thrombosis	◦ Within 24–96 h after cardiogenic shock
	◦ From splenic sequestration

Abbreviation: DIC, disseminated intravascular thrombosis.
[a] Re-exposure within three months of prior heparin therapy.

Thrombocytopenia in HIT can present as an absolute drop in platelet count less than the normal range (platelet count <150 × 10^9/L) or as a relative decrease of 30% to 50% from the baseline counts. Absolute thrombocytopenia results in a moderate thrombocytopenia, with mean platelet counts of 50 to 70 × 10^9/L. In the postoperative period, when platelet counts typically rebound to a higher number than the preoperative count, the immediate postoperative platelet count should be considered as the baseline platelet count for determining the change in platelet count. This revised definition of thrombocytopenia has been shown to be sensitive and specific for diagnosing HIT.[31]

Less than 5% of patients with HIT will have a platelet count less than 20 × 10^9/L.[29] The presence of petechiae or extensive ecchymoses in the absence of disseminated intravascular coagulation (DIC) should prompt a search for an alternative diagnoses (see **Table 1**).[29] Severe thrombocytopenia as a manifestation of HIT is associated with a high risk of thrombotic complications, likely because of platelet consumption.[28] In a retrospective series of 408 patients, patients with severe thrombocytopenia (defined as >90% decline from baseline counts) were noted to have an 8-fold higher risk for thrombotic complications as compared with patients with a less than 30% platelet count decline.[28]

Several retrospective and prospective studies have shown that isolated thrombocytopenia is a harbinger of subsequent thromboses in patients (20%–50%).[28,32–34] In one-third of patients, the thromboembolic complication (TEC) can occur concurrently or precede the development of thrombocytopenia.[28,35,36] Because of the therapeutic implications of finding a VTE in patients with HIT with isolated thrombocytopenia, patients diagnosed with isolated HIT should undergo routine screening for subclinical TEC, such as lower extremity ultrasound.[34]

Thrombosis in HIT

Thrombosis is the most feared complication of HIT. In prospective and retrospective series, thrombotic complications have been reported to occur in 29% to 57%[28,37] of patients with HIT. In one registry, 25% of patients developed 3 or more thromboembolic complications.[28] Before the availability of current therapies, 16% of all thrombotic complications were fatal and 9% of all thrombotic events resulted in limb amputation.[37] In relation to thrombocytopenia, a large retrospective study of patients with HIT found that in 34% of patients, thrombotic complications will precede or occur concurrently with a major decrease in platelets.[28]

Thrombotic events involving the venous circulation occur far more commonly than arterial thrombotic events, with reported frequencies of 2.4:1.0 to 4:1.[28,33] Lower limb deep venous thrombosis (DVT) and pulmonary embolism compose most of the venous thrombotic events.[28] Upper limb DVTs are also common but are reported to occur almost exclusively at central venous catheter sites.[38] The postoperative period has also been strongly associated with venous thrombosis in HIT.[33,37,39]

Arterial thromboses occur in 7% to 14%[33,37] of patients affected with HIT. In one series of patients with HIT, a history of cardiovascular events, including myocardial infarction, and a history of cardiovascular surgery were associated with a significantly increased incidence of arterial thrombosis.[39] In order of decreasing frequency, common sites of arterial thrombosis include limb artery thrombosis, thrombotic stroke, and myocardial infarction.[28] Atypical sites of presentation including bilateral adrenal hemorrhage,[40] venous limb gangrene, cerebral venous thrombosis,[41] spinal ischemia,[41] and skin necrosis should warrant consideration of HIT in the differential diagnosis.[42]

Presently, there are no definitive means for predicting the risk of thrombosis in patients who develop isolated thrombocytopenia in HIT. Studies have shown that established risk factors for hypercoagulability, such as protein C, protein S, antithrombin clotting factor mutations, and/or platelet polymorphisms, do not contribute significantly to thrombotic tendency.[39,43] Certain common serologic features occur at a higher frequency among patients with thrombotic HIT as compared with those with isolated thrombocytopenia in HIT, including IgG isotype,[44] antibodies capable of platelet activation,[44–46] and high antibody levels (as gauged by optical density [OD] and/or titer).[47–49] Risk factors for thrombosis development are outlined in **Table 2**.

Despite the risk associated with certain serologic features, the presence of platelet-activating IgG antibodies in some patients with asymptomatic PF4/H antibodies[50] or the occurrence of low titer antibodies in other patients with a clinically confirmed diagnosis of thrombotic HIT[47] does not permit unambiguous segregation of patients with and without HIT. Discontinuing heparin therapy after early recognition of HIT does not seem to lower the risk of subsequent thrombosis.[51]

Establishing the Temporal Course of Thrombocytopenia Relative to Heparin Exposure

In heparin-naïve patients, platelet counts classically decline within 5 to 10 days of heparin initiation. As shown in a recent study of the evolution of the HIT immune response, 12 patients with HIT were examined serially for PF4/H antibody levels and platelet counts. As shown in **Fig. 1**, seroconversions occurred at a median of 4 days from the start of heparin therapy, with a decrease in platelet count occurring 2 days after seroconversion (~6 days from the start of heparin therapy). The interval time to when the platelet count decline met diagnostic criteria for HIT in this study (>50% platelet count decrease) occurred 4 days after seroconversion (median time interval of 8 days from the start of heparin). Thrombosis also occurred after seroconversion but was often coincident with changes in platelet counts.[36] These observations, coupled with studies of murine models,[52] suggest that patients' PF4/H seroconversions must precede thrombocytopenia and/or thrombosis, and clinical events predating seroconversion are unlikely to be related to HIT.[36] In 30% of patients with HIT, an atypical, rapid decrease in the platelet count, occurring at a median of 10 hours after beginning heparin therapy, can occur from preexisting, circulating PF4/H antibodies caused by recent heparin exposure (within 3–6 months).[26] Another clinical variant of HIT presentation is delayed-onset HIT, in which platelet counts fall 10 to 14 days after last heparin exposure.[53] Delayed-onset HIT is frequently associated with complications of DIC and/or extensive thrombosis[54] and should be considered in patients presenting with new-onset thrombocytopenia within 2 to 4 weeks of a recent hospitalization.

Discontinuation of heparin should allow prompt resolution of thrombocytopenia. In clinical practice, platelet counts typically increase within 48 hours of heparin discontinuation, and thrombocytopenia usually resolves within 4 to 14 days.[29] A prolonged

Table 2	
Risk factors for thrombosis in HIT	
Predictors of Thrombosis in HIT	
Correlated with Thrombotic Risk	**No Correlation with Thrombotic Risk**
• Sites of previous arterial or venous injury[38,39] • Low platelet nadir[28] • High antibody titers[45,47]	• Thrombophilic markers (protein C, protein S, antithrombin III, or factor V Leiden)[39] • FcR H/R (histidine/arginine) 131 and other platelet glycoproteins[43]

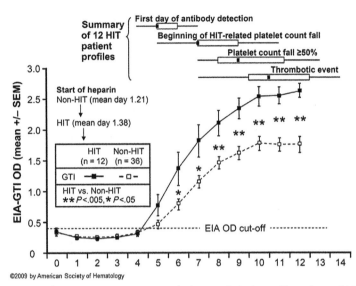

©2009 by American Society of Hematology

Fig. 1. Evolution of the immune response relative to clinical manifestations of HIT. Twelve patients with HIT and 36 seropositive non-HIT control patients were monitored for PF4/H antibodies, thrombocytopenia, and thrombosis after orthopedic surgery. Patients with HIT are indicated by ■, and seropositive non-HIT controls by □. Time course of seroconversions are shown on the x-axis and OD levels between the patients with HIT and the seropositive non-HIT controls (P<.05 by nonpaired t test) are shown on the y-axis. At the top of the figure, summary data for 12 patients with HIT profiles are shown for 4 key events (first day of antibody detection, beginning of HIT-related platelet count decrease, platelet count decrease ≥50%, and thrombotic event), summarized as median (*small black squares within rectangles*), interquartile range (*open rectangles*), and range (*ends of thin black lines*). EIA, enzyme immunoassay. GTI, GTI PF4ENHANCED® assay (GTI Diagnostics, Waukesha, WI). (*Adapted from* Warkentin TE, Sheppard JA, Moore JC, et al. Studies of the immune response in heparin-induced thrombocytopenia. Blood 2009;113(20):4963–9; with permission.)

duration of thrombocytopenia (>7 days) after heparin discontinuation has been linked with disease severity.[51] Despite platelet count recovery, thrombotic risk remains high for 4 to 6 weeks because of the presence of circulating PF4/H antibodies[33]; these antibodies likely contribute to the development of delayed-onset HIT.[54] The median time to antibody clearance is 85 to 90 days,[26,49] although in one series, approximately 35% of patients were noted to be seropositive for up to 1 year.[49] To what extent PF4/H seropositivity, in the absence of thrombocytopenia and/or thrombosis, predisposes patients to thrombotic complications remains controversial.[49,55–57] Unlike other drug-induced thrombocytopenias, the risk of recurrent HIT with subsequent heparin reexposure seems to be low; but these findings have not been prospectively investigated. Although several retrospective analyses and case reports suggest that the risk of recurrence may be low in patients who become seronegative for PF4/H antibodies,[58] current guidelines recommend avoiding routine heparin reexposure in these patients.[59]

Excluding Other Causes of Thrombocytopenia

Most patients suspected of HIT are not likely to have disease.[60,61] With the routine implementation of heparin thromboprophylaxis in most hospitals as well as the frequent occurrence of thrombocytopenia in hospitalized patients,[62] the statistical likelihood that these two clinical scenarios will converge is far more likely than the occurrence of HIT. Illustrating this point was a recent study by Oliveira and colleagues[63] of 2420 patients treated with heparin who were assessed for the development of thrombocytopenia (defined as a platelet count less than $150 \times 10^9/L$, reduction in platelet count of 50% or more from the admission level, or both). In this study, 881 patients or 36.4% (95% confidence interval, 34.5%–38.3%) met the definition for thrombocytopenia while receiving heparin therapy; 13% of patients met both criteria of a decreased absolute platelet count as well as a reduction in platelet count of more than 50%. In this study, approximately 0.7% of patients were diagnosed with HIT.[63]

The differential diagnosis of acute thrombocytopenia in hospitalized patients is extensive as shown in **Table 1** ("HIT Unlikely" column). Thrombocytopenia is common in the intensive care units (ICU), occurring in 38% to 46% of patients.[64] Thrombocytopenia is particularly problematic in the cardiac surgery setting, where patients have several risk factors for HIT, including recent heparin exposure, the inflammatory milieu of surgery, and high rates of PF4/H seroconversion.[50,55,65,66] In one recent study of cardiac surgery patients requiring more than 7 days in the cardiac ICU, 21% of patients (70 out of 329) developed thrombocytopenia, with 67 out of 70 patients (95%) having alternative or non–HIT-related causes for thrombocytopenia.[67] Adding to the complexity of the evaluation of cardiac surgery patients is the relatively frequent use of mechanical devices, such as intra-aortic balloon pumps (IABP). Thrombocytopenia is frequently encountered in patients with IABP, occurring at a frequency of 30% to 50% of cases.[68]

CLINICAL ALGORITHMS IN ASSESSING LIKELIHOOD OF HIT

Given the broad differential diagnosis and frequency of thrombocytopenia in hospitalized patients, clinical algorithms have been developed to assist clinicians in tabulating the risk of HIT in a given patient.

4Ts Scoring System

The most widely used clinical scoring system is the 4Ts developed by Dr Warkentin at McMaster University. The 4Ts scoring system assesses the clinical diagnostic elements discussed earlier and assigns a score (0, 1, or 2; maximum total score of 8) for the following features: the magnitude of thrombocytopenia, timing of platelet count decrease or complication in relation to heparin use, thrombosis or other HIT-associated sequelae, and the absence of another explanation for thrombocytopenia.[29] A 4T score of 6 to 8 is consistent with a high pretest probability of HIT, a score of 4 to 5 is consistent with an intermediate probability of HIT, and a score of 0 to 3 is consistent with a low probability of HIT.[29] The diagnostic utility of the 4T score has been examined in numerous prospective and retrospective studies.[46,69–73] In all studies to date, the 4Ts has consistently demonstrated excellent negative predictive value (NPV), with a 4T score less than 3 reliably translating into a low likelihood of serologically confirmed HIT.[46,69–74] On the other hand, the positive predictive value (PPV) of the 4T scoring system is variable and highly dependent on the practitioner's background.[69] To demonstrate the effect of a practitioner's experience in using the 4Ts scoring system, Lo and colleagues[69] tested this algorithm at 2 medical centers (Hamilton, Canada and Greifswald, Germany [GW]). The practitioner applying the 4Ts at the Hamilton General Hospital (HGH) was Dr Warkentin, the developer of the 4Ts scoring system. In GW, the general practitioners used the 4Ts for diagnosing HIT. When the clinical scores were correlated with laboratory testing, the NPV was high at both medical centers (98% at HGH and 100% at GW). However, the predictive value of intermediate scores (HGH: 8 out of 28 [28.6%], GW: 11 out of 139 [7.9%]) and high scores (HGH: 8 out of 8 [100%], GW: 9 out of 42 [21.4%]) markedly differed by institution. The clinical utility of the 4Ts in predicting the likelihood of HIT was low in Germany, where primary care providers were using the algorithm, but much higher in Canada in the hands of an experienced HIT diagnostician. This study, as well as others,[70–73] confirms that the PPV of intermediate and high scores is far less reliable than the NPV.

HIT Expert Probability Score

In an effort to improve on the specificity and the PPV of the 4Ts, the HIT Expert Probability (HEP) score was developed using expert opinion to refine the clinical scoring system. In this model, 26 experts were asked to assign points to 8 clinical features of HIT based on diagnostic relevance (magnitude of the decrease in platelet count, timing of the decrease in platelet count, nadir platelet count, thrombosis, skin necrosis, acute systemic reaction, bleeding, and other causes of thrombocytopenia).[75] Based on the median score, each clinical feature was then assigned a point ranging from −3 to +3 and the HEP score, a pretest probability model, was created. In a validation study at a single institution, the HEP score demonstrated improved interobserver agreement and improved correlation with serologic HIT testing when compared with the 4Ts score. In this study, the HEP score was 100% sensitive and 60% specific for diagnosing HIT.[75] However, unlike the 4Ts, which is fairly simple to perform, the HEP score is more complex to use. Additional prospective studies are needed to validate the HEP scoring system.

Cardiac Surgery (Lillo-Le Louet) Scoring System

Nowhere is the challenge of distinguishing HIT from other causes of thrombocytopenia more difficult than in the clinical setting of cardiac surgery. Cardiac surgery is associated with several comorbidities that confound the diagnosis of HIT, including several risk factors for thrombocytopenia (dilutional effect, infection/DIC, cardiogenic shock, mechanical devices, multiple medications), increased rates of thrombosis (20% in one recent retrospective study of non-HIT patients),[76] and a high prevalence of PF4/H seroconversion (see "Laboratory Elements of Diagnosis"). Despite the high-risk features of this clinical setting, retrospective and prospective series have demonstrated that the postoperative risk of HIT after cardiac surgery is low (0.6%–2.0%).[77,78] Because of the difficulty in recognizing HIT after cardiac surgery, Lillo-Le Louet and colleagues[79] identified 3 independent clinical variables (platelet count pattern, time from cardiopulmonary bypass [CPB] to suspicion of HIT, and CPB duration) based on a clinical cohort suspected of HIT. In patients with HIT, a characteristic biphasic pattern of platelet count recovery was observed. Platelet counts initially decline for 2 to 4 days after surgery, then rebound into the normal range or beyond, and then decrease once again[79] because of antibody development and HIT. Based on these observations, scores were assigned for platelet count, time course, or pattern (biphasic = 2, persistent thrombocytopenia = 1); time from CPB to date of HIT suspicion (≥5 days = 2, <5 days = 0); and CPB duration (≤118 minutes = 1, >118 minutes = 0). In their retrospective study, a score of 2 or more was associated with a high probability of HIT (PPV of 62%), whereas a score 5 or more was associated with a markedly higher PPV of 95%.[79] In a recent prospective study of 1722 patients undergoing cardiac surgery, the Lillo-Le Louet scoring system was compared with that of the 4Ts in predicting the likelihood of HIT.[78] In this study, both scoring systems were found to have a low PPV (56% for the 4Ts and 41% for Lillo-Le Louet) and low concordance (kappa coefficient = 0.39). The Lillo-Le Louet scoring system also had a lower NPV (78%) than the 4Ts (91%). The investigators concluded that the diagnostic performance of both scoring systems were low. However, the investigators found that the biphasic pattern of platelet count recovery in the post–cardiac surgery setting remained a strong predictor for HIT.[78]

LABORATORY ELEMENTS OF DIAGNOSIS

In clinical practice, most of the patients suspected of HIT are likely to have an intermediate clinical probability for HIT. In these patients, establishing the presence or absence of PF4/H antibodies by laboratory methods comprises an essential element of the diagnostic evaluation. This section discusses the types of immunologic and functional assays for diagnosing HIT.

Immunoassays

Immunoassays for the detection of PF4/H antibodies are widely available. These assays detect binding of antibodies from plasma or serum to immobilized PF4/H complexes. Bound antibody is then detected by secondary labeled antibodies using a colorimetric endpoint. Detailed descriptions or comparisons of the strengths and limitations of the various assays are beyond the scope of this article. The reader is referred to **Table 3** with test-specific information and references.

Commercial immunoassays are routinely used at most medical centers because of the technical ease, rapid turnaround time, and high sensitivity of these assays (>99%[44,72,80,81]). However, the main shortcoming of these assays is their lack of specificity (40%–70%[44,65]) caused by the frequency of asymptomatic seroconversions. Seropositivity, without HIT, can be seen in approximately 8% to 17% of general medical and surgical patients treated with UFH,[82–85] 2% to 8% of those treated with LMWH,[19,82] and 1% to 2% of patients treated with fondaparinux.[19,21] Heparin exposure during cardiac surgery remains the highest risk factor for asymptomatic seroconversions. Depending on the immunoassay, asymptomatic seroconversions can be demonstrated in 27% to 61% of patients after cardiac surgery.[55,83,86]

Because of these constraints in specificity, several test modifications have been introduced to improve the diagnostic performance of immunoassays. These modifications include the use of IgG-specific assays, quantitative measurement of OD, and the utilization of high heparin concentration to demonstrate heparin-dependent binding. Several studies have shown that the IgG-specific enzyme-linked immunoassays (ELISAs) improve diagnostic specificity.[87–89] In a pooled analysis of studies examining the sensitivity and specificity of the polyclonal versus IgG-specific ELISAs, Cuker and Ortel[87] showed that the specificity of the IgG ELISA was increased compared with the polyspecific ELISA (94% for the IgG-specific versus 89% for the polyclonal ELISA) but occurred at a small expense to the sensitivity of the assay (96% for the IgG-specific vs 98% for the polyclonal ELISA).[87] This finding translates into a small number of patients who truly have HIT but who will have a false-negative result based on the IgG-specific ELISA. Studies have also shown that the quantitative assessment of ODs or expression of titers in particle-based ELISAs also improves the diagnostic accuracy of the ELISAs. These studies confirm a strong correlation of the OD/titers with platelet-activating properties[48,90] and thrombotic risk.[47,56] Several investigators have examined the utility of using higher OD cutoffs in ELISAs for determining the likelihood of HIT.[72,91] In these studies, based on the type of immunoassay and the cutoff values, a change in the cutoff value was uniformly associated with a loss in sensitivity (17%–91% sensitivity reported using an IgG-specific ELISA with a cutoff OD >1).[72,91]

Table 3
Immunoassays available for the detection of PF4/H Abs

Assay[a]	Vendor[a]	Polyclonal Versus IgG Specific	Principle	Sensitivity (%)	Specificity (%)
Asserachrom IgGAM	Diagnostica Stago	Polyclonal	ELISA	100[71,89]	64–86[71,89]
GTI PF4 IgG	GTI Diagnostics	IgG specific	ELISA	100[89,123]	42–96[89,123]
HemosIL AcuStar HIT-Ab (PF4-H)	Instrumentation laboratory	Polyclonal	Latex-enhanced immunoturbidimetric assay	100[124]	81[124]
HemosIL AcuStar HIT-IgG (PF4/H)	Instrumentation laboratory	IgG specific	Latex-enhanced immunoturbidimetric assay	100[124]	96[124]
ID-heparin/PF4 PaGIA	Diamed	Polyclonal	Particle gel immunoassay	94–100[71,72,125]	61–95[71,72,125]
Poly-ELISA	GTI Diagnostics	Polyclonal	ELISA	100[72]	81[72]
Zymutest HIA IgG	Hyphen Biomed Research	IgG specific	ELISA	100[89,123]	44–96[89,123]
Zymutest HIA IgGAM	Hyphen Biomed Research	Polyclonal	ELISA	100[89]	87[89]

Abbreviation: ELISA, enzyme-linked immunoassay.
[a] Names of assay and vendor as listed in citations.

HIT antibodies show heparin-dependent binding over a range of physiologic heparin concentrations (0.1–1.0 U/mL). The presence of excess heparin (10–100 U/mL) significantly attenuates the binding of HIT antibodies to antigen. This principle is the basis of using high heparin concentrations in serologic and functional assays to confirm the presence of heparin-dependent antibodies. Studies have shown that the use of a high heparin step improves the specificity from 72% to 89%.[91,92] The high heparin step, however, can fail to show inhibition in instances when the OD is extremely high.[91,92] Recent studies have also shown that combining the use of 2[91,92] or all 3 maneuvers (IgG, ODs, and high heparin step) improves the diagnostic utility of the ELISAs. Although such an approach, theoretically, should markedly improve the assay's specificity, there are many examples/reports of patients with HIT whose serologic profiles do not conform to these criteria.[47,87,91] Until prospective evaluation and validation of these laboratory modifications occurs, it should be stressed that laboratory testing must accompany a clinical evaluation to avoid serious adverse outcomes from underdiagnosis or overdiagnosis of HIT.

Functional Assays

Functional assays, such as the serotonin release assay (SRA; in North America) and the heparin-induced platelet activation test (in Europe), use washed platelets to measure HIT antibody-induced platelet activation.[93] A positive result is established when heparin-dependent platelet activation is demonstrated along with the inhibition of platelet activation in the presence of excess heparin (100 U/mL) and/or in the presence of an antibody that blocks platelet Fc receptors.[29]

Functional assays are more specific for HIT[44] and more predictive for thrombocytopenia when compared with ELISA-based testing. Although functional assays, particularly the SRA, have high specificity (>95%)[44] and are associated with a high PPV (89%–100%),[21] the sensitivity of functional assays are less robust (62%–100%)[44,65,94,95] because of several technical variables affecting platelet reactivity.[96] Other important drawbacks to these assays include lack of standardization,[97] complexity of the assays, and the use of radioactive isotopes with the SRA. For these reasons, many medical centers do not offer this test on site; testing is often referred to specialized commercial laboratories. Consequently, functional assays are rarely available to clinicians at the time of initial evaluation and are often used to confirm the diagnosis of HIT post hoc.

Normalization of Laboratory Testing

After discontinuing heparin, the median time to platelet recovery is approximately 4 days, although it can take up to 4 weeks for platelets to fully recover to more than $150 \times 10^9/L$.[29] However, both ELISA testing for HIT antibodies and functional assays, such as the SRA, require longer to normalize. In a retrospective study of 243 patients with serologically confirmed HIT, the median time for the antigen assay to normalize was 85 days and the median time for the activation assay to normalize was 50 days.[26]

THERAPEUTIC OPTIONS AND PROGNOSIS
General Principles

The management of HIT requires that the clinician navigate between the Scylla of overdiagnosis/overtreatment and Charybdis of withholding therapy in patients with true HIT. With the widespread use of ELISAs and high false-positive rates of PF4/H antibodies in many clinical settings, current clinical practices have leaned toward the overdiagnosis of HIT.[60] Overtreatment with potent nonheparin anticoagulants, such as the direct thrombin inhibitors (DTIs), is associated with a high risk of bleeding (1% risk for major bleeding per treatment day).[98] Similarly, disastrous consequences can be expected if the clinical manifestations of HIT are not promptly recognized (5%–10% daily risk of thrombosis).[11] To avoid these extremes, physicians need to apply clinical algorithms (described earlier) and initiate treatment based on the strength of the clinical suspicion of HIT, even before availability of laboratory results.

Patients with a low clinical suspicion of HIT should not undergo laboratory testing or have their heparin discontinued because the NPV of clinical scoring systems approaches 100% in numerous studies.[46,69–74] Patients who are deemed to have an intermediate or high clinical suspicion for HIT should have all heparin products (including heparin flushes) discontinued and have an alternative anticoagulant started, ideally a parenteral DTI. Simply discontinuing heparin alone or starting a vitamin K antagonist alone is not adequate to prevent the development or progression of thrombotic complications. In a retrospective review of patients with serologically confirmed HIT, 48% of patients who had heparin substituted for warfarin suffered a subsequent thrombosis.[33]

Of the 3 agents available in the United States for the treatment of HIT, 2 belong to the DTI family (argatroban and bivalirudin; lepirudin production has been discontinued by the manufacturer as of May 2013) and the other, fondaparinux, a synthetic pentasaccharide, belongs to the heparin family but has minimal cross-reactivity with heparin. Refer to **Table 4** for recommendations on dosing and monitoring of the alternative anticoagulants.

Argatroban

Argatroban is the only DTI approved by the US Food and Drug Administration (FDA) for the prevention and treatment of thrombosis in patients with HIT as well as for patients undergoing percutaneous coronary intervention with, or at risk for, HIT. Argatroban was approved based on 2 prospective, open-label, multicenter studies enrolling a total of 373 patients with HIT.[32,99] In these trials, patients treated with argatroban were compared with historical controls and were found to have a reduced incidence of new thrombosis, the need for amputation, and death (34%–35%) as compared with controls (43%).[32,99] More rapid platelet recovery was also seen in the argatroban arm, and major bleeding rates were not different between the two study arms.[99]

In patients with normal hepatic function, argatroban should be infused at an initial rate of 1.5 to 2.0 mcg/kg/min without an initial bolus. Initial infusion rates should be reduced to 0.5 to 1.2 mcg/kg/min for patients with heart failure, anasarca, or other conditions resulting in hepatic dysfunction.[100] An activated partial thromboplastin time (aPTT) should be obtained 2 hours after starting the infusion, and the infusion should be adjusted by 0.25 to 0.5 mcg/kg/min to achieve a goal aPTT 1.5 to 3.0 times the baseline aPTT value, with a maximum goal aPTT of 100 seconds. The infusion rate should not exceed 10 mcg/kg/min.[100] Argatroban is hepatically cleared and, therefore, is the agent of choice for patients with HIT and renal insufficiency.[59]

Once patients are stably anticoagulated on argatroban and the platelet count has fully recovered (>150 × 10^9/L), warfarin can be initiated at a low dose (≤5 mg) and overlapped with argatroban for at least 5 days.[59] Because argatroban prolongs the international normalized ratio (INR),[101] the transition to warfarin requires close monitoring of factor X levels, as measured by chromogenic assays. A chromogenic factor X level 45% or less at the time of argatroban discontinuation has been shown to be predictive of a therapeutic INR.[102]

Reported major bleeding rates with argatroban range from 0% to 10%.[103,104] Identified risk factors for major bleeding on argatroban include the presence of a

HIT-associated TEC, pulmonary impairment, and an aPTT more than 100 seconds.[105] If bleeding occurs, the infusion rate should be decreased or the infusion should be entirely discontinued. Once argatroban is discontinued, the aPTT will typically normalize within 2 to 4 hours.[106] No specific antidote for argatroban is available at this time. The reported wholesale acquisition cost of one vial of argatroban (100 mg/mL, 2.5-mL vial) required for 1 day's treatment is $1313.[107]

Bivalirudin

Bivalirudin is a DTI approved for use by the FDA only in patients who have or are at risk of developing HIT during percutaneous coronary intervention (PCI), a setting where its safety and efficacy have been demonstrated.[108] Bivalirudin has not been approved by the FDA for other clinical settings of HIT, but several case series have reported the safety of this agent for HIT in non-PCI settings.[109,110]

If used for treatment of HIT, bivalirudin should be given without a bolus and infused at an initial rate of 0.15 to 0.2 mg/kg/h for a goal aPTT, which is 1.5 to 2.5 times the patients' baseline aPTT.[59] Bivalirudin has a short half-life of 25 minutes and is cleared by both renal (20%) and plasma enzymatic (80%) mechanisms.[109] For patients with renal insufficiency, bivalirudin should be dose reduced (0.08–0.1 mg/kg/h for creatinine clearance 30–60 mL/min; 0.03–0.05 mg/kg/h for creatinine clearance less than 30 mL/min or for patients receiving renal replacement therapy).[109] The reported wholesale acquisition cost of one vial bivalirudin (250-mg vial) required for 1 day's treatment is $742.[107]

Fondaparinux

Fondaparinux belongs to the heparin family and is a long-acting (half-life = 17 hours), selective inhibitor of factor Xa.[93] This drug has not received FDA approval for use in HIT. However, emerging data suggests a role for fondaparinux in HIT because HIT antibodies show minimal cross-reactivity with this agent in vitro (less than 5%).[111] In several small series of patients with HIT treated with fondaparinux (n = 55), no recurrent TECs were reported.[112–115] Therapy with fondaparinux was well tolerated; only 1 patient, who had developed renal dysfunction, developed a major bleed.[115] These studies demonstrated that fondaparinux may be an effective anticoagulant for the treatment of HIT.

If used for the treatment of HIT, guidelines for therapeutic dosing should be followed (see **Table 4**). A dosage of 5 mg subcutaneously (SC) daily should be given for patients who weigh less than 50 kg, 7.5 mg SC daily for patients who weigh 50 to 100 kg, and 10 mg SC daily for patients who weigh more than 100 kg.[59] Fondaparinux is primarily eliminated in the urine as unchanged drug (77%).[116] Therefore, the use of fondaparinux is contraindicated in patients with severe renal impairment (creatinine clearance <30 mL/min) because of the increased risk of bleeding in patients when renal clearance is reduced.[116] The reported wholesale acquisition cost of 1 vial of generic fondaparinux (7.5-mg vial) required for 1 day's treatment is $103.[107]

Warfarin Therapy

Once patients are stably anticoagulated on an alternative, nonheparin anticoagulant and the platelet count has fully recovered (>150 × 10⁹/L), warfarin can be initiated at a low dose (≤5 mg).[59] Administration of the alternative anticoagulant and warfarin should overlap for at least 5 days because premature discontinuation of the alternative anticoagulant may lead to thrombotic events.[117] Up to 4 weeks of anticoagulation with warfarin have been recommended for patients with isolated HIT who do not have a

Table 4
Alternative anticoagulants for treatment of HIT

	Argatroban	Bivalirudin	Fondaparinux
Approval	HIT or patients with HIT undergoing PCI with or at risk for HIT	Patients with or at risk of developing HIT during PCI	Has not received FDA approval for use in HIT
Bolus	None	None	N/A
Initial dose for isolated HIT or HIT with thrombosis	1.5–2.0 mcg/kg/min[100]	0.15–0.2 mg/kg/h[59]	<50 kg: 5 mg SC daily 50–100 kg: 7.5 mg SC daily >100 kg: 10 mg SC daily[59]
Initial dose for renal impairment	No adjustment necessary[126]	0.08–0.1 mg/kg/h (CrCl 30–60 mL/min) 0.03–0.05 mg/kg/h (CrCl <30 mL/min or for patients receiving renal replacement therapy)[109]	Use with caution if CrCl 30–50 mL/min Contraindicated if CrCl <30 mL/min[116]
Initial dose for hepatic impairment	0.5–1.2 mcg/kg/min[100]	No adjustment necessary[127]	No adjustment necessary[116]
Monitoring	Obtain baseline aPTT and 2 h after starting infusion[126]	Obtain baseline aPTT and 2–3 h after starting infusion	Anti-FXa activity can be monitored in renal insufficiency[115]
Target	aPTT 1.5–3.0 times the baseline aPTT; max goal aPTT = 100 s[100]	aPTT 1.5–2.5 times the baseline aPTT[59]	N/A
Dosage adjustment	Adjust infusion by 0.25–0.5 mg/kg/min to achieve goal aPTT; recheck aPTT 2–4 h after each dosage change[126]	Adjust infusion by 20%–25% to achieve goal aPTT; recheck aPTT 2 h after each dosage change	N/A

Maximum dose	10 mcg/kg/min	0.25 mg/kg/h[127]	10 mg daily[116]
Transition to warfarin	Monitor chromogenic FXa level while on combined therapy[101] Chromogenic FXa 24%–45% (INR 2–3) 15%–35% (INR 2.5–3.5) Confirm INR 4–6 h after infusion is stopped	Monitor INR and/or chromogenic FXa while on combined therapy Chromogenic FXa 24%–45% (INR 2–3) 15%–35% (INR 2.5–3.5)	Monitor INR while on combined therapy Discontinue therapy when INR ≥2 for 2 consecutive days[116]
Cost of daily therapy[107]	$1313	$742	$103
Special considerations	No antidote is available[126]	No antidote is available[127] HIT in PCI 0.75 mg/kg bolus followed by a 1.75 mg/kg/h infusion for the duration of the procedure (all subgroups) After PCI 1.75 mg/kg/h (CrCl ≥30 mL/min) 1 mg/kg/h (CrCl <30 mL/min) 0.25 mg/kg/h (hemodialysis) Optional infusion after PCI 0.2 mg/kg/h for 20 h[127]	No antidote is available[116]

Abbreviations: aPTT, activated partial thromboplastin time; CrCl, creatinine clearance; FDA, Food and Drug Administration; FX, factor Xa; INR, international normalized ratio; max, maximum; N/A, not applicable; PCI, percutaneous coronary intervention; SC, subcutaneously.

TEC.[21,59] For patients with HIT who develop a thrombotic complication, extending anticoagulation with warfarin for a total of 3 to 6 months is recommended.[59]

Platelet Transfusions

Despite the frequency of thrombocytopenia in patients with HIT, bleeding complications remain very rare[29]; historically, routine platelet transfusions were not advised because of concern for an increased risk of thrombosis.[118] Although recent reports indicate that platelet transfusions may be safe and are not associated with TEC,[119] there is considerable theoretical concern that platelet transfusions may heighten the prothrombotic state in HIT because of the high concentrations of the antigen PF4 in platelets.[120] Thus, at this time, platelet transfusions are only recommended for patients with HIT who have active bleeding or for those patients who need to undergo procedures associated with a high risk of bleeding.[59]

Heparin Reexposure

HIT is thought to be a self-limited disorder, based on the transience of circulating PF4/H antibodies[26]; isolated case series of inadvertent exposure demonstrate a lack of disease recurrence. In a small case series, 7 patients with a history of HIT who were serologically negative did not experience recurrent thrombocytopenia or thrombotic events after subsequent courses of heparin.[26] Likewise, patients with a history of HIT who become seronegative for PF4/H antibodies have been successfully and safely anticoagulated with heparin during hemodialysis[121] and during cardiopulmonary bypass surgery.[58,122]

In the absence of prospective studies examining the safety of heparin reexposure in patients with HIT, current guidelines recommend avoidance of heparin in patients with recent HIT who still have detectable PF4/H antibodies because they are at risk for developing rapid-onset HIT and thrombosis.[59] However, once HIT antibodies become undetectable by serologic assays, short-term reexposure to heparin can be considered.[59] In this scenario, administration of heparin should be restricted to the procedure itself, and unnecessary heparin exposure should be avoided.[59]

SUMMARY

HIT is a prothrombotic disorder caused by antibodies to PF4/H complexes. It classically presents with declining platelet counts 5 to 14 days after heparin administration and results in a predisposition to arterial and venous thrombosis. Establishing the diagnosis of HIT can be extremely challenging, especially in patients with multiple medical comorbidities. Therefore, it is essential to conduct a thorough clinical evaluation in addition to laboratory testing to confirm the presence of PF4/H antibodies. Multiple clinical algorithms have been developed to aid the clinician in predicting the likelihood of HIT. Once HIT is recognized, an alternative anticoagulant (DTI or fondaparinux) should be initiated to prevent further complications.

REFERENCES

1. Kahn SR, Lim W, Dunn AS, et al. Prevention of VTE in nonsurgical patients: antithrombotic therapy and prevention of thrombosis, 9th ed: American College of Chest Physicians evidence-based clinical practice guidelines. Chest 2012;141: e195S–226S.
2. Cuker A, Cines DB. How I treat heparin-induced thrombocytopenia. Blood 2012; 119:2209–18.

3. Weismann RE, Tobin RW. Arterial embolism occurring during systemic heparin therapy. AMA Arch Surg 1958;76:219–25 [discussion: 25–7].

4. Rhodes GR, Dixon RH, Silver D. Heparin induced thrombocytopenia: eight cases with thrombotic-hemorrhagic complications. Ann Surg 1977;186:752–8.

5. Amiral J, Bridey F, Dreyfus M, et al. Platelet factor 4 complexed to heparin is the target for antibodies generated in heparin-induced thrombocytopenia. Thromb Haemost 1992;68:95–6.

6. Suvarna S, Espinasse B, Qi R, et al. Determinants of PF4/heparin immunogenicity. Blood 2007;110:4253–60.

7. Kelton JG, Sheridan D, Santos A, et al. Heparin-induced thrombocytopenia: laboratory studies. Blood 1988;72:925–30.

8. Rauova L, Hirsch JD, Greene TK, et al. Monocyte-bound PF4 in the pathogenesis of heparin-induced thrombocytopenia. Blood 2010;116:5021–31.

9. Kasthuri RS, Glover SL, Jonas W, et al. PF4/heparin-antibody complex induces monocyte tissue factor expression and release of tissue factor positive microparticles by activation of FcgammaRI. Blood 2012;119:5285–93.

10. Xiao Z, Visentin GP, Dayananda KM, et al. Immune complexes formed following the binding of anti-platelet factor 4 (CXCL4) antibodies to CXCL4 stimulate human neutrophil activation and cell adhesion. Blood 2008;112:1091–100.

11. Greinacher A, Eichler P, Lubenow N, et al. Heparin-induced thrombocytopenia with thromboembolic complications: meta-analysis of 2 prospective trials to assess the value of parenteral treatment with lepirudin and its therapeutic aPTT range. Blood 2000;96:846–51.

12. Prandoni P, Siragusa S, Girolami B, et al. The incidence of heparin-induced thrombocytopenia in medical patients treated with low-molecular-weight heparin: a prospective cohort study. Blood 2005;106:3049–54.

13. Stein PD, Hull RD, Matta F, et al. Incidence of thrombocytopenia in hospitalized patients with venous thromboembolism. Am J Med 2009;122:919–30.

14. Francis JL, Palmer GJ 3rd, Moroose R, et al. Comparison of bovine and porcine heparin in heparin antibody formation after cardiac surgery. Ann Thorac Surg 2003;75:17–22.

15. Ban-Hoefen M, Francis C. Heparin induced thrombocytopenia and thrombosis in a tertiary care hospital. Thromb Res 2009;124:189–92.

16. Martel N, Lee J, Wells PS. Risk for heparin-induced thrombocytopenia with unfractionated and low-molecular-weight heparin thromboprophylaxis: a meta-analysis. Blood 2005;106:2710–5.

17. Zhou A, Winkler A, Emamifar A, et al. Is the incidence of heparin-induced thrombocytopenia affected by the increased use of heparin for the prevention of deep venous thrombosis? Chest 2012;142(5):1175–8.

18. Rothberg MB, Pekow PS, Lahti M, et al. Comparative effectiveness of low-molecular-weight heparin versus unfractionated heparin for thromboembolism prophylaxis for medical patients. J Hosp Med 2012;7:457–63.

19. Warkentin TE, Cook RJ, Marder VJ, et al. Anti-platelet factor 4/heparin antibodies in orthopedic surgery patients receiving antithrombotic prophylaxis with fondaparinux or enoxaparin. Blood 2005;106:3791–6.

20. Warkentin TE, Maurer BT, Aster RH. Heparin-induced thrombocytopenia associated with fondaparinux. N Engl J Med 2007;356:2653–5 [discussion: 2653–5].

21. Arepally GM, Ortel TL. Clinical practice. Heparin-induced thrombocytopenia. N Engl J Med 2006;355:809–17.

22. Warkentin TE, Sheppard JA, Sigouin CS, et al. Gender imbalance and risk factor interactions in heparin-induced thrombocytopenia. Blood 2006;108:2937–41.

23. Gruel Y, Pouplard C, Lasne D, et al. The homozygous FcgammaRIIIa-158V genotype is a risk factor for heparin-induced thrombocytopenia in patients with antibodies to heparin-platelet factor 4 complexes. Blood 2004;104:2791–3.

24. Rollin J, Pouplard C, Gratacap MP, et al. Polymorphisms of protein tyrosine phosphatase CD148 influence FcgammaRIIA-dependent platelet activation and the risk of heparin-induced thrombocytopenia. Blood 2012;120:1309–16.

25. Pouplard C, Cornillet-Lefebvre P, Attaoua R, et al. Interleukin-10 promoter microsatellite polymorphisms influence the immune response to heparin and the risk of heparin-induced thrombocytopenia. Thromb Res 2012;129:465–9.

26. Warkentin TE, Kelton JG. Temporal aspects of heparin-induced thrombocytopenia. N Engl J Med 2001;344:1286–92.

27. Warkentin TE. Heparin-induced thrombocytopenia: pathogenesis and management. Br J Haematol 2003;121:535–55.

28. Greinacher A, Farner B, Kroll H, et al. Clinical features of heparin-induced thrombocytopenia including risk factors for thrombosis. A retrospective analysis of 408 patients. Thromb Haemost 2005;94:132–5.

29. Warkentin TE, Greinacher A. Heparin-induced thrombocytopenia. 3rd edition. New York: Marcel Dekker Inc.; 2004.

30. Schindewolf M, Lindhoff-Last E, Ludwig RJ, et al. Heparin-induced skin lesions. Lancet 2012;380(9856):1867–79.

31. Warkentin TE, Roberts RS, Hirsh J, et al. An improved definition of immune heparin-induced thrombocytopenia in postoperative orthopedic patients. Arch Intern Med 2003;163:2518–24.

32. Lewis BE, Wallis DE, Leya F, et al. Argatroban anticoagulation in patients with heparin-induced thrombocytopenia. Arch Intern Med 2003;163:1849–56.

33. Warkentin TE, Kelton JG. A 14-year study of heparin-induced thrombocytopenia. Am J Med 1996;101:502–7.

34. Tardy B, Tardy-Poncet B, Fournel P, et al. Lower limb veins should be systematically explored in patients with isolated heparin-induced thrombocytopenia. Thromb Haemost 1999;82:1199–200.

35. Warkentin TE, Levine MN, Hirsh J, et al. Heparin-induced thrombocytopenia in patients treated with low-molecular-weight heparin or unfractionated heparin. N Engl J Med 1995;332:1330–5.

36. Warkentin TE, Sheppard JA, Moore JC, et al. Studies of the immune response in heparin-induced thrombocytopenia. Blood 2009;113:4963–9.

37. Nand S, Wong W, Yuen B, et al. Heparin-induced thrombocytopenia with thrombosis: incidence, analysis of risk factors, and clinical outcomes in 108 consecutive patients treated at a single institution. Am J Hematol 1997;56:12–6.

38. Hong AP, Cook DJ, Sigouin CS, et al. Central venous catheters and upper-extremity deep-vein thrombosis complicating immune heparin-induced thrombocytopenia. Blood 2003;101:3049–51.

39. Boshkov LK, Warkentin TE, Hayward CP, et al. Heparin-induced thrombocytopenia and thrombosis: clinical and laboratory studies. Br J Haematol 1993;84:322–8.

40. Ernest D, Fisher MM. Heparin-induced thrombocytopaenia complicated by bilateral adrenal haemorrhage. Intensive Care Med 1991;17:238–40.

41. Pohl C, Harbrecht U, Greinacher A, et al. Neurologic complications in immune-mediated heparin-induced thrombocytopenia. Neurology 2000;54:1240–5.

42. Warkentin TE, Roberts RS, Hirsh J, et al. Heparin-induced skin lesions and other unusual sequelae of the heparin-induced thrombocytopenia syndrome: a nested cohort study. Chest 2005;127:1857–61.

43. Carlsson LE, Lubenow N, Blumentritt C, et al. Platelet receptor and clotting factor polymorphisms as genetic risk factors for thromboembolic complications in heparin-induced thrombocytopenia. Pharmacogenetics 2003;13:253–8.

44. Warkentin TE, Sheppard JA, Moore JC, et al. Laboratory testing for the antibodies that cause heparin-induced thrombocytopenia: how much class do we need? J Lab Clin Med 2005;146:341–6.

45. Alberio L, Kimmerle S, Baumann A, et al. Rapid determination of anti-heparin/platelet factor 4 antibody titers in the diagnosis of heparin-induced thrombocytopenia. Am J Med 2003;114:528–36.

46. Pouplard C, Gueret P, Fouassier M, et al. Prospective evaluation of the '4Ts' score and particle gel immunoassay specific to heparin/PF4 for the diagnosis of heparin-induced thrombocytopenia. J Thromb Haemost 2007;5:1373–9.

47. Zwicker JI, Uhl L, Huang WY, et al. Thrombosis and ELISA optical density values in hospitalized patients with heparin-induced thrombocytopenia. J Thromb Haemost 2004;2:2133–7.

48. Warkentin TE, Sheppard JI, Moore JC, et al. Quantitative interpretation of optical density measurements using PF4-dependent enzyme-immunoassays. J Thromb Haemost 2008;6:1304–12.

49. Mattioli AV, Bonetti L, Zennaro M, et al. Heparin/PF4 antibodies formation after heparin treatment: temporal aspects and long-term follow-up. Am Heart J 2009;157:589–95.

50. Bauer TL, Arepally G, Konkle BA, et al. Prevalence of heparin-associated antibodies without thrombosis in patients undergoing cardiopulmonary bypass surgery. Circulation 1997;95:1242–6.

51. Wallis DE, Workman DL, Lewis BE, et al. Failure of early heparin cessation as treatment for heparin-induced thrombocytopenia. Am J Med 1999;106:629–35.

52. Reilly MP, Taylor SM, Hartman NK, et al. Heparin-induced thrombocytopenia/thrombosis in a transgenic mouse model requires human platelet factor 4 and platelet activation through FcgammaRIIA. Blood 2001;98:2442–7.

53. Warkentin TE, Kelton JG. Delayed-onset heparin-induced thrombocytopenia and thrombosis. Ann Intern Med 2001;135:502–6.

54. Rice L, Attisha WK, Drexler A, et al. Delayed-onset heparin-induced thrombocytopenia. Ann Intern Med 2002;136:210–5.

55. Everett BM, Yeh R, Foo SY, et al. Prevalence of heparin/platelet factor 4 antibodies before and after cardiac surgery. Ann Thorac Surg 2007;83:592–7.

56. Baroletti S, Hurwitz S, Conti NA, et al. Thrombosis in suspected heparin-induced thrombocytopenia occurs more often with high antibody levels. Am J Med 2012; 125:44–9.

57. Yusuf AM, Warkentin TE, Arsenault KA, et al. Prognostic importance of preoperative anti-PF4/heparin antibodies in patients undergoing cardiac surgery. A systematic review. Thromb Haemost 2012;107:8–14.

58. Potzsch B, Klovekorn WP, Madlener K. Use of heparin during cardiopulmonary bypass in patients with a history of heparin-induced thrombocytopenia. N Engl J Med 2000;343:515.

59. Linkins LA, Dans AL, Moores LK, et al. Treatment and prevention of heparin-induced thrombocytopenia: antithrombotic therapy and prevention of thrombosis, 9th ed: American College of Chest Physicians evidence-based clinical practice guidelines. Chest 2012;141:e495S–530S.

60. Cuker A. Heparin-induced thrombocytopenia (HIT) in 2011: an epidemic of overdiagnosis. Thromb Haemost 2011;106:993–4.

61. Lo GK, Sigouin CS, Warkentin TE. What is the potential for overdiagnosis of heparin-induced thrombocytopenia? Am J Hematol 2007;82:1037–43.
62. Stephan F, Hollande J, Richard O, et al. Thrombocytopenia in a surgical ICU. Chest 1999;115:1363–70.
63. Oliveira GB, Crespo EM, Becker RC, et al. Incidence and prognostic significance of thrombocytopenia in patients treated with prolonged heparin therapy. Arch Intern Med 2008;168:94–102.
64. Baughman RP, Lower EE, Flessa HC, et al. Thrombocytopenia in the intensive care unit. Chest 1993;104:1243–7.
65. Pouplard C, May MA, Iochmann S, et al. Antibodies to platelet factor 4-heparin after cardiopulmonary bypass in patients anticoagulated with unfractionated heparin or a low-molecular-weight heparin: clinical implications for heparin-induced thrombocytopenia. Circulation 1999;99:2530–6.
66. Trossaert M, Gaillard A, Commin PL, et al. High incidence of anti-heparin/platelet factor 4 antibodies after cardiopulmonary bypass surgery. Br J Haematol 1998;101:653–5.
67. Selleng S, Selleng K, Wollert HG, et al. Heparin-induced thrombocytopenia in patients requiring prolonged intensive care unit treatment after cardiopulmonary bypass. J Thromb Haemost 2008;6:428–35.
68. Bream-Rouwenhorst HR, Hobbs RA. Heparin-dependent antibodies and thrombosis without heparin-induced thrombocytopenia. Pharmacotherapy 2008;28:1401–7.
69. Lo GK, Juhl D, Warkentin TE, et al. Evaluation of pretest clinical score (4 T's) for the diagnosis of heparin-induced thrombocytopenia in two clinical settings. J Thromb Haemost 2006;4:759–65.
70. Crowther MA, Cook DJ, Albert M, et al. The 4Ts scoring system for heparin-induced thrombocytopenia in medical-surgical intensive care unit patients. J Crit Care 2010;25:287–93.
71. Denys B, Stove V, Philippe J, et al. A clinical-laboratory approach contributing to a rapid and reliable diagnosis of heparin-induced thrombocytopenia. Thromb Res 2008;123:137–45.
72. Bakchoul T, Giptner A, Najaoui A, et al. Prospective evaluation of PF4/heparin immunoassays for the diagnosis of heparin-induced thrombocytopenia. J Thromb Haemost 2009;7:1260–5.
73. Nellen V, Sulzer I, Barizzi G, et al. Rapid exclusion or confirmation of heparin-induced thrombocytopenia: a single-center experience with 1,291 patients. Haematologica 2012;97:89–97.
74. Bryant A, Low J, Austin S, et al. Timely diagnosis and management of heparin-induced thrombocytopenia in a frequent request, low incidence single centre using clinical 4T's score and particle gel immunoassay. Br J Haematol 2008;143:721–6.
75. Cuker A, Arepally G, Crowther MA, et al. The HIT Expert Probability (HEP) score: a novel pre-test probability model for heparin-induced thrombocytopenia based on broad expert opinion. J Thromb Haemost 2010;8:2642–50.
76. Trehel-Tursis V, Louvain-Quintard V, Zarrouki Y, et al. Clinical and biological features of patients suspected or confirmed to have heparin-induced thrombocytopenia in a cardiothoracic surgical ICU. Chest 2012;142(4):837–44.
77. Kuitunen A, Suojaranta-Ylinen R, Kukkonen S, et al. A comparison of the haemodynamic effects of 4% succinylated gelatin, 6% hydroxyethyl starch (200/0.5) and 4% human albumin after cardiac surgery. Scand J Surg 2007;96:72–8.

78. Piednoir P, Allou N, Provenchere S, et al. Heparin-induced thrombocytopenia after cardiac surgery: an observational study of 1,722 patients. J Cardiothorac Vasc Anesth 2012;26:585–90.
79. Lillo-Le Louet A, Boutouyrie P, Alhenc-Gelas M, et al. Diagnostic score for heparin-induced thrombocytopenia after cardiopulmonary bypass. J Thromb Haemost 2004;2:1882–8.
80. Greinacher A, Juhl D, Strobel U, et al. Heparin-induced thrombocytopenia: a prospective study on the incidence, platelet-activating capacity and clinical significance of antiplatelet factor 4/heparin antibodies of the IgG, IgM, and IgA classes. J Thromb Haemost 2007;5:1666–73.
81. McFarland J, Lochowicz A, Aster R, et al. Improving the specificity of the PF4 ELISA in diagnosing heparin-induced thrombocytopenia. Am J Hematol 2012; 87:776–81.
82. Amiral J, Peynaud-Debayle E, Wolf M, et al. Generation of antibodies to heparin-PF4 complexes without thrombocytopenia in patients treated with unfractionated or low-molecular-weight heparin. Am J Hematol 1996;52:90–5.
83. Warkentin TE, Sheppard JA, Horsewood P, et al. Impact of the patient population on the risk for heparin-induced thrombocytopenia. Blood 2000;96:1703–8.
84. Arepally G, Reynolds C, Tomaski A, et al. Comparison of PF4/heparin ELISA assay with the 14C-serotonin release assay in the diagnosis of heparin-induced thrombocytopenia. Am J Clin Pathol 1995;104:648–54.
85. Schmitt BP, Adelman B. Heparin-associated thrombocytopenia: a critical review and pooled analysis. Am J Med Sci 1993;305:208–15.
86. Visentin GP, Malik M, Cyganiak KA, et al. Patients treated with unfractionated heparin during open heart surgery are at high risk to form antibodies reactive with heparin: platelet factor 4 complexes. J Lab Clin Med 1996;128:376–83.
87. Cuker A, Ortel TL. ASH evidence-based guidelines: is the IgG-specific anti-PF4/heparin ELISA superior to the polyspecific ELISA in the laboratory diagnosis of HIT? Hematology Am Soc Hematol Educ Program 2009;250–2.
88. Denys B, Devreese K. A clinical-laboratory approach contributing to a rapid and reliable diagnosis of heparin-induced thrombocytopenia: an update. Thromb Res 2009;124:642–3.
89. Morel-Kopp MC, Aboud M, Tan CW, et al. Heparin-induced thrombocytopenia: evaluation of IgG and IgGAM ELISA assays. Int J Lab Hematol 2011;33: 245–50.
90. Pouplard C, Leroux D, Regina S, et al. Effectiveness of a new immunoassay for the diagnosis of heparin-induced thrombocytopenia and improved specificity when detecting IgG antibodies. Thromb Haemost 2010;103:145–50.
91. Althaus K, Strobel U, Warkentin TE, et al. Combined use of the high heparin step and optical density to optimize diagnostic sensitivity and specificity of an anti-PF4/heparin enzyme-immunoassay. Thromb Res 2011;128:256–60.
92. Whitlatch NL, Kong DF, Metjian AD, et al. Validation of the high-dose heparin confirmatory step for the diagnosis of heparin-induced thrombocytopenia. Blood 2010;116:1761–6.
93. Warkentin TE. How I diagnose and manage HIT. Hematology Am Soc Hematol Educ Program 2011;2011:143–9.
94. Walenga JM, Jeske WP, Wood JJ, et al. Laboratory tests for heparin-induced thrombocytopenia: a multicenter study. Semin Hematol 1999;36:22–8.
95. Tomer A, Masalunga C, Abshire TC. Determination of heparin-induced thrombocytopenia: a rapid flow cytometric assay for direct demonstration of antibody-mediated platelet activation. Am J Hematol 1999;61:53–61.

96. Walenga JM, Jeske WP, Fasanella AR, et al. Laboratory tests for the diagnosis of heparin-induced thrombocytopenia. Semin Thromb Hemost 1999;25(Suppl 1): 43–9.

97. Price EA, Hayward CP, Moffat KA, et al. Laboratory testing for heparin-induced thrombocytopenia is inconsistent in North America: a survey of North American specialized coagulation laboratories. Thromb Haemost 2007;98:1357–61.

98. Warkentin TE, Greinacher A, Koster A, et al. Treatment and prevention of heparin-induced thrombocytopenia: American College of Chest Physicians evidence-based clinical practice guidelines (8th edition). Chest 2008;133: 340S–80S.

99. Lewis BE, Wallis DE, Berkowitz SD, et al. Argatroban anticoagulant therapy in patients with heparin-induced thrombocytopenia. Circulation 2001;103: 1838–43.

100. Hursting MJ, Soffer J. Reducing harm associated with anticoagulation: practical considerations of argatroban therapy in heparin-induced thrombocytopenia. Drug Saf 2009;32:203–18.

101. Hursting MJ, Zehnder JL, Joffrion JL, et al. The international normalized ratio during concurrent warfarin and argatroban anticoagulation: differential contributions of each agent and effects of the choice of thromboplastin used. Clin Chem 1999;45:409–12.

102. Arpino PA, Demirjian Z, Van Cott EM. Use of the chromogenic factor X assay to predict the international normalized ratio in patients transitioning from argatroban to warfarin. Pharmacotherapy 2005;25:157–64.

103. Bartholomew JR, Pietrangeli CE, Hursting MJ. Argatroban anticoagulation for heparin-induced thrombocytopenia in elderly patients. Drugs Aging 2007;24: 489–99.

104. Hoffman WD, Czyz Y, McCollum DA, et al. Reduced argatroban doses after coronary artery bypass graft surgery. Ann Pharmacother 2008;42:309–16.

105. Hursting MJ, Verme-Gibboney CN. Risk factors for major bleeding in patients with heparin-induced thrombocytopenia treated with argatroban: a retrospective study. J Cardiovasc Pharmacol 2008;52:561–6.

106. Swan SK, Hursting MJ. The pharmacokinetics and pharmacodynamics of argatroban: effects of age, gender, and hepatic or renal dysfunction. Pharmacotherapy 2000;20:318–29.

107. Choice of drugs for heparin-induced thrombocytopenia. Med Lett Drugs Ther 2012;54:43–4.

108. Mahaffey KW, Lewis BE, Wildermann NM, et al. The anticoagulant therapy with bivalirudin to assist in the performance of percutaneous coronary intervention in patients with heparin-induced thrombocytopenia (ATBAT) study: main results. J Invasive Cardiol 2003;15:611–6.

109. Kiser TH, Burch JC, Klem PM, et al. Safety, efficacy, and dosing requirements of bivalirudin in patients with heparin-induced thrombocytopenia. Pharmacotherapy 2008;28:1115–24.

110. Dang CH, Durkalski VL, Nappi JM. Evaluation of treatment with direct thrombin inhibitors in patients with heparin-induced thrombocytopenia. Pharmacotherapy 2006;26:461–8.

111. Savi P, Chong BH, Greinacher A, et al. Effect of fondaparinux on platelet activation in the presence of heparin-dependent antibodies: a blinded comparative multicenter study with unfractionated heparin. Blood 2005;105:139–44.

112. Lobo B, Finch C, Howard A, et al. Fondaparinux for the treatment of patients with acute heparin-induced thrombocytopenia. Thromb Haemost 2008;99:208–14.

113. Grouzi E, Kyriakou E, Panagou I, et al. Fondaparinux for the treatment of acute heparin-induced thrombocytopenia: a single-center experience. Clin Appl Thromb Hemost 2010;16:663–7.
114. Goldfarb MJ, Blostein MD. Fondaparinux in acute heparin-induced thrombocytopenia: a case series. J Thromb Haemost 2011;9:2501–3.
115. Warkentin TE, Pai M, Sheppard JI, et al. Fondaparinux treatment of acute heparin-induced thrombocytopenia confirmed by the serotonin-release assay: a 30-month, 16-patient case series. J Thromb Haemost 2011;9:2389–96.
116. GlaxoSmithKline. Arixtra prescribing information. Available at: http://us.gsk.com/products/assets/us_arixtra.pdf. Accessed March 27, 2013.
117. Bartholomew JR, Hursting MJ. Transitioning from argatroban to warfarin in heparin-induced thrombocytopenia: an analysis of outcomes in patients with elevated international normalized ratio (INR). J Thromb Thrombolysis 2005;19:183–8.
118. Babcock RB, Dumper CW, Scharfman WB. Heparin-induced immune thrombocytopenia. N Engl J Med 1976;295:237–41.
119. Refaai MA, Chuang C, Menegus M, et al. Outcomes after platelet transfusion in patients with heparin-induced thrombocytopenia. J Thromb Haemost 2010;8:1419–21.
120. Zucker MB, Katz IR. Platelet factor 4: production, structure, and physiologic and immunologic action. Proc Soc Exp Biol Med 1991;198:693–702.
121. Wanaka K, Matsuo T, Matsuo M, et al. Re-exposure to heparin in uremic patients requiring hemodialysis with heparin-induced thrombocytopenia. J Thromb Haemost 2010;8:616–8.
122. Nuttall GA, Oliver WC Jr, Santrach PJ, et al. Patients with a history of type II heparin-induced thrombocytopenia with thrombosis requiring cardiac surgery with cardiopulmonary bypass: a prospective observational case series. Anesth Analg 2003;96:344–50, table of contents.
123. Bakchoul T, Giptner A, Bein G, et al. Performance characteristics of two commercially available IgG-specific immunoassays in the assessment of heparin-induced thrombocytopenia (HIT). Thromb Res 2011;127:345–8.
124. Legnani C, Cini M, Pili C, et al. Evaluation of a new automated panel of assays for the detection of anti-PF4/heparin antibodies in patients suspected of having heparin-induced thrombocytopenia. Thromb Haemost 2010;104:402–9.
125. Eichler P, Raschke R, Lubenow N, et al. The new ID-heparin/PF4 antibody test for rapid detection of heparin-induced antibodies in comparison with functional and antigenic assays. Br J Haematol 2002;116:887–91.
126. GlaxoSmithKline. Argatroban prescribing information. Available at: http://www.gsksource.com/gskprm/htdocs/documents/ARGATROBAN.PDF. Accessed March 26, 2013.
127. Company TM. Angiomax prescribing information. Available at: http://www.angiomax.com/downloads/Angiomax%20US%20PI-%20PN%201601-15.pdf. Accessed March 26, 2013.

Thrombotic Thrombocytopenic Purpura and the Atypical Hemolytic Uremic Syndrome

An Update

Han-Mou Tsai, MD

KEYWORDS

- Thrombotic thrombocytopenic purpura • Atypical hemolytic uremic syndrome
- Microangiopathic hemolysis • Shear stress • ADAMTS13 • Complement regulators

KEY POINTS

- Both thrombotic thrombocytopenic purpura (TTP) and atypical hemolytic uremic syndrome (aHUS) are chronic diseases that often present with thrombocytopenia and microangiopathic hemolysis (MAHA), yet they have entirely different pathology and pathogenesis and require different therapeutic approaches.
- Patients presenting with thrombocytopenia and MAHA are started on plasma exchange therapy for presumed TTP unless history and laboratory test results clearly indicate that patients have one of the disorders that do not require plasma therapy.
- Plasma exchange is continued for acquired TTP until clinical remission. The treatment may be switched to plasma infusion for hereditary TTP unless the patient has renal failure. Depending on its course, acquired TTP may require rituximab treatment to prevent relapses.
- Plasma exchange is switched to eculizumab for patients without severe ADAMTS13 (a disintegrin and metalloprotease with thrombospondin type 1 motif, member 13) deficiency and considered to have aHUS.
- Both TTP and aHUS are chronic diseases that require long-term monitoring and management.

A major challenge in the management of patients presenting with thrombocytopenia and microangiopathic hemolytic anemia (MAHA) is making a distinction between TTP and aHUS. The discovery of ADAMTS13 and its deficiency in TTP has provided a pathogenetic definition of TTP.[1] Nevertheless, some investigators continue to view aHUS as a subtype of TTP without severe ADAMTS13 deficiency.[2] Under such schemes, aHUS in adult patients is treated indiscriminately from TTP.

In reality, TTP and aHUS not only differ in pathology, pathogenesis, pathophysiology, and prognosis but also require different therapeutic management. The similarity

iMAH Hematology Associates, New Hyde Park, New York 11040, USA
E-mail address: hmtsai@gmail.com

Hematol Oncol Clin N Am 27 (2013) 565–584
http://dx.doi.org/10.1016/j.hoc.2013.02.006
0889-8588/13/$ – see front matter © 2013 Elsevier Inc. All rights reserved.

between TTP and aHUS in causing thrombocytopenia and microangiopathic hemolysis is an epiphenomenon of microvascular stenosis resulting from entirely different mechanisms.

Fragmentation of the red blood cells occurs in 2 types of clinical conditions: vascular devices, such as prosthetic heart valves, ventricular assist devices, and extracorporeal oxygenator, and microvascular stenosis. These 2 conditions share a common feature of abnormal intravascular shear stress that is sufficient to cause fragmentation of the red blood cells (**Fig. 1**). In the absence of vascular devices, fragmentation of the red blood cells signifies stenosis in the arterioles and capillaries.

Pathologically at least 5 different types of arteriolar stenosis are observed (see **Fig. 1**): (1) von Willebrand factor (VWF) platelet thrombosis, typically observed in patients with TTP due to severe ADAMTS13 deficiency; (2) platelet fibrin thrombosis, as exemplified in patients with disseminated intravascular coagulopathy (DIC); (3) tumor cell invasion of the microvasculature in patients with metastatic neoplasm; (4) microvascular vasculitis complicating autoimmune or certain infectious disorders; and (5) thrombotic microangiopathy, as observed in patients with the typical shiga toxin–associated hemolytic uremic syndrome after certain *Escherichia coli* infection or aHUS due to defective regulation of the alternative complement pathway.

In thrombotic microangiopathy, endothelial changes are prominent. Endothelial cell swelling or disruption, accompanied by intimal expansion and cellular proliferation, may cause microvascular stenosis or occlusion with or without thrombosis. In addition, edema of the brain and other organs and fluid accumulation in cavitary spaces due to abnormal vascular permeability may contribute to organ dysfunction in patients with thrombotic microangiopathy. In TTP, tissue injury results from ischemia of microvascular thrombosis; the endothelium and vessel wall structures are intact and complications of abnormal vascular permeability do not occur.

The various types of microvascular stenosis, in particular types 1 to 4, are often incorrectly referred to as thrombotic microangiopathy without distinction. Furthermore, thrombocytopenia and microangiopathic hemolysis are often equated in practice with thrombotic microangiopathy, ignoring other types of pathology causing microvascular stenosis. Both practices obscure the important differences among the various types of pathology and contribute to the unfounded view of TTP and aHUS as one disease entity.

PATHOGENESIS AND PATHOPHYSIOLOGY OF TTP AND AHUS

The pathogenesis of TTP and aHUS are different. TTP results from severe ADAMTS13 deficiency due to genetic mutations or, more commonly, autoimmune inhibitors,[3] whereas aHUS results from defective regulation of the complement system. Although a recent report describes the activation of the complement system in TTP,[4] presumably by the ADAMTS13-inhibitor complexes, there is no evidence that complement dysregulation contributes to the development of TTP.

ADAMTS13 is a major determinant preventing VWF platelet aggregation in the normal circulation. Inflammation, infection, surgery, or pregnancy may decrease the plasma ADAMTS13 activity level by suppressing the biosynthesis of ADAMTS13 or possibly enhancing its inactivation.[5,6] Although inflammation or pregnancy-mediated decrease in ADAMTS13 per se is insufficient to induce microvascular thrombosis, it may lead to disease exacerbation in patients with preexisting TTP.

In the presence of severe ADAMTS13 deficiency, the propensity of VWF and platelet to form aggregates is affected by multiple other factors, including the platelet count,

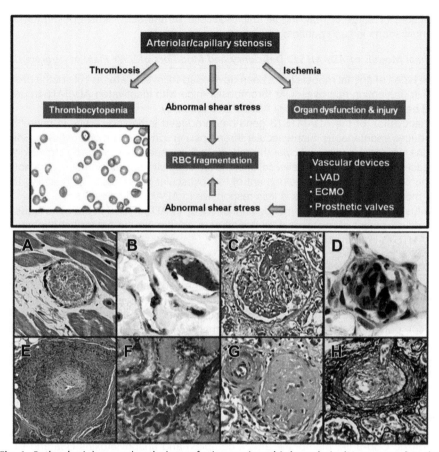

Fig. 1. Pathophysiology and pathology of microangiopathic hemolysis. (*Upper panel*) In the absence of vascular device, fragmentation of the red cell signifies arteriolar/capillary stenosis. Consumptive thrombocytopenia occurs when the microvascular stenosis is due to thrombosis. Organ dysfunction and injury may result from microvascular stenosis, with or without thrombosis. (*Lower panel*) Microvascular stenosis may result from at least 5 different types of pathology: (*A, B*) TTP with arteriolar thrombosis that stains strongly for VWF (*brown*); (*C*) DIC with microvascular thrombosis in renal glomeruli; (*D*) tumor cells in the microvasculature; (*E*) vasculitis with fibrinoid necrosis and inflammatory cell infiltration of the vessel wall; (*F*) thrombotic microangiopathy of shiga toxin–associated HUS with prominent fibrin deposits (*magenta*); and (*G, H*) thrombotic microangiopathy with marked subendothelial expansion of aHUS. All are H & E stain except (*B*) immunochemical stain with anti-VWF, (*F*) platelet and fibrin stain of Carstairs, and (*H*) Jones silver stain. LVAD, left ventricular devices; ECMO, extracorporeal membrane oxygenator.

the conformational responsiveness of VWF to activation by shear stress, and, most importantly, the shear stress profile in the microcirculation.

In vitro, the critical shear stress required for VWF platelet aggregation is near the high end of physiological range (50–90 dyn/cm^2). Therefore, in patients with shear stress profiles that are not sufficient to activate the VWF in their microcirculation, VWF platelet aggregation may not occur even when ADAMTS13 deficiency is severe. This may explain why some patients with severe ADAMTS13 deficiency are asymptomatic and have normal platelet counts. Any condition, however, such as fever, infection, or surgery, may trigger microvascular thrombosis, causing symptomatic complications in such patients.

Animal Models of ADAMTS13 Deficiency and Modifiers of VWF Platelet Aggregation

Two types of animal models have been developed to investigate the role of the protease in preventing microvascular thrombosis: mice with inactivated ADAMTS13 gene and baboons given an inhibitory ADAMTS13 antibody.

Inactivation of the ADAMTS13 gene has produced intriguing results in mice.[7,8] It produces spontaneous microvascular thrombosis in some but not other strains. Shiga toxins may induce microvascular thrombosis in the susceptible strains by inducing the release of VWF from endothelial cells. In the resistant strains, infusion of large amount of human VWF leads to development of microvascular thrombosis,[9] suggesting that the mouse VWF platelet axis is less responsive to ADAMTS13 deficiency.

Infusion of an inactivating monoclonal antibody of ADAMTS13 in baboons leads to the development of microvascular thrombosis, confirming the antithrombotic role of ADAMTS13 in normal circulation.[10]

Pathogenesis and Pathophysiology of aHUS

aHUS results from defects in the regulation of the complement system (**Fig. 2**). Three types of molecular defects or variants are detected in aHUS patients: inactivating mutations of complement factor H (CFH; 25%), membrane cofactor protein (MCP, ie, CD46), complement factor I (CFI), or thrombomodulin (THBD) (approximately 5%–10% each); gain-of-function mutations of complement factor B (CFB) or C3 approximately 5%–10%); and autoantibodies of CFH (approximately 5%–10%). Additionally, certain common variants of CFH, CFH-related protein (CFHR) 2 and other regulators; or their combinations (haplotypes and complotypes) may increase the risk of aHUS.[11–14] Because the list of affected molecules remains incomplete, negative genetic or antibody test results do not exclude the diagnosis of aHUS.

Defective regulation of the complement activation leads to excess generation of cytotoxic C5b-9 (ie, membrane attack complex) and anaphylatoxins C3a and C5a. Membrane attack complex causes cytotoxicity of endothelial cells, leading to endothelial swelling or disruption and intimal swelling and cellular proliferation. Endothelial disruption exposes the prothrombotic components in the subendothelial space, leading to activation of the coagulation system and fibrin deposition (**Fig. 3**).

In aHUS, microvascular stenosis may result not only from thrombosis but also directly from endothelial swelling and subendothelial expansion. Furthermore, abnormal vascular permeability mediated by C3a and C5a may cause interstitial edema of the brain and other vital organs and cavitary fluid accumulation. Therefore, mental changes, seizures, cardiac dysfunction or arrest, pericardial effusion, chest pain, dyspnea, pleural effusion, pulmonary infiltrates, abdominal pain, nausea, vomiting, diarrhea, pancreatitis, ascites, renal failure, and anasarca may occur in aHUS without concurrent worsening of MAHA or thrombocytopenia.

A PATHOGENETIC CLASSIFICATION OF MAHA

Microangiopathic hemolysis may be classified according to its pathogenetic mechanisms or pathology (**Table 1**). This scheme is anchored on group I of TTP with severe ADAMTS13 deficiency due to autoimmune inhibitors or genetic mutations, and group II of aHUS with defective complement regulation due to genetic mutations or autoantibodies of the activators or regulators of the alternative complement pathway. Included in either group I or II are comorbid conditions, such as infection,

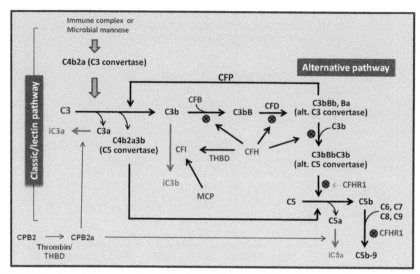

Fig. 2. Activation of the complement system and its regulation. Triggers of the complement system, such as immune complex or microbial lectins, lead to the generation of C3 and C5 convertases of the classic and alternative pathways. The alternative pathway, self-perpetuating via a loop of amplification, is essential for innate immunity. This loop of amplification is regulated by complement factor I (CFI), a serine protease, which, with complement factor H (CFH), membrane cofactor protein (MCP) and thrombomodulin (THBD) as cofactors, cleaves C3b to its inactive form (iC3b). THBD also acts as a cofactor of thrombin to cleave carboxypeptidase B2 (CPB2) to its active form (CPB2a), which cleaves and inactivates C3a and C5a. Complement factor H related protein 1 (CFHR1) may contribute to the regulation at C5 convertase and the formation of the membrane attack complex. Inactivating mutations in CFH, MCP, CFI, or THBD; gain-of-function mutations of CFB or C3; and autoantibodies of CFH are detected in approximately 50% of patients with aHUS. Genomic deletion of CFHR1 is detected in 20% of patients, with mutations of CFI and in 90% of patients with antibodies of CFH. CD55 and CD59 are GPI-anchored proteins on blood cells that are deficient in patients with PNH.

inflammation, surgery, trauma, pregnancy, intravenous contrast agents, and pancreatitis, that may trigger acute presentation in patients with preexisting TTP or aHUS, either by promoting the VWF platelet interaction or by activating the complement system (group IB or IIB). Pregnancy is considered group II comorbidity for aHUS because most pregnant women presenting with hemolytic-uremic syndrome (HUS) have molecular defects in the regulation of the alternative complement pathway.[15]

Group IC or IIC includes secondary TTP or aHUS in which the comorbidity is presumed to induce acquired ADAMTS13 deficiency or complement dysregulation. TTP in patients treated with ticlopidine is believed to result from induction of ADAMTS13 autoimmunity by the drug.[16] HIV infection may cause defective regulation of autoreactive B cells making antibody inhibitors of ADAMTS13 or CFH antibodies. Autoimmune dysregulation may also underlie the TTP that affects patients with adult-onset Still disease or antiglomerular basement membrane nephropathy, which is described in the literature and was present in 1 TTP patient each in the author's series to be discussed later.[17,18] It is suspected that thrombotic microangiopathy in some patients following hematopoietic stem cell therapy or with lupus or other autoimmune diseases may result from immune mediated complement dysregulation.

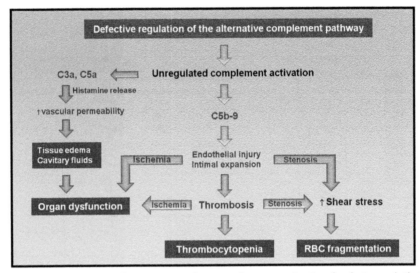

Fig. 3. Pathophysiology of aHUS. Excessive complement activation leads to endothelial injury, which may result in microvascular stenosis by causing endothelial cell swelling and intimal expansion, with or without concurrent thrombosis. Abnormal shear stress created by microvascular stenosis causes red cell fragmentation, which may not be accompanied with severe thrombocytopenia if nonthrombotic stenosis is the predominant mechanism. Organ dysfunction may result from ischemic injury of microvascular stenosis but may also result from abnormal vascular permeability and tissue edema induced by C3a and C5a via release of histamine from basophils or mast cells. Thus, mental changes or seizures due to brain edema may not be accompanied with concurrent worsening of MAHA or thrombocytopenia in aHUS.

Group IV includes diseases with other types of pathology such as fibrin-platelet thrombosis, intravascular cluster of cancer cells, vasculitis and vascular devices. A recent study reveals that mutations of membrane cofactor protein (MCP) or CFI may be more frequent in patients with HELLP.[19] However, the results may be a consequence of misdiagnosis because it is not uncommon in practice to encounter patients who are given the diagnosis of the HELLP syndrome or pre-eclampsia of pregnancy but really have aHUS.

Severe hypertension was believed to be a cause of thrombotic microangiopathy or microangiopathic hemolysis. However, there is increasing evidence to indicate that severe hypertension may be a consequence of aHUS forme fruste. Thrombotic microangiopathy following renal allograft transplantation is often attributed to calcineurin inhibitors. Retrospective studies reveal that some of the patients have aHUS with mutations affecting the complement regulators or activators.

Conceptually, patients with underlying autoimmune connective tissue diseases, such as lupus or scleoderma, may present with microangiopathic hemolysis via one or more mechanisms. Autoimmune diseases may trigger the presentation of TTP or aHUS in patients with preexisting diseases by decreasing the ADAMTS13 level or activating the complement system in (group IB or IIB) or by inducing autoimmunity against ADAMTS13 or the complement components (group IC or IIC). Vasculitis is the most common finding when biopsy is performed in patients with active lupus and microangiopathic hemolysis (group IV).

Antinuclear antibodies and other autoimmune markers are detectable in 10% to 40% of TTP patients; yet, in the few patients with both TTP and lupus, exacerbations

Table 1
A classification of disorders presenting with microangiopathic hemolysis and thrombocytopenia

I. TTP: propensity to VWF-platelet thrombosis due to ADAMTS13 deficiency
- A: Idiopathic TTP
  - Acquired: autoimmune inhibitors of ADAMTS13
  - Genetic: mutations of *ADAMTS13*
- B: Co-morbidity as a trigger: pregnancy, infection, inflammation, surgery, trauma
- C: Co-morbidity as an inducer of inhibitors: ticlopidine, HIV infection, autoimmune diseases, HSCT

II. Atypical HUS: propensity to TMA due to defective regulation of complement activation
- A: Idiopathic aHUS
  - Genetic: mutations or genetic variants of CFH, MCP, CFI, CFB, C3, or THBD
  - Acquired: e.g. autoantibodies of CFH
- B: Co-morbidity as a trigger
  - Pregnancy, intravenous contrasts agents, pancreatitis, infection, inflammation, surgery, trauma, etc.
- C: Co-morbidity as an inducer (e.g. CFH antibodies)
  - Hematopoietic stem cell therapy
  - Suspected but not yet proven: HIV infection, autoimmune disorders, etc.

III. TMA via other mechanisms
- Shiga toxin associated HUS: Shiga toxin producing *Escherichia coli* or *Shigella dysenteriae*
- Microbial neuraminidases causing T-antigen activation (e.g. *S. pneumonia* or *influenza virus*)
- Angiogenesis inhibitors (e.g. bevacizumab)
- Severe hypertension[a]
- Undefined: HIV, HSCT, mitomycin, gemcitabine, quinine, cocaine, calcineurin inhibitors[b]

IV. Other types of pathology
- Fibrin-platelet thrombosis: e.g. DIC, HELLP syndrome, CAPS, HIT, PNH
- Intravascular clusters of neoplastic cells
- Vasculitis of autoimmune diseases or infections (e.g. Rocky Mountain spotted fever, anthrax)
- Vascular devices: e.g. VAD, ECMO, prosthetic heart valves

Abbreviations: aHUS, atypical hemolytic uremic syndrome; CAPS, catastrophic antiphospholipid antibody syndrome; CFB, complement factor B; CFH, complement factor H; CFI, complement factor I; DIC, disseminated intravascular coagulopathy; ECMO, extracorporeal membrane oxygenator; HELLP, hemolysis, elevated liver enzymes and low platelet count of pregnancy; HIT, heparin induced thrombocytopenia; HSCT, hematopoietic stem cell therapy; MCP, membrane cofactor protein (i.e. CD46); PNH, paroxysmal nocturnal hemoglobinuria; THBD, thrombomodulin; TTP, thrombotic thrombocytopenic purpua; VAD, ventricular assist device.

[a] Severe hypertension may be a consequence of forme fruste aHUS rather than a cause of MAHA.
[b] Some patients with presumed calcineurin-inhibitor associated TMA after renal allograft transplantation are found to have aHUS with mutations causing defective complement regulation.

of these 2 diseases usually occur independently (**Fig. 4**), suggesting they result from separate pathways of immune dysregulations.

APPLICATION OF ADAMTS13 IN THE DIFFERENTIAL DIAGNOSIS OF MAHA

Clinically, the ADAMTS13 levels and the presence or absence of comorbidity are the basis for the differential diagnosis of microangiopathic hemolysis and thrombocytopenia.

Correlation of ADAMTS13 Level with the Thrombosis Activity of TTP

VWF platelet aggregation does not occur when the ADAMTS13 activity level is 10% or higher. When the ADAMTS13 level is less than 10%, however, VWF platelet

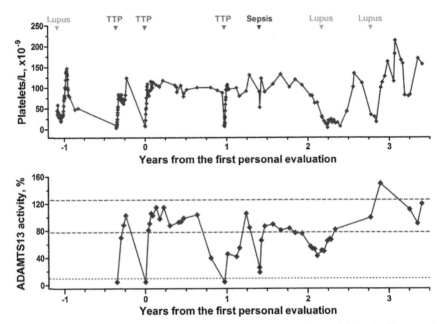

Fig. 4. Independent exacerbation of lupus and TTP in a patient with both diseases. An episode of thrombocytopenia is considered the consequence of TTP exacerbation if the ADAMTS13 activity level decreases to less than 10% of normal without an increase in the antinative DNA and anti-Sm levels; and the consequence of lupus exacerbation if the antinative DNA and anti-Sm antibody levels are increased, the C4 level is decreased, and the ADAMTS13 activity level remains greater than 10%.

aggregation may but does not invariably occur. This is because the process of VWF platelet aggregation is dependent on shear stress and affected by multiple modifiers (discussed previously). The ADAMTS13 levels in TTP at different stages of the disease and their interpretations are summarized in **Table 2**. Persistent thrombocytopenia cannot be due to TTP if the ADAMTS13 level is greater than or equal to 10%. In such cases, other causes should be searched for.

After a TTP patient receives plasma or blood transfusion, the ADAMTS13 level may be less than or greater than or equal to 10%. The platelet count should be rising when the ADAMTS13 is increased to greater than or equal to 10%. An ADAMTS13 level less than 10% does not preclude the possibility that the platelet count may be increasing, because its level immediately after the transfusion may be sufficiently higher to suppress thrombosis and platelet consumption.

Table 2
ADAMTS13 levels in TTP at various clinical stages

Status	ADAMTS13	Platelet Count
Active microvascular thrombosis	<10%	Low or decreasing
After plasma or blood transfusion	<10%	Low, decreasing, or increasing
	≥10%	Increasing
Clinical remission	<10% or ≥10%	Normal

The ADAMTS13 activity may be at any level during clinical remission. A patient is at high risk of relapse anytime if the ADAMTS13 level is persistently less than 10% or exhibits a trend of decrease during remission.

These correlations are based on sodium dodecyl sulfate-polyacrilamide gel electrophoresis assay of VWF fragments and may not be valid when ADAMTS13 activity is measured using other methods.

Patients Without Comorbidity

Laboratory tests are now widely available for demonstration of severe ADAMTS13 deficiency and delineation of its autoimmune inhibitors or genetic basis in patients presenting with comorbidity, although it remains unclear whether the reliability of the assays has been fully validated.

The diagnosis of aHUS is less straightforward. Defining the molecular defects in complement regulation requires sequencing of multiple genes. The tests are not yet readily available with reasonable turnaround time. In some aHUS patients, no molecular defects are detectable and defective complement regulation is inferred by their improvement after anticomplement therapy with eculizumab. Thus, a patient presenting with microangiopathic hemolysis without comorbidity is presumed to have aHUS if there is renal function impairment but no severe ADAMTS13 deficiency.

The ADAMTS13 levels of 335 patients investigated between 1998 and 2007 for MAHA and thrombocytopenia are illustrated in **Fig. 5**. Patients with hereditary TTP or vascular devices are not included in this analysis; 80% of the cases were referral samples and 20% were nonreferral local consecutive patients. TTP accounts for 56% of all the patients presenting with thrombocytopenia and microangiopathic hemolysis and for 76% of the 206 patients without comorbidity ($P<.001$).

The group of 50 (24%) patients without comorbidity or severe ADAMTS13 are considered to have aHUS. Of the 50 patients without severe ADAMTS13 deficiency, all but one (98%) had renal failure with maximal creatinine greater than 2.5 mg/dL. The renal function impairment was minimal in 1 patient without severe ADAMTS13

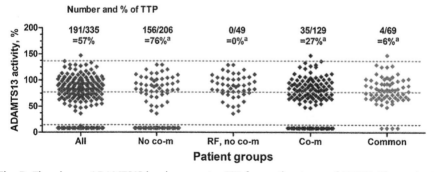

Fig. 5. The plasma ADAMTS13 level segregates TTP from other types of MAHA. The patients without severe ADAMTS13 deficiency in the group without comorbidity are considered to have aHUS. Diagnosis of aHUS in the group of patients with comorbidity is further elaborated in **Table 1**. All, all patients investigated for microangiopathic hemolysis unrelated to vascular devices. Hereditary TTP is also excluded from this analysis, as some of the patients did develop acute or chronic renal failure; No co-m, all patients without comorbidity; RF, no co-m, patients with renal failure (maximum creatinine >2.5 mg/dL) in the no co-m group; Co-m, all patients with comorbidity; Common, all patients with common comorbid conditions, including autoimmune connective tissue disease, hematopoietic stem cell therapy, drugs other than ticlopidine, metastatic cancers, and pregnancy. [a] $P<.001$ compared with the group of all patients.

deficiency. Mild renal function impairment does not exclude the diagnosis of aHUS. None of the acquired TTP patients without comorbidity had advanced renal failure.

In the subgroup of patients without comorbidity, the TTP/aHUS ratio is approximately 3:1. The relative incidence of aHUS is likely to be different in practice.

Comparison of the TTP and the aHUS patients reveals that both TTP and aHUS may present with CNS complications. The presence or absence of neurologic complications does not provide reliable distinction between TTP and aHUS.

Abdominal symptoms due to pancreatitis or intestinal/mesenteric ischemia occur in both disorders, although they are more frequent in aHUS. Diarrhea was the presenting symptom in 30% of the aHUS patients.

Advanced renal failure, hypertension, or complications of abnormal vascular permeability, such as brain edema, pleural or pericardial effusions, pulmonary edema, ascites, or anasarca, are common in aHUS patients but do not occur in acquired TTP without comorbidity. Therefore, the presence of these complications strongly favors the diagnosis of aHUS over acquired TTP.

Unlike acquired TTP, hereditary TTP is prone to acute or chronic renal failure that is not evident in the data of single episodes. Some of the patients with hereditary TTP were given the diagnosis of aHUS before their correct diagnosis was revealed with ADAMTS13 assay and genetic analysis. Among the hereditary TTP patients not receiving maintenance plasma therapy, 10% of them develop at least 1 episode of acute renal failure during their lifetime, and 10% of them have evidence of chronic renal failure.[20] It is speculated that the expression of ADAMTS13 in renal glomeruli[21] may provide protection against VWF platelet aggregation before the protease is neutralized by the circulating inhibitors of acquired TTP. Hereditary TTP is more prone to severe renal injury because the protection by local ADAMTS13 is lost.

Patients with Comorbidity

Most of the comorbid conditions are evident from history, physical findings, and commonly performed laboratory tests. Some of the comorbid conditions in the author's series, such as tumor cells invading microvasculature, PNH, and antiglomerular basement membrane nephropathy, were not clinically evident and required high index of suspicion to reveal their diagnosis.

TTP only accounts for 35 (27%) of the 129 patients with comorbidity (P<.001 vs the entire group). Three patients, 1 with occult metastatic cancer to the bone marrow, 1 with gastric cancer metastatic to a paraspinal mass, and 1 with PNH causing mesenteric microvascular thrombosis, presented with thrombocytopenia and microangiopathic hemolysis without renal function impairment and were initially assumed to have TTP. Extensive search led to the correct diagnosis in these cases after their TTP was excluded by ADAMTS13 assay results.

Further analysis shows that TTP accounted for all the 7 ticlipidine-associated cases and for 20 of the 27 patients with HIV infection. The frequency of TTP was low (6%) among patients with the other most comorbid conditions: autoimmune connective tissue diseases, hematopoietic stem cell therapy, drugs other than ticlopidine, metastatic neoplasm, and pregnancy. Nevertheless, it is obvious that TTP cannot be reliably excluded without ADAMTS13 analysis.

The diagnosis of aHUS is difficult to make in patients with comorbidity. Of the 94 patients with comorbidity but without severe ADAMTS13 deficiency, 65% had renal failure with maximal creatinine greater than 2.5 mg/dL. Unlike its counterpart group of patients without comorbidity, this group of patients is heterogeneous. In practice, the patients may be assumed to have aHUS when TTP is excluded by ADAMTS13 assays and none of the group III or group IV comorbid conditions in **Table 1** is present.

A tissue biopsy may be necessary to make the distinction. Another challenge is to determine whether comorbid conditions, such as autoimmunity, hematopoietic stem cell therapy, drugs, or HIV, causes thrombotic microangiopathy via complement dysregulation (group III) or other (group IV) mechanisms.

CLINICAL COURSE AND MANAGEMENT

Plasma exchange remains the mainstay of treatment of acquired TTP, yet rituximab is assuming increasingly important role for prevention of persistent disease activity or relapse.

Expanding Role of Rituximab in the Management of TTP

Plasma therapy does not address the underlying autoimmunity in TTP patients. Patients are able to achieve sustained remission because the ADAMTS13 autoimmunity wanes spontaneously. Weaning off plasma therapy is impossible in some patients if their ADAMTS13 activity fails to recover above the threshold levels.

Rituximab has been used with high rates (70%–90%) of remission, initially in patients unable to wean off plasma exchange even after therapy with high-dose prednisone, antiplatelet drugs, vincristine, cyclophosphamide, azathioprine, and/or splenectomy.[22] With its efficacy increasingly appreciated, rituximab is used before the other modalities.[23]

To minimize the risk of protracted plasma exchange therapy, rituximab was used preemptively in a prospective phase II trial within 3 days of acute presentation.[24] Compared with historical controls, preemptive rituximab seems to shorten the time to sustained remission and decrease the risk of subsequent relapses. Whether this strategy can be further improved on by an ADAMTS13-guided approach remains to be determined. Except for allergic reactions during administration, rituximab has been associated with few serious side effects.

Without interventions, most TTP patients experience 1 or more relapses in subsequent years (**Fig. 6**). HIV-infected patients had high risk of relapse initially but were relapse-free after 10 months of antiretroviral treatment. Similar impact of HIV infection on TTP has also been reported elsewhere.[25] Patients whose ADAMTS13 levels remain severely decreased during clinical remission should be considered for rituximab therapy.

Normalization of the plasma ADAMTS13 level does not preclude the possibility of subsequent relapses. Serial monitoring of the ADAMTS13 level may detect a trend of decrease before relapse occurs. The period between declining ADAMTS13 and TTP relapse may last for several weeks to months, providing a window for rituximab treatment to avert the impending relapse (**Fig. 7**).

Patients with frequent relapses may consider splenectomy if they fail rituximab or are unable to tolerate the treatment. Cyclosporine[26] is a possible alternative for patients who do not want operation or are not surgical candidates.

The Role of Plasma Exchange Therapy for aHUS

Conventionally aHUS is often treated as TTP with plasma exchange. With plasma therapy, mortality rate is approximately 20% to 30%, which is substantially higher than the 10% mortality rate generally observed in TTP patients. Furthermore, many patients, after initial improvement with plasma exchange, go on to develop progressive renal injury, with or without relapses. Consequently, the dialysis-free survival rate is 40% by 2 years and lower (20%–30%) for patients with CFH mutations or CFI mutation with concurrent CFHR1 deletion.[14]

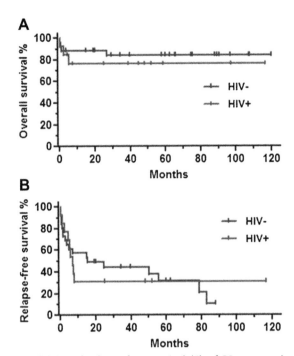

Fig. 6. Overall survival (*A*) and relapse-free survival (*B*) of 39 consecutive nonreferral acquired TTP patients. Acquired TTP is a chronic autoimmune disease that causes relapses in approximately 90% of the patients after 7 years, except those patients with HIV infection and treated with antiretroviral therapy.

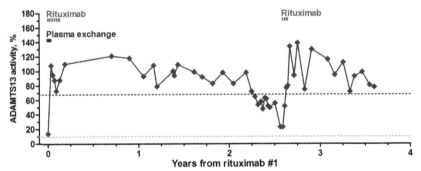

Fig. 7. Preemptive rituximab treatment prevents TTP relapse. This 54-year-old woman had 9 episodes of acute TTP exacerbation during the 12 years before her latest relapse. She was treated with rituximab and her ADAMTS13 recovered to the normal range that lasted for 2 years and 3 months before it began to exhibit staggering but definite decline, reaching 26% at 32 months. After a course of 4 rituximab treatments, her ADAMTS13 activity level returned to the normal or nearly normal range. With this strategy of ADAMTS13-guided preemptive rituximab treatment, she has been free of TTP relapse for more than 3.5 years. The upper dashed line marks the lower limit of the normal range (68%); lower dashed line marks the 10% threshold below which thrombosis may occur.

The nature of the molecular defects may determine whether a patient responds to plasma therapy. Patients with inactivating mutations of the plasma proteins, such as CFH or CFI, but not patients with mutations affecting membrane-bound proteins, such as MCP, are expected to respond to plasma exchange. Patients with gain-of-function mutations of CFB or C3 may respond to intensive plasma exchange therapy, whereas the response of patients with CFH autoantibodies is unpredictable, depending on the antibody levels.

The predictive values of genetics are hampered if patients harbor more than one known or unknown molecular defects. Thus, a therapeutic approach guided by patients' molecular defects remains problematic for individual patients.

Long-term maintenance plasma exchange therapy is effective in preventing relapse of aHUS or progressive renal injury for some patients. Yet, other patients may develop secondary resistance to the treatment after exhibiting an initial improvement. Plasma exchange is a technically demanding procedure and difficult to live with on a long-term basis.

Eculizumab as a Treatment of aHUS

A major advance in the management of aHUS is the use of eculizumab, a humanized monoclonal antibody of complement C5 originally approved in 2007 for the treatment of PNH, another disease due to complement dysregulation.

Two prospective clinical trials have been conducted to assess the efficacy and safety of eculizumab in patients with aHUS.[27,28] One trial included 17 adolescents or adults not responding to plasma exchange therapy and the other included 20 adolescents or adults who were being treated with maintenance plasma therapy.

The eculizumab regimen was 900 mg intravenously each week for 4 doses, followed by 1200 mg on week 5 and every other week thereafter. The plasma therapy was discontinued after eculizumab was started. After a median treatment duration of 38 (range 26–64) or 40 (range 26–52) weeks, respectively, no patients died, relapsed, or required additional plasma therapy. More importantly, improvement in renal function is observed not only in the active disease group (estimated glomerular filtrate rate + 20 mL/min/1.73 m^2, range −1 to 98) but also in the maintenance group, albeit at lower magnitude (estimated glomerular filtration rate + 5 mL/min/1.73 m^2, range −1 to 20).

Eculizumab is generally well tolerated. A major risk is fulminant meningococcal infection. To minimize this risk, patients should be given meningococcal vaccination and take prophylactic antibiotics at least until 2 weeks after vaccination. The vaccination does not prevent group B disease. The risk of meninogococcal disease has been estimated to be 0.9 cases per 100 patient-years in vaccinated PNH patients in the United Kingdom.[29] Patients should be well versed on this risk and carry a medication warning card to facilitate emergent care. Long-term prophylactic antibiotics should also be seriously considered.

Who Should be Treated with Eculizumab and for How Long?

Based on encouraging results of clinical trials and anecdotal case reports, eculizumab is considered the treatment of choice for patients with aHUS (ie, patients presenting with thrombocytopenia and microangiopathic hemolysis but without severe ADAMTS13 deficiency and comorbidity). Eculizumab should also be considered for patients without TTP but with any of the group II or possibly some of the group III comorbid conditions.

The optimal duration of eculizumab treatment has not been determined. aHUS is a chronic disease that often causes subclinical but progressive organ injury. Therefore, eculizumab probably should be continued indefinitely for patients at the edge of requiring renal replacement therapy and patients likely to have recurrent aHUS when eculizumab is discontinued (eg, case 3, discussed later).

For asymptomatic patients with normal or mildly abnormal renal functions (eg, stage 1 or 2) discontinuation of eculizumab may be an option. If eculizumab is discontinued, patients should be closely monitored for clinical symptoms, blood pressures, blood counts, and renal function. Eculizumab should be resumed if patients show evidence of recurrent aHUS disease activity.

Implications for Renal Transplantation

With the exception of those with MCP and possibly THBD mutations, patients with end-stage renal disease due to aHUS have high risk of graft failure after kidney transplantation, primarily due to thrombotic microangiopathy affecting the grafts. Unaware of this risk, some patients have received multiple allografts, all ending in failure.

It was advocated that concurrent liver transplantation might prevent renal graft failure due to thrombotic microangiopathic in patients with CFH mutations.[30] The operation is associated with high rates of perioperative morbidity and mortality, most likely due to activation of the complement system.

Eculizumab therapy is expected to shift the paradigm. With eculizumab started preoperatively and continued postoperatively, preliminary experience suggests that excessive morbidity, mortality, and kidney graft failure may be prevented.[31,32]

Because some patients present with end-stage renal disease without a diagnosis of aHUS, a kidney biopsy and molecular tests for aHUS are recommended for patients with renal failure of undetermined causes if kidney transplantation is considered. Because family members of aHUS patients may be asymptomatic carriers, they should refrain from donating their organs.

BRIEF CASE REPORTS

Three cases of aHUS, 2 after hematopoietic stem cell therapy and 1 with a history of severe and brittle hypertension, are briefly described to illustrate the serious nature of the disease and extend the efficacy of eculizumab to some cases of aHUS after hematopoietic stem cell therapy. All 3 cases presented with gastrointestinal symptoms and renal failure and evidence of abnormal vascular permeability during their course and were initially treated under the incorrect diagnosis of TTP. The patient in case 1 died after exhibiting partial improvement with plasma exchange therapy. The patients in cases 2 and 3 were treated with eculizumab and improved. Their renal function recovery occurred after delay of several weeks and proceeded slowly over many months (**Fig. 8**). Patients with advanced renal failure should not give up hope of coming off dialysis or be rushed prematurely to renal transplantation. Case 3 also illustrates that severe hypertension may be the consequence of aHUS rather than the cause of microangiopathic hemolysis.

In case 1, a 33-year-old man presented with recurrent bouts of abdominal and chest pain and anasarca 3 months after discontinuing immunosuppressive drugs for allogeneic hematopoietic stem cell therapy from a fully matched sibling. His laboratory findings were notable for thrombocytopenia, MAHA, and elevated LDH. His abdominal and chest CT scans revealed pleural and pericardial effusions, mesenteric edema, and focal pancreatitis. The patient was treated with plasma exchange for supposed TTP. His platelet count increased but remained unsteady. His renal function improved but then deteriorated and he required hemodialysis by the 10th week, when his platelet count and LDH were only slightly abnormal. The diagnosis was changed to aHUS on

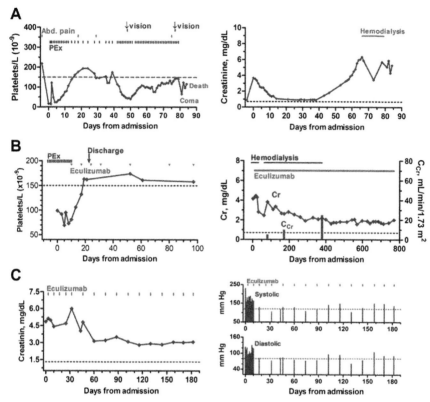

Fig. 8. The courses of 3 aHUS patients. (*A*) Case 1 is notable for relapse of aHUS with development of advanced renal failure and subsequent death on day 85 after exhibiting initial improvement with plasma exchange therapy. During his course, the patient continued to have episodes of abdominal pain and decreased visual acuity due to exudative retinopathy. (*B*) Case 2 is notable for rapid normalization of the platelet count in response to rituximab therapy. The patient's renal function recovered slowly over many months, allowing her to come off hemodialysis at 1 year. (*C*) In case 3, the severe brittle hypertension stabilized after 2 doses of eculizumab therapy. The patient's renal function began to show improvement after 6 weeks of eculizumab treatment. In all 3 cases, mental changes occurred without concurrent severe thrombocytopenia. Dashed lines indicate the lower limit of normal platelet count, the upper limit of serum creatinine concentration, or desired upper limit of systolic blood pressure or diastolic blood pressure.

consultation. Eculizumab was recommended but not immediately available. On day 81, despite plasma exchange and dialysis, the patient was found unconscious. His brain MRI showed posterior reversible encephalopathy syndrome, followed by brain edema, retinal hemorrhage, and central herniation. The patient died soon thereafter. His autopsy findings confirmed thrombotic microangiopathy in the kidneys. In the brain, only cerebral edema with central hermiation but not thrombotic microangiopathy was noted. In this patient, his secondary refractoriness to plasma exchange therapy raises the suspicion of an immune-mediated aHUS.

In case 2, a 54-year-old woman presented with abdominal pain and diarrhea 3 months after undergoing a successful autologous stem cell therapy for her advanced multiple myeloma. Her vomiting worsened and she became confused and anuric, requiring endotracheal intubation. With her platelet count decreasing to 15 × 10^9/L and schistocytes noted on the blood smears, plasma exchange therapy and hemodialysis were started. Her platelet count increased, yet she continued to be confused and tremulous and have recurrent bouts of vomiting. She was transferred and her diagnosis was changed to aHUS. Plasma exchange and hemodialysis were continued until eculizumab was available for the off-label treatment of her aHUS on day 11. Her mental status improved and her platelet count increased to the normal range by the time of her second eculizumab dose, allowing her to be discharged from the hospital before the third dose of eculizumab. Her subsequent course is notable for gradual improvement of her renal function, allowing her to discontinue hemodialysis 1 year later. During the course, she was also treated with a course of rituximab for her CFH autoantibody, resulting in temporary suppression of the antibody

Table 3
Comparison of TTP and aHUS

Disorder	TTP	aHUS

Pathology	• Microvascular thrombosis
	   ○ VWF platelet aggregates
		• Thrombotic microangiopathy
		   ○ Endothelial injury and disruption
		   ○ Intimal expansion and cell proliferation
		• Abnormal vascular permeability
		   ○ Tissue edema
		   ○ Fluid accumulation in cavitary spaces

Molecular defects	• Severe ADAMTS13 deficiency
	   ○ Autoimmune inhibitors
	   ○ Genetic mutations
		• Defective complement regulation
		   ○ Inactivating mutations[a]
		   ○ Gain-of-function mutations[b]
		   ○ Common genetic variants[c]
		   ○ Autoimmune antibody of CFH

Pathophysiology	• Microvascular thrombosis →
	  ischemic tissue injury
		• Endothelial cell injury
		   ○ Stenosis or thrombosis → ischemia
		   ○ Abnormal vascular permeability

Presentation	• Focal neurologic deficits • Mental status change, seizures • Abdominal pain, pancreatitis • Myocardial infarction	• Abdominal pain, vomiting, diarrhea • Chest pain, pulmonary infiltrates • Mental status change, focal deficits, seizures • Renal failure, hypertension • Anasarca
Course	• Quiescent: no progressive organ dysfunction except in patients with genetic ADAMTS13 deficiency • Episodes of exacerbation	• Chronic: progressive organ injury • Episodes of exacerbation
Treatment	• Plasma exchange • Rituximab as indicated • Plasma infusion (hereditary)	• Eculizumab

[a] Complement factor H (CFH), membrane cofactor protein, complement factor I, or thrombomodulin.
[b] Complement factor H or C3.
[c] Polymorphisms or haplotypes of CFH or complement factor H related proteins; combinations of polymorphisms or haplotypes (complotypes).

that lasted for 3 months. She continued eculizumab for more than 2 years without adverse events. The development of CFH antibody in this patient might have resulted from emergence of autoreactive B-cell clones due to defective autoimmune regulation after myeloablation.

In case 3, a 50-year-old man presented to his doctor with gross hematuria after 2 weeks of shortness of breath, abdominal pain, and vomiting. His blood pressure was 200/140 mm Hg and he became intermittently confused. At the emergency service, his blood pressure had decreased to 106/73 mm Hg. His mental status and blood pressures continued to fluctuate after admission. His prior history was notable for severe brittle hypertension for 3.5 years, during which he sought an emergency care several times for bouts of severe abdominal pain with vomiting, headache, or syncope. At some of these visits, laboratory tests showed mild and self-limited elevation of his creatinine and indirect bilirubin that was attributed by the emergency physicians to his severe hypertension as high as 227/155 mm Hg. After the institution of eculizumab therapy on day 3, his mental status improved and his respiratory and digestive symptoms subsided. His blood pressure stabilized in 2 weeks, allowing the

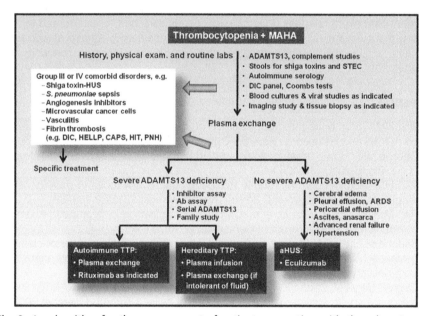

Fig. 9. An algorithm for the management of patients presenting with thrombocytopenia and microangiopathic hemolysis (MAHA). The first steps include history, physical examination, routine laboratory tests, measurement of ADAMTS13, and other tests for the determination of comorbid conditions. Plasma exchange therapy is started to cover the possibility of TTP unless the clinical data and/or ADAMTS13 assay result clearly indicates otherwise. Patients with severe ADAMTS13 should be treated with plasma exchange and possibly rituximab if TTP is autoimmunity-mediated and with plasma infusion if TTP is genetic in nature. Patients without severe ADAMTS13 deficiency are treated as aHUS with eculizumab when shiga toxin and other group III or IV comorbid conditions are excluded as the cause of the patient's MAHA. CAPS, catastrophic antiphospholipid antibody syndrome; DIC, disseminated intravascular coagulopathy; HELLP, the syndrome of hemolysis, elevated liver enzymes and low platelet count; HIT, heparin induced thrombocytopenia; HSCT, hematopoietic stem cell therapy; PNH, paroxysmal nocturnal hemoglobinuria; STEC, shiga toxin producing *Escherichia coli*.

gradual tapering of his hypertension drugs. His kidney biopsy on day 37 showed thrombotic microangiopathy, sclerotic glomeruli, and interstitial fibrosis. His renal function began to show gradual improvement from the 6th week. He continued to experience occasional abdominal pain, nausea, and dizziness on the last 2 to 3 days of his biweekly eculizumab treatment cycle. These symptoms improved when the treatment cycle was shortened to every 12 days.

SUMMARY

Both TTP and aHUS are chronic diseases that often present with thrombocytopenia and microangiopathic hemolysis, yet they have entirely different pathology and pathogenesis and require different therapeutic approaches (**Table 3**). An algorithm for the management of patients presenting with microangiopathic hemolysis is depicted in **Fig. 9**. Patients are started on plasma exchange therapy for presumed TTP unless history and laboratory test results clearly indicate the patient does not require plasma therapy. For acquired TTP, plasma exchange is continued until hematological remission is achieved. The treatment is continued until hematological remission is achieved. Depending on its course, acquired TTP may require rituximab treatment to prevent relapses. Plasma exchange is switched to eculizumab for patients without severe ADAMTS13 deficiency and considered to have aHUS. Both TTP and aHUS are chronic diseases that require long-term monitoring and management.

REFERENCES

1. Tsai HM. Thrombotic thrombocytopenic purpura: a thrombotic disorder caused by ADAMTS13 deficiency. Hematol Oncol Clin North Am 2007;21:609–32, v.
2. George JN. How I treat patients with thrombotic thrombocytopenic purpura: 2010. Blood 2010;116:4060–9.
3. Tsai HM. Autoimmune thrombotic microangiopathy: advances in pathogenesis, diagnosis, and management. Semin Thromb Hemost 2012;38:469–82.
4. Reti M, Farkas P, Csuka D, et al. Complement activation in thrombotic thrombocytopenic purpura. J Thromb Haemost 2012;10:791–8.
5. Sanchez-Luceros A, Farias CE, Amaral MM, et al. von Willebrand factor-cleaving protease (ADAMTS13) activity in normal non-pregnant women, pregnant and post-delivery women. Thromb Haemost 2004;92:1320–6.
6. Cao WJ, Niiya M, Zheng XW, et al. Inflammatory cytokines inhibit ADAMTS13 synthesis in hepatic stellate cells and endothelial cells. J Thromb Haemost 2008;6:1233–5.
7. Motto DG, Chauhan AK, Zhu G, et al. Shigatoxin triggers thrombotic thrombocytopenic purpura in genetically susceptible ADAMTS13-deficient mice. J Clin Invest 2005;115:2752–61.
8. Banno F, Kokame K, Okuda T, et al. Complete deficiency in ADAMTS13 is prothrombotic, but it alone is not sufficient to cause thrombotic thrombocytopenic purpura. Blood 2006;107:3161–6.
9. Schiviz A, Wuersch K, Piskernik C, et al. A new mouse model mimicking thrombotic thrombocytopenic purpura: correction of symptoms by recombinant human ADAMTS13. Blood 2012;119:6128–35.
10. Feys HB, Roodt J, Vandeputte N, et al. Thrombotic thrombocytopenic purpura directly linked with ADAMTS13 inhibition in the baboon (Papio ursinus). Blood 2010;116:2005–10.

11. Ermini L, Goodship TH, Strain L, et al. Common genetic variants in complement genes other than CFH, CD46 and the CFHRs are not associated with aHUS. Mol Immunol 2012;49:640–8.
12. Heurich M, Martinez-Barricarte R, Francis NJ, et al. Common polymorphisms in C3, factor B, and factor H collaborate to determine systemic complement activity and disease risk. Proc Natl Acad Sci U S A 2011;108:8761–6.
13. Dragon-Durey MA, Sethi SK, Bagga A, et al. Clinical features of anti-factor H autoantibody-associated hemolytic uremic syndrome. J Am Soc Nephrol 2010; 21:2180–7.
14. Noris M, Caprioli J, Bresin E, et al. Relative role of genetic complement abnormalities in sporadic and familial aHUS and their impact on clinical phenotype. Clin J Am Soc Nephrol 2010;5:1844–59.
15. Fakhouri F, Roumenina L, Provot F, et al. Pregnancy-associated hemolytic uremic syndrome revisited in the era of complement gene mutations. J Am Soc Nephrol 2010;21:859–67.
16. Tsai HM, Rice L, Sarode R, et al. Antibody inhibitors to von Willebrand factor metalloproteinase and increased binding of von Willebrand factor to platelets in ticlopidine-associated thrombotic thrombocytopenic purpura. Ann Intern Med 2000;132:794–9.
17. Hirata S, Okamoto H, Ohta S, et al. Deficient activity of von Willebrand factor-cleaving protease in thrombotic thrombocytopenic purpura in the setting of adult-onset Still's disease. Rheumatology (Oxford) 2006;45:1046–7.
18. Torok N, Niazi M, Al AY, et al. Thrombotic thrombocytopenic purpura associated with anti-glomerular basement membrane disease. Nephrol Dial Transplant 2010; 25:3446–9.
19. Salmon JE, Heuser C, Triebwasser M, et al. Mutations in complement regulatory proteins predispose to preeclampsia: a genetic analysis of the PROMISSE cohort. PLoS Med 2011;8:e1001013.
20. Tsai HM. Mechanisms of microvascular thrombosis in thrombotic thrombocytopenic purpura. Kidney Int Suppl 2009;(112):S11–4.
21. Manea M, Kristoffersson A, Schneppenheim R, et al. Podocytes express ADAMTS13 in normal renal cortex and in patients with thrombotic thrombocytopenic purpura. Br J Haematol 2007;138:651–62.
22. Gutterman LA, Kloster B, Tsai HM. Rituximab therapy for refractory thrombotic thrombocytopenic purpura. Blood Cells Mol Dis 2002;28:385–91.
23. Elliott MA, Heit JA, Pruthi RK, et al. Rituximab for refractory and or relapsing thrombotic thrombocytopenic purpura related to immune-mediated severe ADAMTS13-deficiency: a report of four cases and a systematic review of the literature. Eur J Haematol 2009;83(4):365–72.
24. Scully M, McDonald V, Cavenagh J, et al. A phase 2 study of the safety and efficacy of rituximab with plasma exchange in acute acquired thrombotic thrombocytopenic purpura. Blood 2011;118:1746–53.
25. Hart D, Sayer R, Miller R, et al. Human immunodeficiency virus associated thrombotic thrombocytopenic purpura–favourable outcome with plasma exchange and prompt initiation of highly active antiretroviral therapy. Br J Haematol 2011;153:515–9.
26. Cataland SR, Jin M, Lin S, et al. Effect of prophylactic cyclosporine therapy on ADAMTS13 biomarkers in patients with idiopathic thrombotic thrombocytopenic purpura. Am J Hematol 2008;83:911–5.
27. Loirat C, Babu S, Furman R, et al. Eculizumab efficacy and safety inpatients with atypical hemolyticuremic syndrome (aHUS) resistanttoplasmaexchange/infusion. Haematologica 2011;96:S2–979.

28. Loirat C, Muus P, Legendre C, et al. A phase II study of eculizumab in patients with atypical hemolyticuremic syndrome receiving chronic plasma exchange/infusion. Haematologica 2011;96:S2–980.

29. Kelly RJ, Hill A, Arnold LM, et al. Long-term treatment with eculizumab in paroxysmal nocturnal hemoglobinuria: sustained efficacy and improved survival. Blood 2011;117:6786–92.

30. Saland JM, Ruggenenti P, Remuzzi G. Liver-kidney transplantation to cure atypical hemolytic uremic syndrome. J Am Soc Nephrol 2009;20:940–9.

31. Weitz M, Amon O, Bassler D, et al. Prophylactic eculizumab prior to kidney transplantation for atypical hemolytic uremic syndrome. Pediatr Nephrol 2011;26:1325–9.

32. Nester C, Stewart Z, Myers D, et al. Pre-emptive eculizumab and plasmapheresis for renal transplant in atypical hemolytic uremic syndrome. Clin J Am Soc Nephrol 2011;6:1488–94.

Inherited Platelet Function Disorders

Overview and Disorders of Granules, Secretion, and Signal Transduction

A. Koneti Rao, MD

KEYWORDS

- Inherited platelet function disorders • Platelet secretion disorders
- Storage pool deficiency • Signal transduction defects • Scott syndrome

KEY POINTS

- Inherited disorders of platelet function are characterized by highly variable mucocutaneous bleeding manifestations that are mild to moderate in most patients.
- The platelet dysfunction in these patients arises by diverse mechanisms, including abnormalities in platelet membrane glycoproteins, granules, signaling and secretion mechanisms, and procoagulant activities.
- In the vast majority of patients suspected to have an inherited platelet function defect, the molecular and genetic mechanisms are unknown.
- Platelet aggregation and secretion studies using platelet-rich plasma form the primary basis for the diagnosis of an inherited platelet dysfunction in most patients.
- The therapeutic options in these patients include platelet transfusions, DDAVP, recombinant factor VIIa, and antifibrinolytic agents.

PLATELET FUNCTION IN HEMOSTASIS

Following injury to the blood vessel, platelets adhere to exposed subendothelium by a process (adhesion) that involves, among other events, the interaction of a plasma protein, von Willebrand factor (vWF), and a specific glycoprotein complex on the platelet surface, glycoprotein (GP) Ib-IX-V (GPIb-IX) (**Fig. 1**). This interaction is particularly important for platelet adhesion under conditions of high shear stress. Adhesion is followed by recruitment of additional platelets that form clumps, a process called aggregation (cohesion). This platelet-platelet interaction involves binding of fibrinogen to

Hematology Section, Department of Medicine and Sol Sherry Thrombosis Research Center, Temple University School of Medicine, 3400 North Broad Street, OMS-300, Philadelphia, PA 19140, USA

E-mail address: koneti@temple.edu

Hematol Oncol Clin N Am 27 (2013) 585–611
http://dx.doi.org/10.1016/j.hoc.2013.02.005
0889-8588/13/$ – see front matter © 2013 Elsevier Inc. All rights reserved.

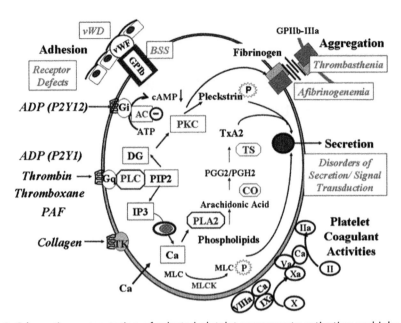

Fig. 1. Schematic representation of selected platelet responses to activation and inherited disorders of platelet function. AC, adenylyl cyclase; ADP, adenosine diphosphate; BSS, Bernard-Soulier syndrome; CO, cyclooxygenase; DAG, diacylglycerol; G, guanosine triphosphate–binding protein; IP3, inositol trisphosphate; MLC, myosin light chain; MLCK, myosin light chain kinase; PAF, platelet activating factor; PIP2, phosphatidylinositol bisphosphate; PKC, protein kinase C; PLA2, phospholipase A2; PLC, phospholipase C; TK, tyrosine kinase; TS, thromboxane synthase; TxA2, thromboxane A2; vWD, von Willebrand disease; vWF, von Willebrand factor. The Roman numerals in the circles represent coagulation factors. (*Modified from* Rao AK. Congenital disorders of platelet function: disorders of signal transduction and secretion. Am J Med Sci 1998;316:69–76; with permission.)

specific platelet surface receptors, a complex composed of GPIIb-IIIa (integrin αIIbβ3). Resting platelets do not bind fibrinogen and platelet activation induces a conformational change in the GPIIb-IIIa complex that leads to fibrinogen binding. Activated platelets release the contents of their granules (secretion), including ADP and serotonin from the dense granules, which causes the recruitment of additional platelets. In addition, contents of the α-granules and other vesicles are also released. Moreover, platelets play a major role in coagulation mechanisms; several key enzymatic reactions occur on the platelet membrane lipoprotein surface. During platelet activation, the negatively charged phospholipids, especially phosphatidylserine, become exposed on the platelet surface, an essential step for accelerating specific coagulation reactions by promoting the binding of coagulation factors involved in thrombin generation (platelet procoagulant activity).

A number of physiologic agonists interact with specific receptors on the platelet surface to induce responses, including a change in platelet shape from discoid to spherical (shape change), aggregation, secretion, and thromboxane A_2 (TxA$_2$) production. Other agonists, such as prostacyclin, inhibit these responses by increasing cyclic AMP levels (cAMP). Binding of agonists to platelet receptors initiates the production or release of several intracellular messenger molecules, including products of hydrolysis of phosphoinositide (PI) by phospholipase C (diacylglycerol and inositol 1,4,5-triphosphate [InsP$_3$]), TxA$_2$, and cyclic nucleotides (cAMP) (see **Fig. 1**). These induce or modulate the various platelet responses of Ca^{2+} mobilization, protein phosphorylation, aggregation, secretion, and thromboxane production. The interaction between the platelet surface receptors and the key intracellular enzymes (eg, phospholipases A_2 and C, adenylyl cyclase) is mediated by a group of proteins that bind and are modulated by guanosine triphosphate (G proteins). As in most secretory cells, platelet activation results in an increase in cytoplasmic ionized calcium concentration; $InsP_3$ functions as a messenger to mobilize Ca^{2+} from intracellular stores. Diacylglycerol activates protein kinase C (PKC), and this results in the phosphorylation of several proteins. PKC activation plays a major role in regulating responses, including platelet secretion and the activation of GPIIb-IIIa. Numerous other mechanisms, such as activation of tyrosine kinases and phosphatases, are also triggered by platelet activation. Inherited or acquired defects in these platelet mechanisms may lead to impairment of the platelet role in hemostasis.

INHERITED DISORDERS OF PLATELET FUNCTION: AN OVERVIEW

Disorders of platelet function are characterized by highly variable mucocutaneous bleeding manifestations and excessive hemorrhage following surgical procedures or trauma. Spontaneous hemarthrosis and deep hematomas are distinctly unusual in patients with platelet defects. In general, most patients have mild to moderate bleeding manifestations. Most patients, but not all, have a prolonged bleeding time. Platelet aggregation and secretion studies using platelet-rich plasma (PRP) provide evidence for platelet dysfunction but are, in general, neither predictive of severity of clinical manifestations nor the molecular mechanisms. Defects in platelet function may be inherited or acquired, with the latter being far more commonly encountered. The platelet dysfunction in these patients arises by diverse mechanisms. In the vast majority of patients suspected to have an inherited platelet function defect based on family studies, the molecular and genetic mechanisms are unknown.

Box 1 provides a classification of inherited disorders associated with impaired platelet function, based on the platelet function or responses that are abnormal (see **Fig. 1**). Of note, not all of them are caused by a defect in the platelets per se. Some, such as von Willebrand disease (vWD) and afibrinogenemia, result from deficiencies of plasma proteins essential for platelet adhesion or aggregation. Some of these disorders are distinctly rare, but they shed enormous light on platelet physiology. Moreover, in many patients with inherited abnormal platelet aggregation responses, the underlying molecular mechanisms remain unknown. In patients with defects in platelet–vessel wall interactions (adhesion disorders), adhesion of platelets to subendothelium is abnormal. The 2 disorders in this group are vWD, in which there is a deficiency or abnormality in plasma vWF, and the Bernard-Soulier syndrome (BSS), in which platelets are deficient in GPIb (and GPV and GPIX); in both disorders, platelet-vWF interaction is compromised. Binding of fibrinogen to the GPIIb-IIIa complex is a prerequisite for platelet aggregation. Disorders characterized by abnormal platelet-platelet interactions (aggregation disorders) arise because of a severe deficiency of plasma fibrinogen (congenital afibrinogenemia) or because of a quantitative or qualitative abnormality of the platelet membrane GPIIb-IIIa complex, which binds fibrinogen (Glanzmann thrombasthenia). Patients with defects in platelet secretion and signal transduction are a heterogeneous group lumped together for convenience of classification rather than based on an understanding of the specific underlying abnormality. The major common characteristics in these patients, as currently perceived, are abnormal aggregation responses and an inability to release intracellular granule (dense) contents on activation of PRP with agonists, such as ADP, epinephrine, and

---

Box 1
Inherited disorders of platelet function

1. Defects in platelet–vessel wall interaction (disorders of adhesion)

   a. von Willebrand disease (deficiency or defect in plasma vWF)

   b. Bernard-Soulier syndrome (deficiency or defect in GPIb)

2. Defects in platelet-platelet interaction (disorders of aggregation)

   a. Congenital afibrinogenemia (deficiency of plasma fibrinogen)

   b. Glanzmann thrombasthenia (deficiency or defect in GPIIb-IIIa)

3. Disorders of platelet secretion and abnormalities of granules

   a. Storage pool deficiency (δ, α, $\alpha\delta$)

   b. Quebec platelet disorder

4. Disorders of platelet secretion and signal transduction

   a. Defects in platelet-agonist interaction (receptor defects) (ADP, thromboxane A_2, collagen, epinephrine)

   b. Defects in G-proteins (Gαq, Gαs, Gαi abnormalities)

   c. Defects in phosphatidylinositol metabolism and protein phosphorylation

   Phospholipase C-β2 deficiency

   PKC-θ deficiency

   d. Abnormalities in arachidonic acid pathways and thromboxane A_2 synthesis

   Phospholipase A2 deficiency

   Cyclooxygenase deficiency

   Thromboxane synthase deficiency

5. Disorders of platelet coagulant-protein interaction (Scott syndrome)

6. Defects related to cytoskeletal/structural proteins

   a. Wiskott-Aldrich syndrome

   b. β1 tubulin deficiency

   c. Kindlin-3 deficiency (leukocyte adhesion defect-III)

7. Abnormalities of transcription factors leading to functional defects

   a. RUNX1 (Familial platelet dysfunction with predisposition to acute myelogenous leukemia);

   b. GATA-1

---

collagen. In general, in platelet studies, the primary wave of aggregation is present but the second wave is blunted or absent. In these patients, the platelet dysfunction arises from diverse mechanisms. A small proportion have a deficiency of dense granule or their stores (storage pool deficiency). In other patients, the impaired secretion results from aberrations in the signal transduction events or other mechanisms, such as in pathways leading to thromboxane synthesis, in mechanisms that govern end-responses of secretion and aggregation. The findings on the aggregation studies are nonspecific and it is difficult to conclude a specific abnormality from the tracings. Another group consists of patients who have an abnormality in interactions of platelets with proteins of the coagulation system; the best described is the Scott syndrome, which is characterized by impaired transmembrane migration of procoagulant–phosphatidylserine during platelet activation. Defects related to platelet cytoskeletal or structural proteins may also be associated with platelet dysfunction. Recent studies document impaired platelet function associated with mutations in transcription factors (eg, RUNX1, GATA1, FLI-1) that regulate expression of important platelet proteins. In addition to these groups, there are patients who have abnormal platelet function associated with systemic disorders, such as Down syndrome and the May-Hegglin anomaly, in which the specific aberrant platelet mechanisms are unclear. The prevalence and relative frequencies of the various platelet abnormalities described previously remain unknown. Disorders related to platelet membrane glycoproteins are described in the article by Drs Reyhan Diz-Kücükkaya and José A. López, elsewhere in this issue. Other inherited platelet disorders are reviewed here.

DISORDERS OF PLATELET SECRETION, GRANULES, AND SIGNAL TRANSDUCTION

Patients lumped in this remarkably heterogeneous group of platelet secretion defects generally manifest decreased aggregation and absence of the second wave of aggregation on stimulation of PRP with ADP and epinephrine, and impaired secretion of dense granule contents; responses to collagen, thromboxane analog (U46619), arachidonic acid, and thrombin receptor peptides may also be impaired. Simplistically in these patients, platelet secretion and function are abnormal either because the granules or their contents are diminished (SPD) or when there are aberrations in the signaling or activation mechanisms that lead to aggregation and secretion on platelet activation (see **Fig. 1**).

During the late 1960s, several investigators described patients with bleeding disorders associated with abnormalities in platelet aggregation induced by collagen, ADP, and epinephrine.[1,2] In some of these patients, the abnormal platelet responses were attributed to a defect in the secretion of ADP. In 1969, Weiss and colleagues[3] reported a family with impaired platelet aggregation whose platelets had decreased amounts of ADP. Holmsen and Weiss[4,5] subsequently established that the defect in this family was a deficiency in the nonmetabolic pool of ADP that is stored in the dense granules, leading to the entity being called "storage pool deficiency" (SPD). In 1982, Rao and colleagues[6] reported 5 patients with a lifelong bleeding diathesis whose platelets had decreased aggregation, and diminished secretion of dense granule and acid hydrolase secretion even though their platelets had normal granule stores and thromboxane production. Such patients without SPD or defective TxA$_2$ production were subsequently referred to as "primary secretion defects"[7,8] and described in several reports.[9–12] Such patients are more common than those with thrombasthenia, BSS, SPD, or defects in TxA$_2$ production. In some of them, there is evidence for abnormalities in the specific signaling proteins or events that precede aggregation and secretion.

DISORDERS OF PLATELET GRANULES
SPD

The term SPD now encompasses patients with deficiencies in the platelet contents of dense granules (δ-SPD), α-granules (α-SPD) (gray platelet syndrome), or both types of granules (αδ-SPD). Another α-granule disorder is the Quebec platelet disorder (QPD), which is associated with abnormal proteolysis of several α-granule proteins.

δ-SPD

Patients with δ-SPD have a mild to moderate bleeding diathesis associated with a prolonged bleeding time.[2,13] In the platelet studies, the second wave of aggregation in response to ADP and epinephrine is absent or blunted, and the collagen response is markedly decreased (**Fig. 2**). Both impaired and normal aggregation responses to arachidonic acid have been noted. These conflicting observations may be related to the severity of platelet ADP deficiency. The responses to epinephrine may also be variable; a second wave of aggregation has been noted in some patients. Interestingly, δ-SPD has been documented[14] in some patients with prolonged bleeding times and normal aggregation responses. Normal bleeding times have also been observed in δ-SPD. Thrombin-induced secretion of acid hydrolases is impaired in SPD platelets; this is corrected by addition of exogenous ADP, suggesting that it is secondary to the ADP deficiency and secretion.

Normal platelets possess 3 to 8 dense granules (each 200–300 nm in diameter). Under the electron microscope, platelet-dense granules are decreased in δ-SPD. Other methods to demonstrate a decrease in the dense granules include fluorescence microscopy after staining platelets with mepacrine (quinacrine) and specific staining by uranyl ions (uranaffin reaction). By direct biochemical measurements, the total platelet and granule ATP and ADP contents are decreased along with other dense granule constituents, calcium, pyrophosphate, and serotonin. Two-thirds of platelet ATP and ADP resides in the dense granules with a smaller amount in the metabolic pool; dense granules have proportionally greater ADP than ATP.[15] Thus, in δ-SPD platelets, the ratio of total ATP to ADP increases (>2.5) compared with normal platelets.

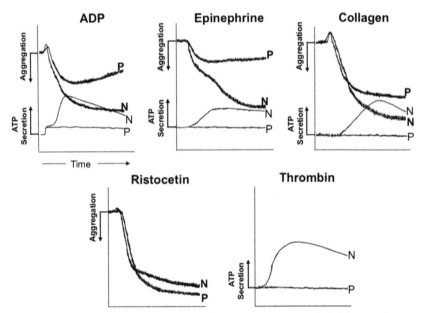

Fig. 2. Aggregation and ATP secretion studies in δ-storage pool deficiency. Shown are responses of the patient (P) and a healthy subject (N) to ADP (7.5 μM), epinephrine (7.5 μM), collagen (1 μg/mL), ristocetin (1.5 μg/mL) and thrombin (2 u/mL). In the patient, only the primary wave of aggregation is noted with ADP and epinephrine; aggregation is blunted with collagen. Secretion is decreased with all agonists except ristocetin. With thrombin only secretion is shown because addition of thrombin induces clotting of fibrinogen and does not permit recording of aggregation. (*Reprinted from* Rao AK, Essex DW. Platelet function in hemostasis and inherited disorders of platelet number and function. In: Schmaier AH, Lazarus HM, editors. Concise Guide to Hematology. Oxford (United Kingdom): Wiley-Blackwell; 2012. p. 140–53.)

Incubation of normal platelets with ^{14}C-serotonin results in its incorporation into dense granules. This serotonin is subsequently secreted on activation, providing a method to assess dense granule secretion. In normal platelets, the incorporated ^{14}C-serotonin remains in the platelet over 4 to 6 hours of incubation, being protected from the mitochondrial monoamine oxidases because of its sequestration in the dense granules. In SPD platelets, the uptake of ^{14}C serotonin is normal; however, this serotonin is metabolized by the cytoplasmic monoamine oxidases to 5-hydroxyindoleacetic acid and 5-hydroxytryptophol, resulting in the loss of the radioactive label from the platelets.

Other Abnormalities in δ-SPD

Other associated abnormalities have been described in some patients, including in synthesis of prostaglandins, thromboxane A2 and malondialdehyde, and in platelet procoagulant activity (prothrombinase activity) in association with an inability of δ-SPD platelets to maintain elevated intracellular Ca^{2+} levels.[1,2] Both the Ca^{2+} defect and the decreased prothrombinase activity are corrected by addition of exogenous ADP, indicating that dense granule constituents may play a role in these responses.

δ-SPD has been reported in association with other inherited disorders, such as the Hermansky-Pudlak syndrome (HPS) (a combination of oculocutaneous albinism, nystagmus, and increased reticuloendothelial ceroid), the Chediak-Higashi syndrome (CHS), the Wiskott-Aldrich syndrome (WAS), the thrombocytopenia-absent-radii (TAR) syndrome, and the Griscelli syndrome.[16–18] The simultaneous occurrence of δ-SPD and defects in skin pigment granules, as in the HPS, point to the interrelatedness of the 2 kinds of granules (dense granules and melanosomes) with respect to genetic control. This concept has been strongly supported by studies in animal models that combine platelet defects with pigment disorders.[16,18]

Pathogenesis

Studies in animal models suggest that dense granule abnormalities may occur by different mechanisms and involve defects at the megakaryocyte level. Dense granules are absent in megakaryocytes of CHS cattle that also have a pigmentary disorder, suggesting defective organelle development. In some mouse models (also having a pigment disorder), platelets have been found to have a substantial or normal number of mepacrine-positive granules, suggesting that there may be functional defect leading to impaired localization of the nucleotides to the granules, rather than a lack of granule formation. In line with this, some patients with HPS and δ-SPD have markedly decreased dense granules, suggesting an abnormality in granule development, whereas some patients without HPS have had the presence of uranaffin and mepacrine-positive granules but with a lack of dense core ("empty granules"), suggesting a more qualitative granule defect. Dense granule membranes possess the lysosomal proteins LAMP2 (lysosomal-associated membrane protein-2) and CD63 (granulophysin or LAMP3), as well as P-selectin and GPIIb-IIIa. Granulophysin has been shown to be deficient in some HPS platelets.[19] Studies with antigranulophysin antibody demonstrated the presence of a normal number of platelet granules in 2 patients with SPD who were not albino[20]; these patients, thus, have the granules but with reduced contents.

A substantial amount of our information in SPD has been obtained from patients with HPS, which is characterized by oculocutaneous albinism, platelet SPD, and lipofuscinosis.[16,17] There is a large group of patients with HPS in northwest Puerto Rico where HPS occurs in 1 of every 1800 individuals (gene frequency 1 in 21). There are at least 9 known HPS-causing genes leading to 9 subtypes of human HPS, with most of the patients being in HPS-1 and from Puerto Rico.[13,16,18] There are more than 15 mouse models of HPS reported to date; many of these constitute models for the human subtypes.[13,16,18] Together, the human and mouse models have been an invaluable source of basic information of vesicle formation and trafficking. The human HPS subtypes are autosomal recessive and the heterozygotes have no clinical findings. In addition to the albinism that is variable among the HPS subtypes, most patients have congenital nystagmus and decreased visual acuities. Moreover, approximately 15% of the patients develop granulomatous colitis,[17] which resembles Crohn disease in pathology and in response to treatment. Another manifestation is pulmonary fibrosis, a crippling end result of an inflammatory process. An antifibrotic agent pirfenidone appears to slow the progression of pulmonary fibrosis. Of the multiple HPS subtypes, HPS-1 is the most severe and prevalent form of HPS. It arises from mutations in the *HPS-1* gene; the most frequent HPS-1 mutation is a 16-bp duplication in exon 15, although other mutations have been noted. In general, with one exception (HPS-2) caused by mutations in *AP3B1,* all of the HPS-causing genes encode novel proteins. The gene defective in HPS-2, *AP3B1,* codes for the β3A subunit of AP3, a heterotetrameric complex responsible for vesicle formation from the trans-Golgi network.[16,18]

CHS is a rare autosomal recessive disorder characterized by SPD, oculocutaneous albinism, immune deficiency, neurologic dysfunction, and the presence of giant cytoplasmic inclusions in different cells.[16,18] Patients with CHS have defective cytotoxic T and NK cell function. CHS arises from mutations in the lysosomal trafficking regulator (*LYST*) gene on chromosome 1. The protein coded by *LYST* interacts with several proteins, including the SNARE complex protein HRS and signaling proteins, and participates in intracellular membrane fusion reactions and vesicle trafficking.

α-granule SPD (Gray Platelet Syndrome)

The rubric "gray-platelet syndrome" (GPS) has been derived from the initial observation by Raccuglia in 1971[21] of a gray appearance of platelets with paucity of granules in peripheral blood smears from a patient with a lifelong bleeding disorder. Patients with GPS have an isolated deficiency of α-granule contents.[22,23] They have a lifelong bleeding diathesis, mostly of autosomal recessive inheritance, mild thrombocytopenia, and prolonged bleeding time. Under the electron microscope, platelets and megakaryocytes reveal absent or markedly decreased α-granules. The platelets are deficient in α-granule proteins: platelet factor-4, β-thromboglobulin, vWF, thrombospondin, fibronectin, factor V, high molecular weight kininogen, and platelet-derived growth factor. Platelet aggregation responses have been variable. Responses to ADP and epinephrine were normal in most patients; in some patients, aggregation responses to thrombin, collagen, and ADP have been impaired. There is increased reticulin in the bone marrow from patients with GPS; this has been attributed to elevated plasma PDGF levels.

GPS is a markedly heterogeneous disorder characterized by thrombocytopenia, large platelet size, and deficiency of α-granules and their contents, which includes proteins synthesized by MK (eg, PF4, β-thromboglobulin) and those incorporated by endocytosis into the granules (eg, albumin, fibrinogen, immunoglobulin [Ig] G).[22,24] The molecular mechanisms leading to α-granule deficiency in GPS and in αδ-SPD are unclear; they have been attributed to multiple mechanisms including failure of α-granule maturation during MK differentiation; of transport or targeting of proteins to α-granules; and synthesis of granule membranes.[22,24] Proteomic studies in a patients with GPS suggested a failure to incorporate endogenously synthesized MK proteins into α-granules.[24] Some patients with GPS have elevated plasma PF4,[22] suggesting that PF4 synthesis was normal and the primary defect was impaired granule biogenesis with leakage of PF4. Several patients with decreased α-granule contents have had a mutation in transcription factor RUNX1,[25,26] and PF4 is a transcriptional target of RUNX1.[27] This suggests that in some patients, decreased platelet PF4 level may be due to a defect in transcriptional regulation and synthesis of PF4. GPS has been reported[28] in a patient with an X-linked thrombocytopenia, thalassemia, and Arg216Gln mutation in GATA-1, a major regulator of megakaryopoiesis. GATA-1 knockdown mice have granule abnormalities with a decrease in PF4 mRNA in primary MK.[29] Moreover, a mutation in VPS33B protein (a member of the Sec1/Munc18 protein family) involved in vesicle trafficking has been associated with human α-granule deficiency in the arthrogryposis multiplex congenital, renal dysfunction, and cholestasis (ARC) syndrome.[30] More recently, a mutation in *VPS16B* gene has also been linked to α-granule deficiency in the ARC syndrome, and it appears that VPS16B and VPS33B interact with each other.[31] Three groups[32–34] have recently reported mutations in *NBEAL2*, a gene that encodes for a protein linked to vesicle transport in neuronal cells. Together, these studies elegantly implicate defective vesicle transport as a major mechanism in GPS. Overall, it appears that the mechanisms are likely different in individual patients with GPS; the inheritance of α-granule deficiency has been autosomal recessive in most reports, and autosomal dominant or sex-linked in some.[22,25,26,28]

Quebec Platelet Disorder

QPD is an autosomal dominant disorder associated with delayed bleeding and abnormal proteolysis of α-granule proteins due to increased amounts of platelet urokinase–type plasminogen activator arising from random duplication of *PLAU* gene.[35,36] These patients have had normal to reduced platelet counts, proteolytic degradation of α-granule proteins, deficiency of α-granule multimerin (a factor V binding protein), and defective aggregation selectively with epinephrine. Platelet factor V, but not plasma factor V, is degraded along with several other α-granule proteins (fibrinogen, vWF, thrombospondin, osteonectin, fibronectin, and P-selectin). The platelets have increased fibrinolytic activity.[36] They appear morphologically normal under the light microscope. Patients with QPD suffer from mucocutaneous bleeding, which is often delayed by 12 to 24 hours following injury and unresponsive to platelet transfusions but responsive to fibrinolytic inhibitors.

DISORDERS OF SECRETION CAUSED BY DEFECTS IN PLATELET SIGNALING MECHANISMS

Signal transduction events encompass processes that are triggered by the interaction of agonists with specific platelet receptors and result in the activation of effectors, such as phospholipase C (PLC) and phospholipase A_2 (PLA2) (see **Fig. 1**), leading ultimately to end responses of aggregation and secretion. The link between the surface receptors for several agonists (eg, ADP, epinephrine, thrombin, and thromboxane A_2) and the effector enzymes is provided by G-proteins. Simplistically, if the key components of platelet signal transduction mechanisms are the surface receptors, the G-proteins, and the effectors, evidence now exists for specific platelet abnormalities at each of these levels.

Defects in Platelet-Agonist Interaction: Receptor Defects

Impaired platelet responses because of an abnormality in platelet surface receptors have been documented for TxA_2, collagen, ADP, epinephrine, and PAF.[1,2] Because ADP and TxA_2 play a synergistic role in amplifying the platelet responses to other agonists, patients with defects in the ADP or TxA$_2$ receptor have impaired responses to other agonists as well, including collagen and thrombin.

Thromboxane A$_2$ receptor defect

Mutations in the platelet TxA$_2$ receptor have been reported by Hirata and colleagues,[37] who described an Arg^{60} to Leu mutation in the first cytoplasmic loop of the TxA$_2$ receptor in 2 unrelated patients. This Arg^{60} corresponds to a highly conserved basic residue among G-protein coupled receptors.[37] These patients had a mild bleeding disorder with an autosomal dominant pattern of inheritance. Aggregation responses to several agonists were impaired with the exception of thrombin.[38] The binding of TxA$_2$ analogs to platelets was normal.[38,39] GTPase activity on activation with a TxA$_2$ analog, but not thrombin, was diminished,[39,40] suggesting a defect in TxA$_2$ receptor–G-protein coupling. TxA$_2$-induced activation of PLC (measured as Ca^{2+} mobilization, and inositol trisphosphate and phosphatidic acid formation) was impaired, whereas PLA$_2$ activation and TxA$_2$ production were normal. Fewer than half the number of TxA$_2$ receptors are sufficient for irreversible aggregation with TxA$_2$ agonist.[41] The finding that the aggregation responses were impaired in the heterozygous family members[37] suggest a dominant negative effect of the mutation. Last, impaired aggregation response to TxA$_2$ has also been observed in patients without evidence for a defect of TxA$_2$ receptor.

Defects in platelet ADP receptors (P2Y1, P2Y2, and P2X1)

At least 3 receptors (P2Y1, P2Y12, P2X1) mediate ADP interaction with platelets (see the review by Brass and colleagues elsewhere in this issue). P2Y$_1$ receptors induce PLC activation, intracellular Ca^{2+} mobilization, and shape change, whereas P2Y$_{12}$ receptors mediate inhibition of cAMP formation by adenylyl cyclase. ADP-induced platelet aggregation requires activation of both P2Y$_1$ and P2Y$_{12}$ receptors. P2X$_1$ receptors function as an ATP-gated and ADP-gated cation channel. Several patients have been described with P2Y$_{12}$ receptor abnormalities, characterized by blunted ADP-induced platelet aggregation responses, impaired ADP suppression of PGE$_1$-induced elevation in cAMP, and normal ADP-stimulated shape change.[42] Patients' symptoms have ranged in severity, with moderately severe hemorrhage in association with surgery and trauma and prolonged bleeding times. Because released ADP potentiates the responses to other agonists, such as collagen and thromboxane A$_2$, platelet aggregation in response to these agonists are also abnormal. Platelet binding of ADP or the ADP analog 2-methylthio-ADP was decreased in almost all of these patients.

The genetic defects have been defined in some of these patients. Three patients have had homozygous deletions in the P2Y$_{12}$ gene, resulting in premature termination and a lack of P2Y$_{12}$ protein.[42,43] A homozygous missense mutation in the translation initiation codon was described in another patient,[44] and another patient was reported to have a 2-nucleotide deletion (at amino acid 240) in one P2Y$_{12}$ gene allele, resulting in a frame shift and a premature stop codon.[45,46] Although this last patient had one P2Y$_{12}$ allele with a normal coding region, the patient's platelets lacked P2Y$_{12}$ receptors, suggesting repression of the normal allele or an unrelated abnormality in its transcriptional regulation. In contrast, platelets from the patient's daughter had an intermediate number of ADP-binding sites, a normal platelet response to ADP, and one frame-shifted allele and one normal allele, suggesting that the mutant allele does not act in a dominant negative manner.[45] Studies in yet another patient with abnormal ADP-induced aggregation revealed a compound heterozygous state encompassing an R256N substitution and an R265W substitution in the 2 alleles.[47] The former mutation was in the sixth transmembrane domain and the latter was in the third extracellular loop of the receptor. Interestingly, platelet binding of ^{33}P-2MeS ADP was normal. In expression studies in Chinese hamster ovary cells, neither mutation affected the translocation of the P2Y$_{12}$ receptor to the cell surface, but ADP-induced inhibition of adenylyl cyclase was partially reduced, indicating a functional abnormality. In another study involving screening 92 patients with type 1 vWD, a heterozygous mutation in the second extracellular loop of P2Y$_{12}$ was identified in one patient and several family members[48]; this was associated with decreased 2MeS-ADP binding and modest defects in ADP-induced platelet aggregation. Thus, in some patients with vWD, the added platelet defect may contribute to the overall bleeding. Another heterozygous mutation, P258T in the third extracellular loop, has been described in association with a bleeding diathesis.[49]

A defect in the P2X$_1$ purinergic receptor has been described in a 6-year-old patient with a history of petechiae, ecchymoses, and severe expistaxis.[50] The patient had isolated impairment of ADP-induced platelet aggregation and was heterozygous for a deletion of a single leucine in a stretch of 4 leucine residues (351–354) in the second transmembrane domain of P2X$_1$. The mutant protein apparently caused a dominant negative effect on P2X$_1$-mediated calcium channel activity.

A preliminary report of one patient with a defect in the P2Y1 platelet receptor, which is coupled to PLC and ADP-induced calcium mobilization, described impaired platelet aggregation in response to ADP and other agonists.[51]

Defects in platelet collagen receptors
Platelet-collagen interaction is important in hemostasis and thrombosis. Collagen is a substrate for platelet adhesion, a binding site for vWF in the extracellular matrix, and an agonist for platelet aggregation and secretion. Two receptors, GPVI[52] and the integrin $\alpha2\beta1$,[53,54] mediate the platelet-collagen interaction.

GPVI, a member of the immunoglobulin gene superfamily, is associated with the Fc receptor γ chain in the platelet plasma membrane. Murine platelets lacking either the γ chain or Syk are unable to respond to collagen and the interaction of GPVI-deficient human platelets with either immobilized and soluble collagen is markedly impaired.

There are several reports of patients with congenital GPVI deficiency.[2] They have had mild to severe mucocutaneous bleeding and their platelets failed to aggregate following stimulation with collagen despite the presence of normal amounts of $\alpha2\beta1$, but retained some ability to adhere to collagen-coated surfaces. GPVI deficiency has also been reported in a patient with GPS.[22] Several patients have been described whose plasma contained autoantibodies against GPVI that inhibited collagen-induced platelet function[2]; platelets of these patients have had little or no detectable GPVI on the platelet surface, and no mutations in GPVI were noted. In some patients, GPVI was restored on platelets following treatment of the immunologic disease. These studies suggest that the autoantibodies selectively deplete platelet GPVI.

The integrin $\alpha2\beta1$ (GPIa-IIa, VLA-2) also serves as a platelet collagen receptor. Current models suggest that the initial platelet tethering of platelets is mediated by platelet GPIb-IX-V binding to vWF bound to collagen and this enables GPVI to bind to collagen and generate "outside-in" signals. These signals increase the affinity of $\alpha2\beta1$ for collagen, resulting in a firm platelet adhesion to collagen. Several patients have been reported whose platelets lacked $\alpha2\beta1$ and impaired interaction with collagen. Of 2 patients with bleeding diatheses, platelets from one contained approximately 15% to 25% of the normal amount of $\alpha2$, failed to aggregate in response to collagen, and failed to adhere to collagen under both static and flow conditions,[55,56] whereas platelets from the second patient lacked $\alpha2$, as well as the α-granule protein thrombospondin, failed to aggregate in response to low concentrations of collagen, and adhered to, but did not spread on, collagen-coated surfaces.[57] In 2 families with auto-somal dominant thrombocytopenia and mild cutaneous bleeding, platelets had 38% to 63% of the normal amount of $\alpha2\beta1$ and adhered poorly to collagen-coated surfaces, whereas collagen-induced platelet aggregation was either normal or only slightly decreased.[58]

Defects in responsiveness to epinephrine

Epinephrine-induced aggregation, mediated by α2-adrenergic receptors (α_2AR), may be decreased in some presumably healthy individuals. In one study, the second wave of aggregation was absent in 10% to 15% of healthy subjects.[59] Studies in twins suggest that platelet α_2AR expression is under genetic control.[60] One family has been described[61] in which several members had impaired aggregation and secretion in response to only epinephrine associated with decreased number of platelet α_2AR. Three family members had a history of easy bruising with minimally prolonged bleeding times. Despite the diminished aggregation response, epinephrine inhibition of adenylate cyclase was normal, indicating that the receptor requirements for these 2 platelet responses are different. Although other families with an epinephrine defect have been reported,[62] the relationship of the selective epinephrine defect to bleeding manifestations needs to be defined. The isolated impaired aggregation response to epinephrine has been reported in Quebec platelet disorder.

Defects in GTP-binding Proteins

GTP-binding proteins (consisting of α, β, and γ subunits) link surface receptors and intracellular enzymes and constitute a potential locus for aberrations leading to platelet dysfunction. Abnormalities involving Gαq, Gαi$_2$, and Gαs have been described in human platelets.

Gαq deficiency

Gabbeta and colleagues[63] described, in a patient with a mild bleeding disorder, abnormal aggregation and secretion in response to several agonists, and diminished GTPase activity (a reflection of α-subunit function) on platelet activation. The binding of ^{35}S-GTPγS to platelet membranes was diminished, and there was a selective decrease in platelet membrane Gαq with normal levels of Gα_{i2}, Gα_{12}, Gα_{13}, and Gα_z. This patient had abnormalities in other downstream events, including activation of the GPIIb-IIIa complex, Ca^{2+} mobilization,[64] and release of arachidonic acid from phospholipids on platelet activation.[65] Gαq coding sequence in this patient was normal and the Gαq mRNA levels are decreased in platelets but not neutrophils, which have normal responses and Gαq protein.[66]

Gαs hyperfunction and genetic variation in extra-large Gαs

Activation of Gαs results in increased platelet cAMP levels and inhibition of platelet responses to activation. Two unrelated families have been described with inducible hyperactivity of Gαs.[67] These patients had a bleeding diathesis, prolonged bleeding times, variable mental retardation, and mild skeletal malformations. Platelet aggregation responses to usual agonists were reportedly normal, but the platelets showed increased sensitivity to inhibition by agents that elevate cAMP levels. Exposure to PGE1, PGI2, or adenosine resulted in an enhanced increase in cAMP associated with an increased platelet Gαs protein. A heterozygous 36–base pair (bp) insertion and 2 bp substitutions were identified in the exon 1 of the extra-large Gαs (XLas) gene in these patients. Because XLas is not activated by activation of the usual platelet Gαs-coupled receptors, the mechanisms leading to the increased cAMP levels and the enhanced expression of Gαs protein in the patients remain unclear.

Interestingly, 2.2% of control subjects also revealed the mutations detected in the patients, along with evidence of inducible $G\alpha s$ hyperfunction and increased platelet $G\alpha s$ protein.

Platelet $G\alpha s$ deficiency has been described[68] in a patient with pseudohypoparathyroidism Ib (PHPIb) in association with disturbed imprinting and altered methylation in the GNAS1 gene. The platelets showed decreased cAMP formation on $G\alpha s$ receptor activation and $G\alpha s$ protein deficiency; the $G\alpha s$ coding sequence was normal. The investigators did not indicate whether the patient had a bleeding diathesis.

$G\alpha i1$ deficiency

The patient described with platelet $G\alpha i1$ deficiency presented with a bleeding disorder, and abnormal aggregation and dense granule secretion on activation with ADP, U46619, collagen, and epinephrine.[69] Additionally, ADP-induced GPIIb-IIIa activation was diminished, indicating a role of $G\alpha i1$ in this response. A major platelet response mediated by $G\alpha i$ is inhibition of adenylyl cyclase and cAMP levels. In the patient's platelets, inhibition of forskolin-stimulated cAMP levels was absent on exposure to ADP, thrombin, or epinephrine. In contrast, $G\alpha q$-mediated responses (activation of PLC-$\beta 2$, Ca^{2+} mobilization, and pleckstrin phosphorylation) were normal. Platelet expression of $G\alpha i1$ was decreased by 75%; other members of the $G\alpha i$ family ($G\alpha i2$, $G\alpha i3$, $G\alpha iz$) and $G\alpha q$ were normal.

PLC-$\beta 2$ Deficiency and Defects in Phospholipase C Activation, Calcium Mobilization and Protein Phosphorylation

Activation of PLC is an early event on platelet stimulation and leads to the formation of intracellular mediators $InsP_3$ and diacylglycerol (see **Fig. 1**) and to mechanisms such as Ca^{2+} mobilization and PKC-induced protein phosphorylation. Defects in some of these specific responses have been documented. PKC-induced pleckstrin phosphorylation and cytoplasmic Ca^{2+} mobilization play a major role in secretion and aggregation on activation. In one study[11] of 8 patients with abnormal aggregation and secretion in response to several different agonists, receptor-mediated Ca^{2+} mobilization and/or pleckstrin phosphorylation were abnormal in 7 of the 8 patients. These studies suggest that the later events of exocytosis or secretion per se are intact in these patients and impaired secretion and aggregation result from upstream abnormalities in early signaling events. True to this supposition, specific human defects at the level of PLC-$\beta 2$,[70,71] $G\alpha q$,[63] and PKC-θ[72] have been documented in these patients.

In another study,[9] 8 patients have been described with decreased initial rates and extents of aggregation in response to weak agonists, ADP, epinephrine, and U44069; the investigators postulated defects in early platelet activation events to explain the abnormal responses. They subsequently demonstrated a defect in phosphatidylinositol hydrolysis and phosphatidic acid formation,[73] and in pleckstrin phosphorylation[74] in one patient.

Cytoplasmic Ca^{2+} mobilization is an early response to platelet stimulation. Attention was, therefore, focused initially on this process to explain the impaired platelet function.[11,64,75] Studies in 2 related patients[75] with impaired aggregation and secretion responses revealed decreased peak Ca^{2+} concentrations following activation with ADP, collagen, PAF, or thrombin, with abnormalities in intracellular release and in the influx of extracellular Ca^{2+}.[64] Formation of InsP3, the key intracellular mediator of Ca^{2+} release, as well as diacylglycerol formation and pleckstrin phosphorylation, were diminished on platelet activation,[70] indicating a defect in PLC activation (see **Fig. 1**). Human platelets contain at least 7 PLC isozymes in the quantitative order PLC-$\gamma 2$ > PLC-$\beta 2$ > PLC-$\beta 3$ > PLC-$\beta 1$ > PLC-$\gamma 1$ > PLC-$\delta 1$ > PLC-$\beta 4$.[71] Studies in one of the patients with impaired PLC activation revealed a selective decrease in only the PLC-β2 isozyme.[71] The decreased platelet PLC-β2 protein levels were associated with a normal coding sequence but with diminished PLC-β2 mRNA levels in platelets but not neutrophils, suggesting a hematopoietic lineage-specific defect in PLC-β2 gene regulation.[76] These studies provide direct validation in human platelets of the importance in hemostasis of PLC-β2.

Abnormalities in these signal transduction pathways, including in phosphatidylinositol metabolism and protein phosphorylation, have been described in other patients,[1,2,73,74,77] although the primary protein abnormality remains unknown. In one patient,[77] the abnormal platelet aggregation was associated with decreased TxA$_2$-induced InsP$_3$ formation but with normal GTPase activity and normal platelet TxA$_2$ receptors (including their cDNA sequence), suggesting that the abnormality in PLC activity was downstream of the surface receptor. Overall, these patients provide evidence for aberrations in the signal transduction pathways in patients with diminished platelet aggregation and secretion.

Defects in Protein Phosphorylation: PKC-θ Deficiency

PKC isozymes are a family of serine and threonine specific protein kinases that phosphorylate numerous proteins involved in signal transduction. PKC activation regulates several platelet responses including GPIIb-IIIa activation and secretion, and megakaryocyte differentiation. Deficiency of a human platelet PKC isozyme (PKC-θ) has been described[72] in a patient previously reported[78] with mucocutaneous bleeding manifestations, mild thrombocytopenia, and markedly abnormal platelet aggregation (including in primary wave) and dense granule secretion in response to multiple agonists. Phosphorylation of pleckstrin and myosin light chain was diminished in the patient's platelets on activation with PAF and thrombin. Signal transduction–dependent activation of GPIIb-IIIa was impaired on stimulation with receptor-mediated agonists. This subject has a heterozygous mutation in a transcription factor, RUNX1 (see also the section on Platelet Function Abnormalities Associated with Transcription Factor Deficiencies).[72] The platelets were specifically deficient in one PKC isozyme, PKC-θ. This deficiency provides one cogent explanation for the impaired protein phosphorylation and abnormal aggregation and secretion.

Protein phosphorylation by other kinases (tyrosine kinases) is important in platelet signaling events. In thrombasthenia[79,80] and the Scott syndrome,[81] tyrosine phosphorylation of several proteins is impaired on platelet activation. In these disorders, this defect is likely secondary to the primary abnormality in the GPIIb-IIIa complex and in phospholipids scrambling, respectively. Interestingly, in patients with the thrombocytopenia with absent radii (TAR) syndrome, thrombopoietin-induced tyrosine phosphorylation is markedly abnormal.[82]

Abnormalities in Arachidonic Acid Pathways and Thromboxane Production

Thromboxane A2 production forms an important positive feedback, enhancing the overall activation process. In the absence of TxA$_2$ synthesis, dense granule secretion is decreased following stimulation of PRP with ADP, epinephrine, and low concentrations of collagen and thrombin. In general, most patients with defects in TxA$_2$ production have had mild to moderate bleeding manifestations.

Defects in the liberation of arachidonic acid from phospholipids

Mobilization of free arachidonic acid from membrane-bound phospholipids by phospholipase A$_2$ is the initial and rate-limiting step in TxA$_2$ synthesis. Defects in this process have been reported in some patients. In 4 such patients,[65] aggregation and secretion were abnormal, and TxA2 production was diminished during stimulation with ADP and thrombin, but was normal with free arachidonic acid. In ^{3}H-arachidonic acid–labeled platelets, thrombin-induced mobilization of free arachidonic acid from phospholipids was impaired in these patients. Subsequent studies in one of the patients showed that the platelet PLA$_2$ levels (both membrane and cytosolic) were normal but agonist-induced Ca^{2+} mobilization[64] was impaired due to a platelet Gαq deficiency.[63] Other reports have also documented patients with an impaired release of arachidonic acid.[1,2] An inherited deficiency in cytosolic phospholipase A$_2$, the principal enzyme that regulates the release of arachidonic acid, has been reported in a patient with recurrent small intestinal ulceration, markedly decreased synthesis of thromboxane, 12-HETE and leukotriene B$_4$, and platelet dysfunction.[83] This patient had 2 heterozygous single base-pair mutations in the PLA$_2$ coding region, leading to S111P and R485H substitutions.

Deficiencies of cyclooxygenase and thromboxane synthetase

In 1975, Malmsten and colleagues[84] reported platelet cyclooxygenase deficiency in a patient with a mild bleeding disorder and impaired aggregation responses to ADP, epinephrine, collagen, and arachidonic acid, but with normal response to PGG2. Subsequently, several other patients have been described with a similar defect in TxA$_2$ synthesis.[1,2] Studies[85] using a radioimmunoassay found normal levels of cyclooxygenase in 5 of 6 patients suspected to have a deficiency, suggesting that these patients have a functionally abnormal molecule. Three patients have been described[86] with impaired platelet responses and markedly decreased ability to convert arachidonic acid, but not of PGH$_2$, to TxA$_2$. The investigators demonstrated decreased platelet cyclooxygenase-1 levels in 2 patients and normal levels in the third; levels of thromboxane synthase were normal in all 3. Two patients have been described with thromboxane synthetase deficiency.[87,88]

DISORDERS OF PLATELET PROCOAGULANT ACTIVITY (SCOTT SYNDROME)

Platelet procoagulant activity refers to the essential role of platelets in supporting the enzymatic reactions of the coagulation system. These reactions occur on the outer platelet membrane surface leading to activation of FX to FXa (tenase) and of prothrombin to thrombin (prothrombinase). Isolated deficiency of platelet procoagulant activity is rare. This entity is named after the first patient described with this entity (Scott syndrome).[89] A few additional patients have been reported.[90–92] The initial patient had spontaneous bleeding and excessive bleeding after procedures. The prothrombin time, partial thromboplastin time, bleeding time, and platelet aggregation studies were normal; however, the serum prothrombin times were short reflecting impaired ability of platelets to express normal procoagulant activity. The patient's platelets had markedly impaired prothrombinase activity, decreased number of factor Xa binding sites and impaired factor X activation by factor IXa and factor VIIIa in the presence of platelets. There was a decreased exposure of anionic phospholipids on the platelet surface and decreased membrane vesiculation. Membrane-associated phospholipid scramblase activity that regulates exposure of anionic phospholipids on cell surfaces was impaired in the patient's platelets, erythrocytes, and lymphocytes.[93]

Activated platelets provide the membrane surface for the assembly of the "tenase" and "prothrombinase" complexes that activate factor X and prothrombin, respectively. In resting platelets, phosphatidylcholine is localized predominantly in the outer membrane leaflet or the plasma membrane and anionic phospholipids, phosphatidylserine, and phosphatidylethanolamine, concentrated in the inner leaflet. This asymmetry is maintained by a "flippase," an ATP-dependent aminophospholipid translocase

(P4 ATPase) directing the inward transport of lipids, and a "floppase," an ATP-requiring transporter encoded by the gene *ABCC1* that directs the transport of the phospholipids to the outer leaflet.[93] Platelet activation leads to exposure of anionic phospholipids on the platelet surface. The Ca^{2+}-induced bidirectional movement of phospholipids between membrane leaflets in platelets and other cells appears to be catalyzed by membrane-associated scramblase activity, attributed to a protein TMEM16F. TMEM16F mutations have been identified in 2 patients with Scott syndrome.[94,95]

OTHER INHERITED DISORDERS OF PLATELET FUNCTION
Defects in Cytoskeletal Assembly and Structural Proteins

Wiskott-Aldrich syndrome
WAS is an X-linked inherited disorder affecting T-lymphocytes and platelets, and characterized by thrombocytopenia, small platelets with decreased survival, eczema, and immunodeficiency. The bleeding manifestations are variable. Several platelet abnormalities have been reported, including δ-SPD; deficiencies of GPIb, GPIa, and GPIIb-IIIa; diminished activation of GPIIb-IIIa; impaired aggregation responses and expression of p-selectin; and abnormalities in platelet energy metabolism.[96,97] In addition, resting cytoplasmic Ca^{2+} levels have been reported to be elevated along with enhanced phosphotidylserine expression on platelet surface and microparticle formation in patients with WAS.[98] WAS arises from mutations of *WASP*, which encodes a 53-kD protein WASp[96,99] which constitutes a link between the cytoskeleton and signal transduction pathways and regulates actin polymerization. Splenectomy usually improves the thrombocytopenia in WAS, and bone marrow transplantation has been curative.

Kindlin-3 deficiency (leukocyte adhesion defect-III)
Kindlin-3 deficiency combines features of both mild leukocyte adhesion deficiency and platelet dysfunction with bleeding symptoms. The etiology is a deficiency or defect in the cytoskeletal linking protein kindlin-3 (*FERMTS3*), which binds to the cytoplasmic domain of the integrin β3 subunit of αIIb and plays a role in the inside-out activation of platelet αIIbβ3, and in leukocyte function.[100,101] The disorder is characterized by a variable predisposition to infections and inflammation without pus formation, poor wound healing, delayed umbilical cord stump detachment, mucosal bleeding, intracranial hemorrhage, and variable osteopetrosis.

Abnormalities of β1-tubulin
Megakaryocytes and platelets express primarily and selectively the β1 isoform of tubulin. Individuals heterozygous for the Q43P polymorphism have been reported to have normal platelet counts, relatively high mean platelet volume values, abnormally rounded platelets with abnormal marginal bands of microtubules, and mild abnormalities of platelet aggregation, secretion, and adhesion to collagen.[101,102]

PLATELET FUNCTION ABNORMALITIES ASSOCIATED WITH TRANSCRIPTION FACTOR DEFICIENCIES

Transcription factors regulate expression of proteins in megakaryocytes and platelets. Several reports have associated platelet function abnormalities with mutations in transcription factor RUNX1 (CBFA2, core binding factor A2), including abnormalities in aggregation and secretion, dense granule deficiency, alpha-granule deficiency, and PKC-θ deficiency.[1,2,26,72,101,103] These subjects were initially recognized by an association between autosomal dominant thrombocytopenia and an increased pre-disposition to leukemia, and subsequently linked to a RUNX1 haplodeficiency.[104]

Most of the mutations of *RUNX1* affected the Runt domain.[26] Detailed studies in one patient with a splice site mutation leading to a frame shift and premature termination in the Runt domain revealed abnormal $\alpha IIb\beta 3$ activation, decreased platelet myosin light chain and pleckstrin phosphorylation, and a selective decrease in platelet protein ki-nase C-θ; the patient also had diminished platelet albumin and IgG, suggesting an α granule abnormality, but normal levels of the α granule proteins fibrinogen and β-thromboglobulin.[72,78] Expression profiling of platelets from this patient revealed downregulation of several genes,[105] including *MYL9* (myosin light chain),[106] *ALOX12* (12-lipoxygenase),[107] and *PF4* (platelet factor 4),[27] PKC-θ,[108] and Mpl,[109] all directly relevant to platelet biology. *ALOX12*,[107] PKC-θ,[108] *PF4*,[27] and *MYL9*[106] have been shown to be direct transcriptional targets of *RUNX1* and provide a mechanism for the observed platelet deficiencies. Patients with *RUNX1* haplodeficiency have been shown to have impaired megakaryopoiesis[110] and decreased platelet thrombopoietin receptors (Mpl).[109]

Patients with transcription factor GATA-1 mutations may have not only X-linked thrombocytopenia, but also large platelets and impaired responses to collagen and ristocetin[111] related to abnormalities in GPIbβ. Aggregation in response to ADP and thrombin were normal. Interestingly, one of the patients also had diminished levels of platelet Gαs protein and mRNA[111] and another had GPS (R216N).[28] Overall, these reports suggest that transcription factor abnormalities are associated with platelet dysfunction in addition to thrombocytopenia.

MISCELLANEOUS INHERITED DISORDERS ASSOCIATED WITH PLATELET FUNCTION DEFECTS

Platelet function abnormalities have been reported in several other inherited disorders, which are reviewed elsewhere.[1,2,101] These include inherited connective tissue disor-ders, such as osteogenesis imperfecta, the Ehlers-Danlos syndrome, and the Marfan syndrome, which are associated with bleeding manifestations more likely due to the underlying connective tissue defect rather than the platelet dysfunction. Abnormal platelet responses have been reported in patients with hexokinase deficiency, glucose-6 phosphatase deficiency, and Down syndrome. Markedly impaired platelet responses have been reported with partial trisomy 18p associated with 3 copies of the PACAP (pituitary adenylate cyclase-activating polypeptide) gene and increased platelet cAMP levels via stimulation of Gαs.

RELATIVE FREQUENCY OF VARIOUS INHERITED PLATELET ABNORMALITIES

There is little information available on this aspect. Thrombasthenia, BSS, and afibrino-genemia are rare disorders. It is generally considered that vWD is the most common congenital platelet function disorder, although the severe forms are rare. Patients currently lumped in the heterogeneous category of defects in platelet secretion and signal transduction are probably the most frequently encountered inherited platelet function abnormalities, excluding vWD. However, in the vast majority, the molecular mechanisms are unknown. Although frequently considered, dense granule SPD and defects in TxA$_2$ production occur in a small proportion of these patients. We have analyzed findings in 62 patients with inherited platelet dysfunction studied in our lab-oratory (Rao AK, unpublished, 1998). All patients had impaired aggregation and ^{14}C-serotonin secretion in studies using PRP; dense granule contents (ATP, ADP) and thromboxane A2 production on activation with thrombin and arachidonic acid were measured in all. Ten patients had a dense granule SPD (16%). Twenty-five patients (40%) had clear-cut abnormalities in the aggregation (generally, absent second wave) and secretion on activation but had normal dense granule stores and thromboxane production. These patients may have defects in the signaling mechanisms. In this highly heterogeneous group, there is a pressing need for detailed studies to delineate the mechanisms. In this series, thrombasthenia was detected in one patient.

DIAGNOSIS OF CONGENITAL PLATELET FUNCTION DEFECTS

The usual reasons for referral for evaluation include mucocutaneous bleeding manifestations, and excessive bleeding following a procedure or surgery. In patients suspected to have a platelet function defect, the main clinically available laboratory studies include a platelet count, the platelet function analyzer (PFA), bleeding time, and studies to assess platelet responses of aggregation and secretion in vitro. The platelet studies are usually performed using PRP harvested from anticoagulated blood and responses are monitored to various agonists including ADP, epinephrine, collagen, thromboxane A_2 analog U46619, arachidonic acid, thrombin receptor peptides, and ristocetin. In addition to aggregation, many laboratories assess secretion or release of dense granule contents, specifically ATP, using a lumi-aggregometer, which records secretion in parallel with aggregation. The recorded tracings of aggregation and secretion may provide clues to the nature of the underlying platelet defect; however, additional specific techniques, largely available in research laboratories, are required to establish the molecular and genetic basis. In patients with thrombasthenia (**Fig. 3**) and afibrinogenemia, both the primary and the secondary waves of aggregation are absent in response to all of the commonly used agonists mentioned previously, excepting ristocetin. One can distinguish these 2 disorders by the prolongation of the prothrombin time and the partial thromboplastin time only in the latter. Impaired or absent aggregation response to ristocetin but with normal response to the other agonists suggests vWD or the Bernard Soulier syndrome. In the latter disorder, the platelet counts are decreased and the platelet size is increased, and plasma levels of vWF and factor VIII are normal, whereas they are abnormal in vWD. Patients with impaired granule secretion or diminished dense granule contents (SPD) generally show diminished or absent second wave of aggregation in response to ADP and epinephrine, and blunted responses to other agonists (collagen, U46619), associated with markedly decreased release of dense granule contents (see **Fig. 2**). In some patients, the primary wave of aggregation may also be blunted. Last, it is relevant to note that some patients may have a combination of defective platelet function and thrombocytopenia. Examples include the Bernard Soulier syndrome and patients with *RUNX1* mutations.

There are several limitations in the current approaches available in clinical laboratories for the evaluation of platelet defects. A normal bleeding time does not exclude a platelet function defect. The PFA is neither sensitive nor specific for detecting platelet function defects.[112] Platelet aggregation and secretion studies using PRP form the primary basis for the diagnosis of an inherited platelet defects in most patients. In studies using light transmission aggregometry, normal responses in PRP to the usually used agonists does not rule out a platelet function defect. For example, they are generally normal or minimally abnormal in patients with the Scott syndrome and the GPS; in QPD, the response only to epinephrine is abnormal. Normal aggregation responses have been reported in some patients with dense granule SPD.[14] Even when abnormal, aggregation studies do not reliably provide definitive insights into the molecular mechanisms in most patients. Simultaneous assessment of secretion along

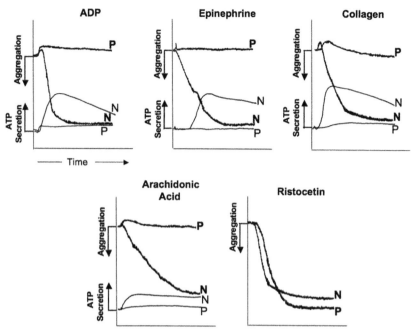

Fig. 3. Aggregation and ATP secretion studies in Glanzmann thrombasthenia performed using a lumi-aggregometer and PRP. Shown are aggregation (*upper tracings in each panel*) and ATP secretion (*lower tracings*) in the patient (P) and a healthy subject (N) in response to ADP (7.5 μM), epinephrine (7.5 μM), collagen (1 μg/mL), ristocetin (1.5 mg/mL), and arachidonic acid (1 mM). With all agonists except ristocetin, neither the primary wave nor the secondary wave of aggregation are noted in the patient, and secretion is decreased. (*Reprinted from* Rao AK, Essex DW. Platelet function in hemostasis and inherited disorders of platelet number and function. In: Schmaier AH, Lazarus HM, editors. Concise Guide to Hematology. Oxford (United Kingdom): Wiley-Blackwell; 2012. p. 140–53.)

with aggregation studies adds invaluable information, but is available only in some clinical laboratories. Some patients have markedly impaired secretion even though aggregation responses are normal or minimally blunted.

In the vast majority of patients with inherited platelet defects, the underlying molecular mechanisms are unknown, and such patients, as a group, are not rare. There is a pressing need to exploit state-of-the-art approaches to unravel the mechanisms in these patients who are an untapped reservoir of new information into platelet physiology and pathology.

THERAPY OF INHERITED PLATELET FUNCTION DEFECTS

Platelet transfusions and 1-desamino-8D-arginine vasopressin (DDAVP) are the mainstays of therapy. Because of the wide disparity in bleeding manifestations therapeutic approaches need to be individualized. Platelet transfusions are effective in controlling the bleeding manifestations but come with the usual potential risks associated with blood products; one additional risk includes alloimmunization to the deficient platelet glycoproteins. A viable alternative is intravenous administration of DDAVP, which shortens the bleeding time in a substantial number of patients with platelet function defects.[113–116] Response to DDAVP appears to be dependent on the abnormalities leading to the platelet dysfunction.[113,115,116] Most patients with thrombasthenia have not responded to DDAVP infusion with a shortening of the bleeding time[113,115–117] with exceptions.[118] However, it is unclear whether DDAVP improves hemostasis in these patients despite a lack of shortening of the bleeding time. Responses in patients with SPD have been variable with a shortening of the bleeding time in some patients[116,119] but not others.[113,115] In uncontrolled studies it has been feasible to manage selected patients with inherited platelet defects undergoing surgical procedures with DDAVP alone.[113,115] However, this approach needs to be individualized based on the nature of the surgery and the intensity of bleeding symptoms, and platelet transfusions need to be readily available for use in the event of excess hemorrhage. The abnormal in vitro platelet aggregation or secretion responses in patients with platelet defects are not corrected by DDAVP.[115]

Several investigators have reported the successful use of recombinant factor VIIa (rFVIIa) in the management of bleeding events in patients with inherited platelet defects, including thrombasthenia, the Bernard Soulier syndrome and SPD.[120–123] Additional larger studies of rFVIIa are warranted in such patients.

The other approaches that have been used to improve hemostasis in patients with inherited platelet defects include a short 3-day to 4-day course of prednisone (20–50 mg)[124] and the administration of antifibrinolytic agents epsilonaminocaproic acid or tranexamic acid, which have been successfully used in patients with coagulation disorders.[114,122,125]

ACKNOWLEDGMENTS

The excellent secretarial assistance of Ms Denise Tierney is gratefully acknowledged. This work was supported by grant award NIH-RO1HL109568.

REFERENCES

1. Rao AK. Hereditary disorders of platelet secretion and signal transduction. In: Colman RW, Marder VJ, Clowes AW, et al, editors. Hemostasis and thrombosis: basic principles and clinical practice. 5th edition. Philadelphia: Lippincott Williams & Wilkins; 2006. p. 961.
2. Bennett JS, Rao AK. Hereditary disorders of platelet function. In: Marder VJ, Aird WC, Bennett JS, et al, editors. Hemostasis and thrombosis: basic principles and clinical practice. 6th edition. Philadelphia: Lippincott Williams & Wilkins; 2013. p. 805–19.
3. Weiss HJ, Chervenick PA, Zalusky R, et al. A familial defect in platelet function associated with impaired release of adenosine diphosphate. N Engl J Med 1969;281:1264.
4. Holmsen H, Weiss HJ. Hereditary defect in the platelet release reaction caused by a deficiency in the storage pool of platelet adenine nucleotides. Br J Haematol 1970;19:643.
5. Holmsen H, Weiss HJ. Further evidence for a deficient storage pool of adenine nucleotides in platelets from some patients with thrombocytopathia—"storage pool disease." Blood 1972;39:197.
6. Rao AK, Willis J, Hassell B, et al. Congenital platelet secretion defects with normal storage pools and arachidonate metabolism. Circulation 1982;66:299.
7. Rao AK, Holmsen H. Congenital disorders of platelet function. Semin Hematol 1986;23:102.
8. Day HJ, Rao AK. Platelet function testing. Semin Hematol 1986;23:89.

9. Lages B, Weiss HJ. Heterogeneous defects of platelet secretion and responses to weak agonists in patients with bleeding disorders. Br J Haematol 1988;68:53.
10. Koike K, Rao AK, Holmsen H, et al. Platelet secretion defect in patients with the attention deficit disorder and easy bruising. Blood 1984;63:427.
11. Yang X, Sun L, Gabbeta J, et al. Platelet activation with combination of ionophore A23187 and a direct protein kinase C activator induces normal secretion in patients with impaired receptor mediated secretion and abnormal signal transduction. Thromb Res 1997;88:317.
12. Cattaneo M, Lombardi R, Zighetti ML, et al. Deficiency of (33)P-2MeS-ADP binding sites on platelets with secretion defect, normal granule stores and normal thromboxane A2 production. Thromb Haemost 1997;77:986.
13. Masliah-Planchon J, Darnige L, Bellucci S. Molecular determinants of platelet delta storage pool deficiencies: an update. Br J Haematol 2013;160:5.
14. Nieuwenhuis HK, Akkerman JWN, Sixma JJ. Patients with a prolonged bleeding time and normal aggregation tests may have storage pool deficiency: studies on one hundred six patients. Blood 1987;70:620.
15. Holmsen H. Secretable storage pools in platelets. Annu Rev Med 1979;30: 119.
16. Gunay-Aygun M, Huizing M, Gahl WA. Molecular defects that affect platelet dense granules. Semin Thromb Hemost 2004;30:537.
17. Gahl WA, Brantly M, Kaiser-Kupfer MI, et al. Genetic defects and clinical characteristics of patients with a form of oculocutaneous albinism (Hermansky-Pudlak syndrome). N Engl J Med 1998;338:1258.
18. Huizing M, Helip-Wooley A, Westbroek W, et al. Disorders of lysosome-related organelle biogenesis: clinical and molecular genetics. Annu Rev Genomics Hum Genet 2008;9:359.
19. Gerrard JM, Lint D, Sims PJ, et al. Identification of a platelet dense granule membrane protein that is deficient in a patient with the Hermansky-Pudlak syndrome. Blood 1991;77:101.
20. McNicol A, Israels SJ, Robertson C, et al. The empty sack syndrome: a platelet storage pool deficiency associated with empty dense granules. Br J Haematol 1994;86:574.
21. Raccuglia G. Gray platelet syndrome: a variety of qualitative platelet disorder. Am J Med 1971;51:818.
22. Nurden AT, Nurden P. The gray platelet syndrome: clinical spectrum of the disease. Blood Rev 2007;21:21.
23. Nurden AT, Nurden P, Bermejo E, et al. Phenotypic heterogeneity in the gray platelet syndrome extends to the expression of TREM family member, TLT-1. Thromb Haemost 2008;100:45.
24. Maynard DM, Heijnen HF, Gahl WA, et al. The alpha granule proteome: novel proteins in normal and ghost granules in gray platelet syndrome. J Thromb Haemost 2010;8:1786.
25. Weiss HJ, Witte LD, Kaplan KL, et al. Heterogeneity in storage pool deficiency: studies on granule-bound substances in 18 patients including variants deficient in alpha-granules, platelet factor 4, beta-thromboglobulin, and platelet-derived growth factor. Blood 1979;54:1296.
26. Michaud J, Wu F, Osato M, et al. In vitro analyses of known and novel RUNX1/AML1 mutations in dominant familial platelet disorder with predisposition to acute myelogenous leukemia: implications for mechanisms of pathogenesis. Blood 2002;99:1364.

27. Aneja K, Jalagadugula G, Mao G, et al. Mechanism of platelet factor 4 (PF4) deficiency with RUNX1 haplodeficiency: RUNX1 is a transcriptional regulator of PF4. J Thromb Haemost 2011;9:383.

28. Tubman VN, Levine JE, Campagna DR, et al. X-linked gray platelet syndrome due to a GATA1 Arg216Gln mutation. Blood 2007;109:3297.

29. Vyas P, Ault K, Jackson CW, et al. Consequences of GATA-1 deficiency in megakaryocytes and platelets. Blood 1999;93:2867.

30. Lo B, Li L, Gissen P, et al. Requirement of VPS33B, a member of the Sec1/Munc18 protein family, in megakaryocyte and platelet alpha-granule biogenesis. Blood 2005;106:4159.

31. Urban D, Li L, Christensen H, et al. The VPS33B binding protein VPS16B is required in megakaryocyte and platelet alpha-granule biogenesis. Blood 2012;120(25):5032–40.

32. Kahr WH, Hinckley J, Li L, et al. Mutations in NBEAL2, encoding a BEACH protein, cause gray platelet syndrome. Nat Genet 2011;43:738.

33. Gunay-Aygun M, Falik-Zaccai TC, Vilboux T, et al. NBEAL2 is mutated in gray platelet syndrome and is required for biogenesis of platelet alpha-granules. Nat Genet 2011;43:732.

34. Albers CA, Cvejic A, Favier R, et al. Exome sequencing identifies NBEAL2 as the causative gene for gray platelet syndrome. Nat Genet 2011;43:735.

35. Hayward CP, Rivard GE. Quebec platelet disorder. Expert Rev Hematol 2011;4:137.

36. Diamandis M, Paterson AD, Rommens JM, et al. Quebec platelet disorder is linked to the urokinase plasminogen activator gene (PLAU) and increases expression of the linked allele in megakaryocytes. Blood 2009;113:1543.

37. Hirata T, Kakizuka A, Ushikubi F, et al. Arg60 to Leu mutation of the human thromboxane A2 receptor in a dominantly inherited bleeding disorder. J Clin Invest 1994;94:1662.

38. Ushikubi F, Okuma M, Kanaji K, et al. Hemorrhagic thrombocytopathy with platelet thromboxane A2 receptor abnormality: defective signal transduction with normal binding activity. Thromb Haemost 1987;57:158.

39. Fuse I, Mito M, Hattori A, et al. Defective signal transduction induced by thromboxane A2 in a patient with a mild bleeding disorder: impaired phospholipase C activation despite normal phospholipase A2 activation. Blood 1993;81:994.

40. Ushikubi F, Ishibashi T, Narumiya S, et al. Analysis of the defective signal transduction mechanism through the platelet thromboxane A2 receptor in a patient with polycythemia vera. Thromb Haemost 1992;67:144.

41. Armstrong RA, Jones RL, Peesapati V, et al. Competitive antagonism at thromboxane receptors in human platelets. Br J Pharmacol 1985;84:595.

42. Cattaneo M. Molecular defects of the platelet P2 receptors. Purinergic Signal 2011;7:333.

43. Cattaneo M. Inherited platelet-based bleeding disorders. J Thromb Haemost 2003;1:1628.

44. Shiraga M, Miyata S, Kato H, et al. Impaired platelet function in a patient with P2Y12 deficiency caused by a mutation in the translation initiation codon. J Thromb Haemost 2005;3:2315.

45. Nurden P, Savi P, Heilmann E, et al. An inherited bleeding disorder linked to a defective interaction between ADP and its receptor on platelets. Its influence on glycoprotein IIb-IIIa complex function. J Clin Invest 1995;95:1612.

46. Hollopeter G, Jantzen HM, Vincent D, et al. Identification of the platelet ADP receptor targeted by antithrombotic drugs. Nature 2001;409:202.

47. Cattaneo M, Zighetti ML, Lombardi R, et al. Molecular bases of defective signal transduction in the platelet P2Y12 receptor of a patient with congenital bleeding. Proc Natl Acad Sci U S A 2003;100:1978.

48. Daly ME, Dawood BB, Lester WA, et al. Identification and characterization of a novel P2Y 12 variant in a patient diagnosed with type 1 von Willebrand disease in the European MCMDM-1VWD study. Blood 2009;113:4110.

49. Remijn JA, Ijsseldijk MJ, Strunk AL, et al. Novel molecular defect in the platelet ADP receptor P2Y12 of a patient with haemorrhagic diathesis. Clin Chem Lab Med 2007;45:187.

50. Oury C, Toth-Zsamboki E, Van Geet C, et al. A natural dominant negative P2X1 receptor due to deletion of a single amino acid residue. J Biol Chem 2000;275:22611.

51. Oury C, Lenaerts T, Peerlinck K, et al. Congenital deficiency of the phospholipase C coupled platelet P2Y1 receptor leads to a mild bleeding disorder [abstract]. Thromb Haemost 1999;(Suppl):20–1.

52. Kehrel B, Wierwille S, Clemetson KJ, et al. Glycoprotein VI is a major collagen receptor for platelet activation: it recognizes the platelet-activating quaternary structure of collagen, whereas CD36, glycoprotein IIb/IIIa, and von Willebrand factor do not. Blood 1998;91:491.

53. Staatz WD, Rajpara SM, Wayner EA, et al. The membrane glycoprotein Ia-IIa (VLA-2) complex mediates the Mg++-dependent adhesion of platelets to collagen. J Cell Biol 1989;108:1917.

54. Inoue O, Suzuki-Inoue K, Dean WL, et al. Integrin alpha2beta1 mediates outside-in regulation of platelet spreading on collagen through activation of Src kinases and PLCgamma2. J Cell Biol 2003;160:769.

55. Nieuwenhuis HK, Akkerman JW, Houdijk WP, et al. Human blood platelets showing no response to collagen fail to express surface glycoprotein Ia. Nature 1985;318:470.

56. Nieuwenhuis HK, Sakariassen KS, Houdijk WP, et al. Deficiency of platelet membrane glycoprotein Ia associated with a decreased platelet adhesion to subendothelium: a defect in platelet spreading. Blood 1986;68:692.

57. Kehrel B, Balleisen L, Kokott R, et al. Deficiency of intact thrombospondin and membrane glycoprotein Ia in platelets with defective collagen-induced aggregation and spontaneous loss of disorder. Blood 1988;71:1074.

58. Noris P, Guidetti GF, Conti V, et al. Autosomal dominant thrombocytopenias with reduced expression of glycoprotein Ia. Thromb Haemost 2006;95:483.

59. Weiss HJ, Lages B. The response of platelets to epinephrine in storage pool deficiency—evidence pertaining to the role of adenosine diphosphate in mediating primary and secondary aggregation. Blood 1988;72:1717.

60. Propping P, Friedl W. Genetic control of adrenergic receptors on human platelets. A twin study. Hum Genet 1983;64:105.

61. Rao AK, Willis J, Kowalska MA, et al. Differential requirements for epinephrine induced platelet aggregation and inhibition of adenylate cyclase. Studies in familial α2-adrenergic receptor defect. Blood 1988;71:494.

62. Tamponi G, Pannocchia A, Arduino C, et al. Congenital deficiency of α-2-adrenoreceptors on human platelets: description of two cases. Thromb Haemost 1987;58:1012.

63. Gabbeta J, Yang X, Kowalska MA, et al. Platelet signal transduction defect with Gα subunit dysfunction and diminished Gαq in a patient with abnormal platelet responses. Proc Natl Acad Sci U S A 1997;94:8750.

64. Rao AK, Disa J, Yang X. Concomitant defect in internal release and influx of calcium in patients with congenital platelet dysfunction and impaired agonist-induced calcium mobilization: thromboxane production is not required for internal release of calcium. J Lab Clin Med 1993;121:52.

65. Rao AK, Koike K, Willis J, et al. Platelet secretion defect associated with impaired liberation of arachidonic acid and normal myosin light chain phosphorylation. Blood 1984;64:914.

66. Gabbeta J, Vaidyula VR, Dhanasekaran DN, et al. Human platelet Gαq deficiency is associated with decreased Gαq gene expression in platelets but not neutrophils. Thromb Haemost 2002;87:129.

67. Freson K, Hoylaerts MF, Jaeken J, et al. Genetic variation of the extra-large stimulatory G protein alpha-subunit leads to Gs hyperfunction in platelets and is a risk factor for bleeding. Thromb Haemost 2001;86:733.

68. Freson K, Thys C, Wittevrongel C, et al. Pseudohypoparathyroidism type Ib with disturbed imprinting in the GNAS1 cluster and Gsalpha deficiency in platelets. Hum Mol Genet 2002;11:2741.

69. Patel YM, Patel K, Rahman S, et al. Evidence for a role for Galphai1 in mediating weak agonist-induced platelet aggregation in human platelets: reduced Galphai1 expression and defective Gi signaling in the platelets of a patient with a chronic bleeding disorder. Blood 2003;101:4828.

70. Yang X, Sun L, Ghosh S, et al. Human platelet signaling defect characterized by impaired production of inositol-1,4,5-triphosphate and phosphatic acid, and diminished Pleckstrin phosphorylation: evidence for defective phospholipase C activation. Blood 1996;88:1676.

71. Lee SB, Rao AK, Lee KH, et al. Decreased expression of phospholipase C-beta 2 isozyme in human platelets with impaired function. Blood 1996;88:1684.

72. Sun L, Mao G, Rao AK. Association of CBFA2 mutation with decreased platelet PKC-θ and impaired receptor-mediated activation of GPIIb-IIIa and pleckstrin phosphorylation: proteins regulated by CBFA2 play a role in GPIIb-IIIa activation. Blood 2004;103:948.

73. Lages B, Weiss HJ. Impairment of phosphatidylinositol metabolism in a patient with a bleeding disorder associated with defects of initial platelet responses. Thromb Haemost 1988;59:175.

74. Speiser-Ellerton S, Weiss HJ. Studies on platelet protein phosphorylation in patients with impaired responses to platelet agonists. J Lab Clin Med 1990;115:104.

75. Rao AK, Kowalska MA, Disa J. Impaired cytoplasmic ionized calcium mobilization in inherited platelet secretion defects. Blood 1989;74:664.

76. Mao GF, Vaidyula VR, Kunapuli SP, et al. Lineage-specific defect in gene expression in human platelet phospholipase C-beta2 deficiency. Blood 2002;99:905.

77. Mitsui T. Defective signal transduction through the thromboxane A2 receptor in a patient with a mild bleeding disorder. Deficiency of the inositol 1,4,5-triphosphate formation despite normal G-protein activation. Thromb Haemost 1997; 77:991.

78. Gabbeta J, Yang X, Sun L, et al. Abnormal inside-out signal transduction-dependent activation of glycoprotein IIb-IIIa in a patient with impaired pleckstrin phosphorylation. Blood 1996;87:1368.

79. Ferrell JE, Martin GS. Tyrosine-specific protein phosphorylation is regulated by glycoprotein IIb-IIIa in platelets. Proc Natl Acad Sci U S A 1989;86:2234.

80. Golden A, Brugge JS, Shattil SJ. Role of platelet membrane glycoprotein IIb-IIIa in agonist-induced tyrosine phosphorylation of platelet proteins. J Cell Biol 1990; 111:3117.

81. Dekkers DW, Comfurius P, Vuist WM, et al. Impaired Ca2+-induced tyrosine phosphorylation and defective lipid scrambling in erythrocytes from a patient with Scott syndrome: a study using an inhibitor for scramblase that mimics the defect in Scott syndrome. Blood 1998;91:2133.

82. Ballmaier M, Schulze H, Cremer M, et al. Defective c-Mpl signaling in the syndrome of thrombocytopenia with absent radii. Stem Cells 1998;16:177.

83. Adler DH, Cogan JD, Phillips JA, et al. Inherited human cPLA(2alpha) deficiency is associated with impaired eicosanoid biosynthesis, small intestinal ulceration, and platelet dysfunction. J Clin Invest 2008;118(6):2121–31.

84. Malmsten C, Hamberg M, Svensson J. Physiological role of an endoperoxide in human platelets: hemostatic defect due to platelet cyclooxygenase deficiency. Proc Natl Acad Sci U S A 1975;72:1446.

85. Roth GJ, Machuga R. Radioimmune assay of human platelet prostaglandin synthetase. J Lab Clin Med 1982;99:187.

86. Matijevic-Aleksic N, McPhedran P, Wu KK. Bleeding disorder due to platelet prostaglandin H synthase-1 (PGHS-1) deficiency. Br J Haematol 1996;92:212.

87. Defryn G, Machin SJ, Carreras LD, et al. Familial bleeding tendency with partial platelet thromboxane synthetase deficiency: reorientation of cyclic endoperoxide metabolism. Br J Haematol 1981;49:29.

88. Mestel F, Oetliker O, Beck E, et al. Severe bleeding associated with defective thromboxane synthetase. Lancet 1980;1:157.

89. Weiss HJ, Vicic WJ, Lages BA, et al. Isolated deficiency of platelet procoagulant activity. Am J Med 1979;67:206.

90. Weiss HJ, Lages B. Family studies in Scott syndrome. Blood 1997;90:475.

91. Toti F, Satta N, Fressinaud E, et al. Scott syndrome, characterized by impaired transmembrane migration of procoagulant phosphatidylserine and hemorrhagic complications, is an inherited disorder. Blood 1996;87:1409.

92. Munnix IC, Harmsma M, Giddings JC, et al. Store-mediated calcium entry in the regulation of phosphatidylserine exposure in blood cells from Scott patients. Thromb Haemost 2003;89:687.

93. Lhermusier T, Chap H, Payrastre B. Platelet membrane phospholipid asymmetry: from the characterization of a scramblase activity to the identification of an essential protein mutated in Scott syndrome. J Thromb Haemost 2011;9:1883.

94. Suzuki J, Umeda M, Sims PJ, et al. Calcium-dependent phospholipid scrambling by TMEM16F. Nature 2010;468:834.

95. Castoldi E, Collins PW, Williamson PL, et al. Compound heterozygosity for 2 novel TMEM16F mutations in a patient with Scott syndrome. Blood 2011;117:4399.

96. Remold-ODonnell E, Rosen FS, Kenney DM. Defects in Wiskott-Aldrich syndrome blood cells. Blood 1996;87:2621.

97. Semple JW, Siminovitch KA, Mody M, et al. Flow cytometric analysis of platelets from children with the Wiskott-Aldrich syndrome reveals defects in platelet development, activation and structure. Br J Haematol 1997;97:747.

98. Shcherbina A, Rosen FS, Remold-O'Donnell E. Pathological events in platelets of Wiskott-Aldrich syndrome patients. Br J Haematol 1999;106:875.

99. Zhu Q, Watanabe C, Liu T, et al. Wiskott-Aldrich syndrome/X-linked thrombocytopenia: WASP gene mutations, protein expression, and phenotype. Blood 1997;90:2680.

100. Malinin NL, Zhang L, Choi J, et al. A point mutation in KINDLIN3 ablates activation of three integrin subfamilies in humans. Nat Med 2009;15:313.

101. Coller BS, French DL, Rao AK. Hereditary qualitative platelet disorders. In: Kaushansky K, Lichtman MA, Beutler E, et al, editors. Williams hematology. 8th edition. New York: McGraw-Hill; 2010. p. 1933.
102. Navarro-Nunez L, Lozano ML, Rivera J, et al. The association of the beta1-tubulin Q43P polymorphism with intracerebral hemorrhage in men. Haematologica 2007;92:513.
103. Ho CY, Otterud B, Legare RD, et al. Linkage of a familial platelet disorder with a propensity to develop myeloid malignancies to human chromosome 21q22.1–22.2. Blood 1996;87:5218.
104. Song WJ, Sullivan MG, Legare RD, et al. Haploinsufficiency of CBFA2 causes familial thrombocytopenia with propensity to develop acute myelogenous leukaemia. Nat Genet 1999;23:166.
105. Sun L, Gorospe JR, Hoffman EP, et al. Decreased platelet expression of myosin regulatory light chain polypeptide (MYL9) and other genes with platelet dysfunction and CBFA2/RUNX1 mutation: insights from platelet expression profiling. J Thromb Haemost 2007;5:146.
106. Jalagadugula G, Mao G, Kaur G, et al. Regulation of platelet myosin light chain (MYL9) by RUNX1: implications for thrombocytopenia and platelet dysfunction in RUNX1 haplodeficiency. Blood 2010;116:6037.
107. Kaur G, Jalagadugula G, Mao G, et al. RUNX1/core binding factor A2 regulates platelet 12-lipoxygenase gene (ALOX12): studies in human RUNX1 haplodeficiency. Blood 2010;115:3128.
108. Jalagadugula G, Mao G, Kaur G, et al. Platelet PKC-θ deficiency with human RUNX1 mutation: PRKCQ is a transcriptional target of RUNX1. Arterioscler Thromb Vasc Biol 2011;31:921.
109. Heller PG, Glembotsky AC, Gandhi MJ, et al. Low Mpl receptor expression in a pedigree with familial platelet disorder with predisposition to acute myelogenous leukemia and a novel AML1 mutation. Blood 2005;105:4664.
110. Walker LC, Stevens J, Campbell H, et al. A novel inherited mutation of the transcription factor RUNX1 causes thrombocytopenia and may predispose to acute myeloid leukaemia. Br J Haematol 2002;117:878.
111. Freson K, Devriendt K, Matthijs G, et al. Platelet characteristics in patients with X-linked macrothrombocytopenia because of a novel GATA1 mutation. Blood 2001;98:85.
112. Hayward CP, Harrison P, Cattaneo M, et al. Platelet function analyzer (PFA)-100 closure time in the evaluation of platelet disorders and platelet function. J Thromb Haemost 2006;4:312.
113. Mannucci PM. Desmopressin (DDAVP) in the treatment of bleeding disorders; the first 20 years. Blood 1997;90:2515.
114. Mannucci PM. Hemostatic drugs. N Engl J Med 1998;339:245.
115. Rao AK, Ghosh S, Sun L, et al. Effect of mechanism of platelet dysfunction on response to DDAVP in patients with congenital platelet function defects. A double-blind placebo-controlled trial. Thromb Haemost 1995;74:1071.
116. Kobrinsky NL, Israels ED, Gerrard JM, et al. Shortening of bleeding time by 1-deamino-8-D-arginine vasopressin in various bleeding disorders. Lancet 1984;1:1145.
117. Schulman S, Johnson H, Egberg N, et al. DDAVP-induced correction of prolonged bleeding time in patients with congenital platelet function defects. Thromb Res 1987;45:165.
118. DiMichele DM, Hathaway WE. Use of DDAVP in inherited and acquired platelet dysfunction. Am J Hematol 1990;33:39.

119. Nieuwenhuis HK, Sixma JJ. 1-Desamino-8-d-arginine vasopressin (Desmopressin) shortens the bleeding time in storage pool deficiency. Ann Intern Med 1988; 108:65.
120. Almeida AM, Khair K, Hann I, et al. The use of recombinant factor VIIa in children with inherited platelet function disorders. Br J Haematol 2003;121:477.
121. Poon MC, d'Oiron R. Recombinant activated factor VII (NovoSeven) treatment of platelet-related bleeding disorders. International Registry on Recombinant Factor VIIa and Congenital Platelet Disorders Group. Blood Coagul Fibrinolysis 2000;11(Suppl 1):S55.
122. Kickler TS. Alternatives to platelet transfusions in the management of platelet dysfunction or thrombocytopenia. Transfus Altern Transfus Med 2006;2:127.
123. del Pozo Pozo AI, Jimenez-Yuste V, Villar A, et al. Successful thyroidectomy in a patient with Hermansky-Pudlak syndrome treated with recombinant activated factor VII and platelet concentrates. Blood Coagul Fibrinolysis 2002;13:551.
124. Mielke CH Jr, Levine PH, Zucker S. Preoperative prednisone therapy in platelet function disorders. Thromb Res 1981;21:655.
125. Seligsohn U. Treatment of inherited platelet disorders. Haemophilia 2012; 18(Suppl 4):161.

Inherited Disorders of Platelets
Membrane Glycoprotein Disorders

Reyhan Diz-Kücükkaya, MD[a],*, José A. López, MD[b,c,d]

KEYWORDS

- Platelet glycoproteins • Bernard-Soulier syndrome • Glanzmann thrombasthenia
- Inherited bleeding tendency • Platelet disorders

KEY POINTS

- Platelet membrane glycoproteins play key roles in various aspects of platelets functions and their deficiency can produce bleeding.
- Bleeding can be severe and manifest during childhood, or mild and only manifested in adulthood after trauma or surgery.
- These disorders can mimic acquired disorders and require careful histories and detailed laboratory evaluation. Management requires both preventive measures and treatment of specific bleeding episodes according to severity.
- The study of platelet membrane disorders also has yielded important insights into the functions of affected proteins, information that has produced some of the most successful antithrombotic drugs currently in use.

Inherited platelet disorders are rare, and chiefly produce defects in primary hemostasis. The severity of symptoms primarily depends on 2 variables: (1) the identity of the deficient or defective protein, and (2) the extent of the deficiency or functional defect. Severe deficiencies manifest themselves early during childhood, with frequent episodes of mucocutaneous bleeding, such as purpura, gingival bleeding, epistaxis, menorrhagia, and prolonged bleeding after trauma or surgery. Hematuria and gastrointestinal bleeding, and rarely intracranial hemorrhage may occur spontaneously. Mild deficiencies may not be diagnosed until adulthood or until the hemostatic system is stressed by surgery or trauma. Inherited platelet disorders can also be associated with other clinical features, such as skeletal abnormalities and mental retardation in velo-cardiofacial syndrome, hearing loss, or renal disorders. In some patients, the

[a] Division of Hematology, Department of Internal Medicine, Hematology and Oncology Clinic, Avrupa Florence Nightingale Hospital, Bedrettin Mahallesi, Bedii Gorbon sokak, No:1, 34420, Sishane, Istanbul, Turkey; [b] Puget Sound Blood Center Research Institute, Puget Sound Blood Center, 1551 Eastlake Avenue East, Suite 100, Seattle, WA 98102, USA; [c] Division of Hematology, University of Washington Medical Center, Box 357710, 1705 North East Pacific Street, Seattle, WA 98195-7710, USA; [d] Department of Biochemistry, University of Washington, Box 357350, 1705 NE Pacific Street, Seattle, WA 98195-7350, USA
* Corresponding author.
E-mail address: rkucukkaya@hotmail.com

Hematol Oncol Clin N Am 27 (2013) 613–627
http://dx.doi.org/10.1016/j.hoc.2013.03.005
0889-8588/13/$ – see front matter © 2013 Elsevier Inc. All rights reserved.
hemonc.theclinics.com

presence of thrombocytopenia with large platelets may lead to the misdiagnosis of immune thrombocytopenia (ITP) and lead to unnecessary treatments. Family history, platelet aggregation tests, flow cytometric analysis of platelet surface glycoproteins, and genetic analysis discriminate inherited disorders from acquired ones, although not always with 100% certainty.

Inherited platelet disorders are a large and heterogeneous group of diseases caused by genetic mutations of a large number genes, some expressed exclusively on platelets and megakaryocytes, and some having more widespread distribution. An overview of inherited platelet function disorders and a review of disorders of platelet granules and secretion is presented elsewhere in this issue. Inherited thrombocytopenias are described in a separate review. This review primarily focuses on inherited defects of platelet membrane glycoproteins.

DISORDERS OF THE GLYCOPROTEIN IB-IX-V COMPLEX

The glycoprotein (GP) Ib-IX-V complex is constitutively expressed on platelets and megakaryocytes and mediates several important platelet interactions with other molecules. The GPIb-IX-V complex contains 4 distinct polypeptide subunits in a stoichiometry of 2 GPIbα, 4 GPIbβ, 2 GPIX, and 1 molecule of GPV.[1,2] Although this stoichiometry has been established, the exact number of subunits in a functional complex has not been. Each subunit has the structure of a type I transmembrane protein, with a single transmembrane domain separating an extracellular N-terminus from an intracellular C-terminus. Each also belongs to the leucine-rich repeat (LRR) superfamily of proteins that includes, prominently, the toll-like receptors.[3] Whether this shared ancestry implies anything about the functions of the GPIb-IX-V complex is not clear. The LRRs reside in the extracellular portion of the polypeptides, where they are flanked by disulfide loops at the N- and C-termini. In GPIbα, the polypeptide that contains the binding sites for all of the known ligands of the complex, the LRR-containing ligand-binding domain is separated from the platelet plasma membrane by a extended, highly glycosylated mucin core. Each polypeptide also has a cytoplasmic domain through which the polypeptides associate with cytoskeletal elements, such as filamin A, and adapter and signaling proteins, such as 14-3-3ζ, calmodulin, and phosphoinositide-3 kinase.[4] The 4 subunits are encoded by different genes. After transcription and translation of the polypeptides, they associate to produce the receptor complex in the endoplasmic reticulum.[5] Posttranslational modifications of the molecule are very important for the functions of the receptor and include extensive N- and O-glycosylation, palmitoylation of GPIbβ and GPIX,[6] and tyrosine sulfation.[7,8] Approximately 15,000 to 25,000 copies of GPIb-IX-V complex are expressed on human platelets.[1,9,10]

The GPIb-IX-V complex mediates several interactions of importance in thrombosis and hemostasis. GPIbα binds von Willebrand Factor (VWF),[11] thrombin,[12] P-selectin,[13] Mac-1,[14] factor XI,[15] factor XII,[16] high molecular weight kininogen,[17] thrombospondin,[18] and β-2 glycoprotein I.[19] Of these, the interaction with VWF, and possibly thrombin, appear to be the most important, as judged by the phenotype of the deficiency syndrome. Binding of GPIbα to VWF is the key event in the adhesion of platelets to the subendothelium, which is exposed with traumatic vessel injury or rupture of atherosclerotic plaques. Matrix-bound VWF, unlike VWF circulating in blood, expresses a normally cryptic GPIbα binding site, allowing platelets from the blood to adhere and spread at the site of injury, with subsequent aggregation mediated by other membrane glycoproteins. Two other circumstances in addition to being immobilized on the subendothelial surface also allow VWF to bind GPIbα: (1) exposure of plasma

VWF to very high shear stresses, where the force unfolds VWF and exposes the GPIbα binding site; and (2) acute release and defective removal of ultralarge VWF multimers from the endothelial surface, as occurs in thrombotic thrombocytopenic purpura.[20,21] Recent data indicate that the GPIbα–VWF interaction may also be important in the pathogenesis of venous thrombosis.[22] Interactions between GPIbα and coagulation proteins, such as thrombin, factor XI, and factor XII, may also influence the activity of the coagulation cascade on the platelet surface. The GPIb-IX-V complex also has a role in inflammatory reactions, as indicated by its ability to bind both P-selectin[13] and Mac-1,[14] and the anti-inflammatory effects of blocking those interactions in experimental models.[23–25]

Inherited mutations of the platelet GPIb-IX-V complex either prevent its expression on the platelet surface or create a dysfunctional receptor. Absence of the receptor on the cell surface, or mutations that interfere with VWF binding, produce Bernard-Soulier syndrome.[9] GPIbα can also be affected by mutations that increase the affinity of the interaction with VWF, producing the bleeding disorder platelet-type von Willebrand disease.

Bernard-Soulier Syndrome

This disorder, originally described by the French physicians Jean Bernard and Jean-Pierre Soulier in 1948, is characterized by a bleeding tendency, thrombocytopenia, giant platelets, and the absence of ristocetin-induced platelet agglutination.[9,10] It is an orphan disease, with an estimated prevalence of fewer than 1 in 1 million.

Patients with BSS generally present with manifestations of mucocutaneous bleeding (purpura, gingival bleeding, epistaxis, menorrhagia) and prolonged and excessive bleeding after trauma or surgery, usually beginning in early childhood. Spontaneous gastrointestinal or urogenital bleeding may occur; intracranial bleeding and intraperitoneal hematomas are very rare.[9,10] Bleeding signs and symptoms may vary considerably among affected individuals, even within the same family.

Thrombocytopenia and giant platelets on the blood smear are important features of the disease. Platelet counts range from 10 to 200 × 10^9. The reason that GPIb-IX-V complex deficiency causes thrombocytopenia and large platelets is not understood, but it has been speculated that the large platelets are a consequence of defective attachment of the plasma membrane to the membrane skeleton, an association largely mediated by the GPIb-IX-V complex. Some of the thrombocytopenia is accounted for by the fact that giant platelets may not be recognized by automatic cell counters, which may count them as leukocytes instead. Although some studies showed platelet survival time to be decreased in patients with BSS, the results are inconsistent and some patients have normal platelet half-lives.[26,27] The difficulty of isolating giant platelets from blood samples may affect the survival studies.[27] Animal models and some studies with patients with BSS have shown that the absence of the GPIb-IX-V complex impairs megakaryocyte membrane development, alters tubulin distribution, and causes abnormal proplatelet formation with production of giant platelets.[27–29] Thrombocytopenia and defective platelet adhesion together account for the hemostatic defect. Prolonged closure times using the platelet function analyzer (PFA)-100, which measures shear-dependent platelet functions in vitro using both collagen/ADP and collagen/epinephrine embedded cartridges, is sensitive in detecting the hemostatic defect of BSS.[30]

Iron deficiency anemia may occur in patients with BSS who experience severe bleeding, especially women with menorrhagia. The erythrocytes are otherwise normal. Leukocyte counts and morphology should be carefully evaluated in patients with giant platelets for discrimination of MYH9-related diseases. Coagulation tests are also normal, including clot retraction, prothrombin time, activated partial thromboplastin time, and levels of VWF and factor VIII. Although they are not routinely tested, prothrombin consumption and thrombin generation are decreased in BSS.[9] The defect in thrombin consumption can be mimicked by treating normal platelets with a GPIbα antibody that blocks VWF binding.[31]

Unfortunately, routine tests cannot differentiate BSS from other inherited and acquired giant platelet syndromes. BSS is most often misdiagnosed as immune thrombocytopenia (ITP), because macrothrombocytopenia is often found in patients with ITP. This is especially true in carriers of BSS mutations. A family history of bleeding and personal history of bleeding signs and symptoms since early childhood weigh against a diagnosis of ITP. Platelet aggregation tests and platelet surface glycoprotein analysis are crucial for diagnosis of BSS. In aggregation studies, BSS platelets characteristically show lack of ristocetin-induced agglutination, but have normal or near-normal responses to collagen, ADP, and epinephrine. Aggregation is defective at low concentrations of thrombin, but normal at higher concentrations. Flow cytometric analysis of platelet surface glycoproteins by immunostaining usually reveals severe deficiency or absence of the GPIb-IX-V complex. Other specific tests, such as immunoblotting after sodium dodecyl sulfate (SDS)-polyacrylamide gel electrophoresis may show absence of specific fragments of the receptor. In a special subtype, the Bolzano variant, GPIb-IX-V complex is present on the platelet surface in normal quantities, but the receptor cannot bind VWF because of mutation of Ala 156 to Val in GPIbα.[28]

BSS is almost always inherited as an autosomal recessive trait, and often associated with consanguinity. Autosomal dominant inheritance has also been reported, but much less frequently.[32,33] Mutations responsible for BSS are usually specific to a particular patient or family. Heterozygous individuals have reduced GPIb-IX-V complex on the platelet surface, and usually do not have bleeding symptoms, but may manifest macrothrombocytopenia. In Italy, heterozygosity for BSS is the most common cause of inherited macrothrombocytopenia.[34,35]

Mutations responsible for BSS are highly heterogeneous and include nonsense mutations, missense mutations, and frameshift insertions or deletions involving the genes encoding GPIbα, GPIbβ, or GPIX. Mutations of the *GPV* gene have not been described in BSS, and its gene product is unnecessary for expression of a functional complex in transfected cells.[36]

Platelet-type von Willebrand disease

Platelet-type von Willebrand disease (VWD) (also called pseudo-VWD) is caused by dominantly inherited gain-of-function mutations in GPIbα. Four point mutations (G233V, G233S, D235Y, M239V) and a 27–base pair deletion have been described in patients with platelet-type VWD.[37,38] These mutations increase the affinity of GPIbα for VWF, allowing VWF to bind spontaneously to platelets (no modulator required), resulting in clearance of the highest-molecular-weight and hemostatically most active multimers of VWF from the plasma and producing a bleeding diathesis. Bleeding symptoms are usually mild to moderate but can become life threatening after surgery, during pregnancy, or with the use of antiplatelet drugs. The blood smear usually displays mild thrombocytopenia and large platelets. Platelet-type VWD is often misdiagnosed as ITP or type 2B VWD. The presence of increased ristocetin-induced platelet aggregation (RIPA), decreased ristocetin cofactor activity of the plasma, and normal or mildly decreased VWF antigen levels help to exclude ITP. On the other hand, discrimination of platelet-type VWD from type 2B VWD can be complicated. The RIPA mixing assay,[39] flow cytometry,[40] and genetic analysis of VWF (for type 2B

VWD) and GPIbα (for platelet-type VWD) are used for the exact diagnosis. In the RIPA mixing assay, combining patient platelets with normal plasma yields RIPA results similar to those with patient platelet-rich plasma.[39] Management of these 2 diseases is also different: bleeding is controlled by platelet transfusions in patients with platelet-type VWD, whereas VWF-containing preparations are used in patients with type 2B VWD.[37,40]

Velo-cardiofacial syndrome

BSS-like functional defects may be seen in patients with velo-cardiofacial syndrome (VCFS). VCFS is a developmental disorder characterized by abnormal development of the pharyngeal arch. Multiple abnormalities, such as craniofacial defects, cardiac abnormalities, immune deficiencies, and mental problems are present in different variants. VCFS is caused by deletions in chromosome 22q11. Because this region contains the gene encoding GPIbβ, patients with VCFS may have increased platelet size, thrombocytopenia, and reduced aggregation with ristocetin.[41]

GPIbα polymorphisms

Several polymorphisms of GPIbα have been described. Because GPIbα is the receptor that mediates platelet adhesion, these polymorphisms have been studied extensively to examine their link with arterial thrombosis.

The GPIbα variable number of tandem repeat polymorphism The GPIbα variable number of tandem repeat (VNTR) polymorphism affects the region encoding the macroglycopeptide of GPIbα, which contains a variable number of 39–base pair tandem repeats, each encoding identical 13–amino acid sequences. Four polymorphic variants have been identified. In order of decreasing size these are: A, B, C, and D, with 4, 3, 2, and 1 repeat, respectively. The number of repeats affects the length of the macroglycopeptide and the degree to which the ligand-binding domain protrudes above the plasma membrane, and thereby may change the ability of GPIbα to bind VWF.[42,43] The GPIbα VNTR polymorphism has been extensively studied in patients with arterial thrombosis, with inconsistent results.[44,45]

HPA-2 (Ko$^{a/b}$) polymorphism of GPIbα Human platelet allo-antigen HPA-2, also known as the Ko polymorphism, is a threonine/methionine dimorphism at position 145 of GPIbα. Threonine is the most prevalent amino acid at this position in all populations tested. The HPA-2 polymorphism is associated with platelet transfusion refractoriness and neonatal alloimmune thrombocytopenia. The polymorphic site is located near the VWF and thrombin binding sites of GPIbα. The HPA-2 polymorphism is in linkage disequilibrium with the GPIbα VNTR polymorphism.[46,47]

Kozak sequence polymorphism of the GPIBA gene The Kozak sequence polymorphism of the GPIBA gene is based on the presence of either thymine or cytosine at position −5 from the initiator ATG codon and therefore does not change the amino acid sequence of the polypeptide. The frequency of the less prevalent C allele ranges from 8% to 17% in different ethnic groups.[48] The presence of the C allele correlated with increased mRNA translation and higher surface expression of GPIbα in affected individuals.[48] The impact of the Kozak polymorphism has been investigated in patients with arterial thrombosis with different results. Some investigators showed an association of the C allele with coronary thrombosis and stroke[49–51]; others found no association.[52] An increased risk of thrombosis linked to the Kozak polymorphism was reported in postmenopausal women taking hormone replacement therapy[53] and in patients with antiphospholipid syndrome.[54]

DISORDERS OF INTEGRIN $\alpha_{IIb}\beta_3$

Integrin $\alpha_{IIb}\beta_3$ (GPIIb-IIIa, CD 41/61) is a receptor for fibrinogen and VWF, and also can bind fibrin, fibronectin, thrombospondin, and vitronectin. This receptor promotes stable platelet adhesion and spreading on the extracellular matrix of the damaged vessel wall and is the primary receptor mediating platelet aggregation to stimulation by all agonists. Integrin $\alpha_{IIb}\beta_3$ is abundantly expressed on platelets, with between 50,000 and 80,000 copies per platelet, representing approximately 1% to 2% of total platelet protein.[55,56]

$\alpha_{IIb}\beta_3$ is a heterodimer composed of 2 subunits: α_{IIb} and β_3, which are encoded by different genes located on chromosome 17. In humans, the α_{IIb} gene (ITGA2B) is expressed only in the megakaryocytic lineage; the β_3 gene (ITGB3) is widely expressed on nonplatelet cells (including on leukocytes and endothelial cells) as a part of integrin $\alpha_v\beta_3$. Both subunits have large extracellular domains, single transmembrane domains, and short cytoplasmic tails. The extracellular domains have a complex 3-dimensional structure that is altered dramatically when platelets are activated and the integrin assumes a ligand-binding conformation.[57] In resting platelets, the cytoplasmic tails and transmembrane domains of the 2 polypeptides are close to each other (clasped form), and the extracellular domains are bent in a manner that prevents access of the ligand-binding region to ligands. Activation of the platelets induces binding of cytoplasmic proteins (such as talin) to the integrin cytoplasmic tails, leading to "unclasping" of the cytoplasmic and transmembrane domains, allowing the ligand-binding domain to straighten and assume a ligand-competent conformation. The integrin then bridges adjacent platelets into aggregates by binding bivalent fibrinogen or multivalent VWF, the latter being more important in regions of high shear stress. After ligand binding, $\alpha_{IIb}\beta_3$ produces outside-in signals that are important for several platelet functions, including procoagulant activity and clot retraction.[58]

The critical role of $\alpha_{IIb}\beta_3$ in hemostasis and thrombosis also makes it an attractive target for antithrombotic drugs. Parenteral $\alpha_{IIb}\beta_3$ inhibitors, which include abciximab, eptifibatide, and tirofiban, decrease mortality in patients undergoing percutaneous interventions, and are widely used for this purpose. Interestingly, oral $\alpha_{IIb}\beta_3$ inhibitors do not have this effect, sometimes even increasing mortality.[59]

Glanzmann Thrombasthenia

Inherited quantitative or qualitative abnormalities affecting $\alpha_{IIb}\beta_3$ cause defective platelet aggregation and produce the bleeding diathesis Glanzmann thrombasthenia (GT), named after Eduard Glanzmann, who first described this entity in 1918 as "hereditary hemorrhagic thrombasthenia." Although it is accepted that GT is the most common integrin disorder, its exact prevalence is not known. It is an autosomal recessive disorder and consanguinity of the parents of affected individuals is frequent. Bleeding symptoms are expected only in individuals who are homozygotes or compound heterozygotes for mutations affecting the genes encoding either subunit.

The primary clinical manifestation of the disorder is mucocutaneous bleeding. Facial purpura may be seen in newborns with GT. Prolonged menstrual bleeding is an important problem in female patients. Spontaneous life-threatening hemorrhage is rare. Surgery, major trauma, and pregnancy will increase the bleeding risk, as does the presence of other acquired or inherited hemostatic defects, such as liver disease or VWD.

Unlike in BSS, the blood smear in GT is unremarkable and the platelet count is normal. A prolonged bleeding time or prolonged closure time on PFA-100 analysis suggests an abnormal platelet function; clot retraction is also defective. Because of the central role of $\alpha_{IIb}\beta_3$ in platelet aggregation, GT platelets fail to aggregate to all agonists; however, GT platelets have a normal agglutination curve with ristocetin, which, together with normal-sized platelets in the blood smear, discriminates GT from BSS. GT patients with severe $\alpha_{IIb}\beta_3$ deficiency (expression levels less than 5%, impaired aggregation responses with no clot retraction) are classified as having type I disease; patients with moderate deficiency (10%–20% expression, abnormal aggregation with residual clot reaction) are classified as having type II GT. A variant form of GT has been described in which a dysfunctional $\alpha_{IIb}\beta_3$ is expressed on the platelet surface.[60–62]

The α_{IIb} gene (ITGA2B) has 30 exons and the β_3 gene (ITGB3) has 15 exons. More than 100 mutations (deletions, insertions, missense and nonsense mutations, splicing defects, frameshift mutations) have been reported in these genes in association with GT. Interestingly, the severity of bleeding does not correlate with the quantity of platelet surface $\alpha_{IIb}\beta_3$ or with the measured functional impairment.[60] Mice genetically deficient in β_3 become osteosclerotic because of osteoclast dysfunction,[63] and are at increased risk of malignancies caused by elevated signaling from vascular endothelial growth factor receptor-2 (VEGFR-2) and enhanced angiogenesis.[64] Both of these phenotypes are likely consequences of deficiency of the related β_3 integrin $\alpha_v\beta_3$, and have not been reported in humans lacking the β_3 subunit.

Integrin $\alpha_{IIb}\beta_3$ (GPIIb-IIIa) Polymorphisms

Several known $\alpha_{IIb}\beta_3$ polymorphisms affect the complex's antigenicity and functions.[65] Antibodies against different epitopes of the receptor may cause immune thrombocytopenia, posttransfusion purpura, refractoriness to platelet transfusions, and neonatal alloimmune thrombocytopenia. It has also been suggested that some polymorphisms, such as the PL[A1/A2] polymorphism, with either a Leu or a Pro residue at position 33 of β_3, alter the function of the receptor, with the hyperfunctional allele associated with increased risk of arterial thrombosis.[66]

The prevalence of the PL[A1] allele (encoding Leu at position 33) varies widely in different ethnic groups: 0.84 in whites to more than 0.99 in east Asians. Platelets expressing PL[A2] were shown to have increased alpha granule secretion and P-selectin expression, increased activation and aggregation, and shortened bleeding time.[67,68] Studies investigating the association between PL[A2] and coronary thrombosis did not produce consistent results.[67,69] The recently reported study of the atherosclerosis risk in communities (ARIC) cohort suggested that only individuals homozygous for PL[A2] are at increased risk of atherosclerotic plaque rupture.[68]

DISORDERS OF PLATELET COLLAGEN RECEPTORS

After the rupture of atherosclerotic plaques, platelet attachment to the injury site is initiated by an interaction between the GPIb-IX-V complex and VWF. This reaction, however, is reversible and may not produce stable adhesion under medium and high shear stresses. After the initial platelet capture, however, subendothelial collagen supports stable platelet adhesion, activates platelets, and induces procoagulant activity. Four collagen receptors have been identified on the platelet surface: integrin $\alpha_2\beta_1$ (GPIa/IIa) and GPVI can bind to collagen directly, whereas others (integrin $\alpha_{IIb}\beta_3$ and GPIb) bind collagen indirectly through VWF. Of these, GPVI elicits the most potent activation response.[70,71] GPVI is a 62-kDa membrane glycoprotein and a member of the immunoglobulin (Ig) receptor superfamily. The receptor has 2 Ig-C2-like domains with internal disulfide bonds, a mucinlike region, a transmembrane domain, and a short cytoplasmic tail. On the platelet surface, GPVI is associated with the

Fc receptor γ chain, which contributes cytoplasmic signaling motifs. After platelets bind collagen, GPVI signals through the Syk/SLP-76/PLCγ2 pathway, inducing calcium mobilization and platelet degranulation, and eventually activating integrins ($\alpha_2\beta_1$ and $\alpha_{IIb}\beta_3$) and thereby mediating adhesion and aggregation. Nieswandt and colleagues[70] demonstrated that treatment of mice with a monoclonal antibody (JAQ1) against GPVI depleted GPVI from the platelet surface. Genetic ablation of GPVI in mice protected against thrombosis without producing major bleeding.[72] These studies indicated that platelet GPVI might be a good antithrombotic target.

Genetic deficiency of GPVI in humans is extremely rare. Some cases of acquired GPVI deficiency produced by autoantibodies have also been described, with the deficiency presumably being produced by a mechanism similar to that in the antibody-treated mice. Although most patients with GPVI defects have slightly elevated bleeding times and usually normal platelet counts, some of the reported cases had severe bleeding requiring red blood cell transfusions.[71] In humans, at least 10 polymorphisms have been described in the *GP6* gene. Some of these polymorphisms may be associated with increased acute myocardial infarction risk, but there are no data on their functional consequences.[71,73]

Other platelet surface receptors participate in the firm adhesion of platelets to the subendothelium, including integrins $\alpha_2\beta_1$ (GPIa-IIa), $\alpha_5\beta_1$ (VLA-5), $\alpha_6\beta_1$ (VLA-6), and $\alpha_V\beta_3$. In humans, inherited deficiencies of these molecules have no significant effect on hemostasis (**Table 1**), although in one report, acquired deficiency of $\alpha_2\beta_1$ in a patient with myelodysplastic syndrome was associated with bleeding and platelet unresponsiveness to collagen.[74]

DIAGNOSIS OF INHERITED PLATELET MEMBRANE GLYCOPROTEIN DISORDERS

Inherited disorders of platelet membrane glycoproteins have clinical manifestations similar to those of other acquired and inherited platelet disorders: spontaneous mucocutaneous bleeding, increased bleeding after trauma or ingestion of antiplatelet

Table 1
Inherited platelet membrane glycoprotein disorders

Platelet Receptor	Ligands	Functions	Inherited Deficiencies
GP Ib-IX-V	VWF, thrombin, P-selectin, HMWK thrombospondin, Mac-1, FXI, FXII	Adhesion	Bernard-Soulier syndrome Platelet-type VWD Velo-cardiofacial syndrome
Integrin $\alpha_{IIb}\beta_3$ (GP IIb-IIIa)	Fibrinogen, collagen, fibrin, vitronectin, VWF	Aggregation, firm adhesion	Glanzmann thrombasthenia
GP VI	Collagen	Adhesion	Inherited deficiency is extremely rare: mild/no bleeding?
Integrin $\alpha_2\beta_1$ (GP Ia/IIa)	Collagen	Firm adhesion	No significant hemostatic defect?
Integrin $\alpha_5\beta_1$ (VLA-5)	Fibronectin	Firm adhesion	No significant hemostatic defect?
Integrin $\alpha_6\beta_1$ (VLA-6)	Laminin	Firm adhesion	No significant hemostatic defect?
Integrin $\alpha_V\beta_3$	Vitronectin, fibronectin, osteopontin	Firm adhesion	No significant hemostatic defect

Abbreviations: VWD, von Willebrand disease; VWF, von Willebrand factor.

medications, and rarely, life-threatening bleeding into the cranial cavity or gastrointestinal tract. Bleeding-score systems have been proposed to quantitatively evaluate the number and severity of bleeding episodes in patients with inherited bleeding disorders.[75] These may help predict who is at risk for bleeding, independent of functional defects identified through laboratory evaluation.

A family history of bleeding strongly suggests an inherited disorder. Clues to the diagnosis include coexisting skeletal and mental abnormalities (velo-cardiofacial syndrome, thrombocytopenia with absent radius [TAR] syndrome, Paris-Trousseau syndrome), hearing loss and/or renal problems (MYH9-related disorders), and recurrent infections (Wiskott-Aldrich syndrome).

The diagnosis of inherited platelet membrane glycoprotein disorders requires detailed laboratory investigation. Because automated blood counts usually produce artifactual results in patients with macrothrombocytopenia, platelet counts should be estimated by examination of the blood smear. Although the presence of giant platelets may suggest inherited platelet disorders, such as BSS, platelet-type VWD, and MYH9-related diseases, they can also be seen in acquired platelet disorders, including immune thrombocytopenia. Pale platelets with no granules suggest gray platelet syndrome. The presence of atypical cells (myelodysplastic syndrome), inclusion bodies in the leukocyte cytoplasm (MYH9-related diseases), and red cell abnormalities are against the diagnosis of inherited platelet membrane disorders.[76–79]

Although the Ivy bleeding time is sensitive to changes in platelet number and function, it is nonspecific, unreliable, and invasive. In most laboratories, PFA-100 analysis has replaced the skin bleeding time. The PFA-100 measures platelet functions at high shear stress using collagen/ADP and collagen/epinephrine embedded cartridges. The system is not sensitive to coagulation factor deficiencies, and PFA is normal in patients with isolated coagulation disorders. However, it is sensitive to thrombocytopenia and anemia. Therefore, platelet counts should be more than 100×10^9 and the hematocrit should be more than 30% to ascertain that abnormal responses are attributable to platelet dysfunction. Prolonged closure times (>300 seconds) in both collagen/ADP and collagen/epinephrine cartridges are typically seen in patients with BSS and GT. This test can thus be used for screening of these 2 inherited platelet disorders.[76,77]

Light transmission aggregometry with whole blood or platelet-rich plasma measures platelet aggregation in response to various agonists, and may produce specific profiles characteristic of individual disorders. Whole blood is preferable in patients with giant platelets because of the artificially low platelet count produced during preparation of platelet-rich plasma. Spontaneous aggregation of platelets in whole blood or platelet-rich plasma may be observed in patients with platelet-type VWD or Montreal platelet syndrome. Absence of ristocetin-induced agglutination, with normal responses to collagen, ADP, and epinephrine, are characteristic features of BSS. Absence of aggregation with ADP, collagen, and arachidonic acid, but normal aggregation with ristocetin is highly suggestive of GT. Increased aggregation with low-dose ristocetin suggests platelet type-VWD, and this syndrome can be differentiated from type 2B VWD with the mixed RIPA assay (see earlier in this article).

Flow cytometry can be used to measure the quantity of membrane glycoproteins on the platelet surface using specific antibodies conjugated to fluorescent probes. These assays can be performed on whole blood or platelet suspensions, and they are not influenced by platelet size or hematocrit. Both homozygous and heterozygous forms of BSS and GT can be diagnosed by flow cytometry. The molecular mass of the platelet receptor can be evaluated by SDS-gel and immunoblotting. Electron microscopy, measurement of platelet nucleotides, and nucleotide release can be used to discriminate membrane glycoprotein disorders from other inherited platelet defects such as storage pool disease, MYH9-related disorders, and Hermansky-Pudlak syndrome. Although sequencing of affected genes provides accurate diagnosis of the molecular defects, it is available only in specialized laboratories.

MANAGEMENT OF PATIENTS WITH INHERITED PLATELET DISORDERS

The management of bleeding in patients with inherited platelet disorders requires both preventive measures and the treatment of individual bleeding episodes according to their severity. Local bleeding, such as gingival bleeding and epistaxis, can be controlled by compression and use of gelatin sponges, fibrin sealants, or tranexaminic acid-embedded gauze. Patient education is vital and should include information about maintaining dental hygiene, avoiding activities such as sports in which trauma is frequent, and avoiding the use of antiplatelet drugs, including those contained in over-the-counter medications and dietary supplements.

Menorrhagia is a common problem; oral contraceptives, hormonal intrauterine devices, and antifibrinolytic drugs may decrease uterine bleeding. Desmopressin increases the plasma concentrations of VWF, and may help decrease bleeding in patients with BSS and GT, perhaps through mechanisms other than those generally believed to be the hemostatic functions of VWF.

Patients who bleed chronically may become anemic from iron deficiency and require iron supplementation. In cases with severe bleeding or in patients who require surgery, platelet and erythrocyte transfusions are indicated, although the risk of these patients developing antibodies to platelets is increased. Recombinant factor VIIa can be used in patients with life-threatening bleeding, or in patients with platelet alloantibodies.[80]

It is generally believed that patients with inherited platelet disorders, such as BSS and GT, should be protected from thrombotic events, but this assumption cannot be verified epidemiologically because of the rarity and heterogeneity of these disorders. One very recent article reviewed cases of thrombosis occurring in BSS and GT.[33] Nine patients with GT (ages 2 through 72) and 3 patients with BSS (ages 51, 62, and 66) have been reported in the literature to have thrombosis. All 3 patients with BSS had arterial thrombosis (acute coronary syndromes), with no reports of venous thrombosis. Two of these patients were cousins and had mild bleeding tendency, arguing for a coinherited thrombotic tendency. Eight patients with GT had venous thrombosis (6 had deep vein thrombosis, 1 had pulmonary embolism, and 1 cerebral vein thrombosis), and 1 had arterial thrombosis (a 6-year-old boy with fatal restrictive cardiomyopathy). The reported cases are very heterogeneous in terms of severity of platelet dysfunction, associated clinical problems, and the ages of the patients. It is not possible to make any firm conclusions on thrombotic risk in these patients. It seems that effective management of patients with inherited platelet disorders allows longer life expectancy, which in turn may increase the risk of thrombosis.

SUMMARY

Although disorders of platelet membrane glycoproteins are rare, their effects on the lives of those affected are very important. It is therefore important that these disorders be appropriately diagnosed, understood, and treated. Study of these disorders also has yielded important insights into the functions of the affected proteins, information that has produced some of the most successful antithrombotic drugs currently in use. Thus, the value of continuing to study these disorders is for the benefit of both those afflicted with the disorder and those suffering from much more common thrombotic disorders.

REFERENCES

1. Modderman PW, Admiraal LG, Sonnenberg A, et al. Glycoproteins V and Ib-IX form a noncovalent complex in the platelet membrane. J Biol Chem 1992;267: 364–9.
2. Luo SZ, Mo X, Afshar-Kharghan V, et al. Glycoprotein Ibα forms disulfide bonds with 2 glycoprotein Ibβ subunits in the resting platelet. Blood 2007;109(2): 603–9.
3. Botos I, Segal DM, Davies DR. The structural biology of Toll-like receptors. Structure 2011;19(4):447–59.
4. Du X. Signaling and regulation of the platelet glycoprotein Ib-IX-V complex. Curr Opin Hematol 2007;14(3):262–9.
5. Dong JF, Gao S, López JA. Synthesis, assembly, and intracellular transport of the platelet glycoprotein Ib-IX-V complex. J Biol Chem 1998;273(47):31449–54.
6. Schick PK, Walker J. The acylation of megakaryocyte proteins: glycoprotein IX is primarily myristoylated while glycoprotein Ib is palmitoylated. Blood 1996;87(4): 1377–84.
7. Dong JF, Li CQ, López JA. Tyrosine sulfation of the GP Ib-IX complex: identification of sulfated residues and effect on ligand binding. Biochemistry 1994;33: 13946–53.
8. Ward CM, Andrews RK, Smith AI, et al. Mocarhagin, a novel cobra venom metalloproteinase, cleaves the platelet von Willebrand factor receptor glycoprotein Ibα. Identification of the sulfated tyrosine/anionic sequence Tyr-276–Glu-282 of glycoprotein Ibα as a binding site for von Willebrand factor and α-thrombin. Biochemistry 1996;35:4929–38.
9. López JA, Andrews RK, Afshar-Kharghan V, et al. Bernard-Soulier syndrome. Blood 1998;91(12):4397–418.
10. Lanza F. Bernard-Soulier syndrome (hemorrhagiparous thrombocytic dystrophy). Orphanet J Rare Dis 2006;1:46.
11. López JA. The platelet glycoprotein Ib-IX complex. Blood Coagul Fibrinolysis 1994;5:97–119.
12. Harmon JT, Jamieson GA. The glycocalicin portion of platelet glycoprotein Ib expresses both high and moderate affinity receptor sites for thrombin. A soluble radioreceptor assay for the interaction of thrombin with platelets. J Biol Chem 1986;261:13224–9.
13. Romo GM, Dong JF, Schade AJ, et al. The glycoprotein Ib-IX-V complex is a platelet counter-receptor for P-selectin. J Exp Med 1999;190:803–13.
14. Simon DI, Chen Z, Xu H, et al. Platelet glycoprotein Ibα is a counterreceptor for the leukocyte integrin Mac-1 (CD11b/CD18). J Exp Med 2000;192(2):193–204.
15. Baglia FA, Badellino KO, Li CQ, et al. Factor XI binding to the platelet glycoprotein Ib-IX-V complex promotes factor XI activation by thrombin. J Biol Chem 2002;277(3):1662–8.
16. Bradford HN, Pixley RA, Colman RW. Human factor XII binding to the glycoprotein Ib-IX-V complex inhibits thrombin-induced platelet aggregation. J Biol Chem 2000;275(30):22756–63.
17. Joseph K, Nakazawa Y, Bahou WF, et al. Platelet glycoprotein Ib: a zinc-dependent binding protein for the heavy chain of high-molecular-weight kininogen. Mol Med 1999;5(8):555–63.
18. Jurk K, Clemetson KJ, de Groot PG, et al. Thrombospondin-1 mediates platelet adhesion at high shear via glycoprotein Ib (GPIb): an alternative/backup mechanism to von Willebrand factor. FASEB J 2003;17(11):1490–2.

19. Hulstein JJ, Lenting PJ, de LB, et al. β2-Glycoprotein I inhibits von Willebrand factor dependent platelet adhesion and aggregation. Blood 2007;110(5):1483–91.

20. Moake JL, Rudy CK, Troll JH, et al. Unusually large plasma factor VIII:von Willebrand factor multimers in chronic relapsing thrombotic thrombocytopenic purpura. N Engl J Med 1982;307(23):1432–5.

21. Dong JF, Moake JL, Nolasco L, et al. ADAMTS-13 rapidly cleaves newly secreted ultralarge von Willebrand factor multimers on the endothelial surface under flowing conditions. Blood 2002;100(12):4033–9.

22. Brill A, Fuchs TA, Chauhan AK, et al. von Willebrand factor-mediated platelet adhesion is critical for deep vein thrombosis in mouse models. Blood 2011; 117(4):1400–7.

23. Katayama T, Ikeda Y, Handa M, et al. Immunoneutralization of glycoprotein Ibα attenuates endotoxin-induced interactions of platelets and leukocytes with rat venular endothelium in vivo. Circ Res 2000;86(10):1031–7.

24. Ehlers R, Ustinov V, Chen Z, et al. Targeting platelet-leukocyte interactions: identification of the integrin Mac-1 binding site for the platelet counter receptor glycoprotein Ibα. J Exp Med 2003;198(7):1077–88.

25. Wang Y, Sakuma M, Chen Z, et al. Leukocyte engagement of platelet glycoprotein Ibα via the integrin Mac-1 is critical for the biological response to vascular injury. Circulation 2005;112(19):2993–3000.

26. Heyns AD, Badenhorst PN, Wessels P, et al. Kinetics, in vivo redistribution and sites of sequestration of indium-111-labelled platelets in giant platelet syndromes. Br J Haematol 1985;60(2):323–30.

27. Strassel C, Eckly A, Leon C, et al. Intrinsic impaired proplatelet formation and microtubule coil assembly of megakaryocytes in a mouse model of Bernard-Soulier syndrome. Haematologica 2009;94(6):800–10.

28. Balduini A, Malara A, Pecci A, et al. Proplatelet formation in heterozygous Bernard-Soulier syndrome type Bolzano. J Thromb Haemost 2009;7(3):478–84.

29. Poujol C, Ware J, Nieswandt B, et al. Absence of GPIbα is responsible for aberrant membrane development during megakaryocyte maturation: ultrastructural study using a transgenic model. Exp Hematol 2002;30(4):352–60.

30. Harrison P, Robinson M, Liesner R, et al. The PFA-100: a potential rapid screening tool for the assessment of platelet dysfunction. Clin Lab Haematol 2002;24(4):225–32.

31. Coller BS, Peerschke EI, Lesley E, et al. Studies with a murine monoclonal antibody that abolishes ristocetin-induced binding of von Willebrand factor to platelets: additional evidence in support of GPIb as a platelet receptor for von Willebrand factor. Blood 1983;61(1):99–110.

32. Miller JL, Lyle VA, Cunningham D. Mutation of leucine-57 to phenylalanine in a platelet glycoprotein Ibα leucine tandem repeat occurring in patients with an autosomal dominant variant of Bernard-Soulier disease. Blood 1992;79:439–46.

33. Girolami A, Vettore S, Vianello F, et al. Myocardial infarction in two cousins heterozygous for ASN41HIS autosomal dominant variant of Bernard-Soulier syndrome. J Thromb Thrombolysis 2012;34(4):513–7.

34. Savoia A, Balduini CL, Savino M, et al. Autosomal dominant macrothrombocytopenia in Italy is most frequently a type of heterozygous Bernard-Soulier syndrome. Blood 2001;97(5):1330–5.

35. Noris P, Perrotta S, Bottega R, et al. Clinical and laboratory features of 103 patients from 42 Italian families with inherited thrombocytopenia derived from the monoallelic Ala156Val mutation of GPIbalpha (Bolzano mutation). Haematologica 2012;97(1):82–8.

36. Li CQ, Dong JF, Lanza F, et al. Expression of platelet glycoprotein (GP) V in heterologous cells and evidence for its association with GP Ibα in forming a GP Ib-IX-V complex on the cell surface. J Biol Chem 1995;270(27):16302-7.
37. Othman M, López JA, Ware J. Platelet-type von Willebrand disease update: the disease, the molecule and the animal model. Expert Rev Hematol 2011;4(5): 475-7.
38. Enayat S, Ravanbod S, Rassoulzadegan M, et al. A novel D235Y mutation in the GP1BA gene enhances platelet interaction with von Willebrand factor in an Iranian family with platelet-type von Willebrand disease. Thromb Haemost 2012;108(5):946-54.
39. Favaloro EJ, Patterson D, Denholm A, et al. Differential identification of a rare form of platelet-type (pseudo-) von Willebrand disease (VWD) from Type 2B VWD using a simplified ristocetin-induced-platelet-agglutination mixing assay and confirmed by genetic analysis. Br J Haematol 2007;139(4):623-6.
40. Giannini S, Cecchetti L, Mezzasoma AM, et al. Diagnosis of platelet-type von Willebrand disease by flow cytometry. Haematologica 2010;95(6):1021-4.
41. Liang HP, Morel-Kopp MC, Curtin J, et al. Heterozygous loss of platelet glyco-protein (GP) Ib-V-IX variably affects platelet function in velocardiofacial syn-drome (VCFS) patients. Thromb Haemost 2007;98(6):1298-308.
42. López JA, Ludwig EH, McCarthy BJ. Polymorphism of human glycoprotein Ibα results from a variable number of tandem repeats of a 13-amino acid sequence in the mucin-like macroglycopeptide region. Structure/function implications. J Biol Chem 1992;267:10055-61.
43. Li CQ, Dong JF, López JA. The mucin-like macroglycopeptide region of glyco-protein Ibα is required for cell adhesion to immobilized von Willebrand factor (VWF) under flow but not for static VWF binding. Thromb Haemost 2002; 88(4):673-7.
44. Gonzalez-Conejero R, Lozano ML, Rivera J, et al. Polymorphisms of platelet membrane glycoprotein Ibα associated with arterial thrombotic disease. Blood 1998;92(8):2771-6.
45. Afshar-Kharghan V, Matijevic-Aleksic N, Ahn C, et al. The variable number of tandem repeat polymorphism of platelet glycoprotein Ibalpha and risk of coro-nary heart disease. Blood 2004;103(3):963-5.
46. Murata M, Furihata K, Ishida F, et al. Genetic and structural characterization of an amino acid dimorphism in glycoprotein Ibα involved in platelet transfusion refractoriness. Blood 1992;79:3086-90.
47. Simsek S, Bleeker PM, van der Schoot CE, et al. Association of variable number of tandem repeats (VNTR) in glycoprotein Ibα and HPA-2 alloantigens. Thromb Haemost 1994;72(5):757-61.
48. Afshar-Kharghan V, Li CQ, Khoshnevis-Asl M, et al. Kozak sequence polymor-phism of the glycoprotein (GP) Ibα gene is a major determinant of the plasma membrane levels of the platelet GP Ib- IX-V complex. Blood 1999;94(1):186-91.
49. Baker RI, Eikelboom J, Lofthouse E, et al. Platelet glycoprotein Ibα Kozak poly-morphism is associated with an increased risk of ischemic stroke. Blood 2001; 98(1):36-40.
50. Meisel C, Afshar-Kharghan V, Cascorbi I, et al. Role of Kozak sequence poly-morphism of platelet glycoprotein Ibα as a risk factor for coronary artery disease and catheter interventions. J Am Coll Cardiol 2001;38(4):1023-7.
51. Maguire JM, Thakkinstian A, Sturm J, et al. Polymorphisms in platelet glycopro-tein 1bα and factor VII and risk of ischemic stroke: a meta-analysis. Stroke 2008; 39(6):1710-6.

52. Chevalier J, Nurden AT, Thiery JM, et al. Freeze-fracture studies on the plasma membranes of normal human, thrombasthenic, and Bernard-Soulier platelets. J Lab Clin Med 1979;94:232–45.

53. Bray PF, Howard TD, Vittinghoff E, et al. Effect of genetic variations in platelet glycoproteins Ibα and VI on the risk for coronary heart disease events in post-menopausal women taking hormone therapy. Blood 2007;109(5):1862–9.

54. Yonal I, Hindilerden F, Hancer VS, et al. The impact of platelet membrane glycoprotein Ibα and Ia/IIa polymorphisms on the risk of thrombosis in the antiphospholipid syndrome. Thromb Res 2012;129(4):486–91.

55. Phillips DR, Charo IF, Parise LV, et al. The platelet membrane glycoprotein IIb-IIIa complex. Blood 1988;71:831–43.

56. Wagner CL, Mascelli MA, Neblock DS, et al. Analysis of GPIIb/IIIa receptor number by quantification of 7E3 binding to human platelets. Blood 1996;88(3): 907–14.

57. Bennett JS, Berger BW, Billings PC. The structure and function of platelet integrins. J Thromb Haemost 2009;7(Suppl 1):200–5.

58. Shattil SJ, Newman PJ. Integrins: dynamic scaffolds for adhesion and signaling in platelets. Blood 2004;104(6):1606–15.

59. Armstrong PC, Peter K. GPIIb/IIIa inhibitors: from bench to bedside and back to bench again. Thromb Haemost 2012;107(5):808–14.

60. George JN, Caen JP, Nurden AT. Glanzmann's thrombasthenia: the spectrum of clinical disease. Blood 1990;75(7):1383–95.

61. Nurden AT. Glanzmann thrombasthenia. Orphanet J Rare Dis 2006;1:10.

62. Salles II, Feys HB, Iserbyt BF, et al. Inherited traits affecting platelet function. Blood Rev 2008;22(3):155–72.

63. McHugh KP, Hodivala-Dilke K, Zheng MH, et al. Mice lacking β3 integrins are osteosclerotic because of dysfunctional osteoclasts. J Clin Invest 2000;105(4): 433–40.

64. Reynolds AR, Reynolds LE, Nagel TE, et al. Elevated Flk1 (vascular endothelial growth factor receptor 2) signaling mediates enhanced angiogenesis in β3-integrin-deficient mice. Cancer Res 2004;64(23):8643–50.

65. Metcalfe P. Platelet antigens and antibody detection. Vox Sang 2004;87(Suppl 1): 82–6.

66. Weiss EJ, Bray PF, Tayback M, et al. A polymorphism of a platelet glycoprotein receptor as an inherited risk factor for coronary thrombosis. N Engl J Med 1996; 334(17):1090–4.

67. Vijayan KV, Liu Y, Sun W, et al. The Pro33 isoform of integrin β3 enhances outside-in signaling in human platelets by regulating the activation of serine/threonine phosphatases. J Biol Chem 2005;280(23):21756–62.

68. Kucharska-Newton AM, Monda KL, Campbell S, et al. Association of the platelet GPIIb/IIIa polymorphism with atherosclerotic plaque morphology: the Atherosclerosis Risk in Communities (ARIC) Study. Atherosclerosis 2011;216(1): 151–6.

69. Zhu MM, Weedon J, Clark LT. Meta-analysis of the association of platelet glycoprotein IIIa PlA1/A2 polymorphism with myocardial infarction. Am J Cardiol 2000;86(9):1000–5 A8.

70. Nieswandt B, Schulte V, Bergmeier W, et al. Long-term antithrombotic protection by in vivo depletion of platelet glycoprotein VI in mice. J Exp Med 2001;193(4): 459–69.

71. Arthur JF, Dunkley S, Andrews RK. Platelet glycoprotein VI-related clinical defects. Br J Haematol 2007;139(3):363–72.

72. Kato K, Kanaji T, Russell S, et al. The contribution of glycoprotein VI to stable platelet adhesion and thrombus formation illustrated by targeted gene deletion. Blood 2003;102(5):1701–7.
73. Shaffer JR, Kammerer CM, Dorn J, et al. Polymorphisms in the platelet-specific collagen receptor GP6 are associated with risk of nonfatal myocardial infarction in Caucasians. Nutr Metab Cardiovasc Dis 2011;21(8):546–52.
74. Handa M, Watanabe K, Kawai Y, et al. Platelet unresponsiveness to collagen: involvement of glycoprotein Ia-IIa ($\alpha2\beta1$ integrin) deficiency associated with a myeloproliferative disorder. Thromb Haemost 1995;73(3):521–8.
75. Tosetto A, Castaman G, Rodeghiero F. Bleeding scores in inherited bleeding disorders: clinical or research tools? Haemophilia 2008;14(3):415–22.
76. Bolton-Maggs PH, Chalmers EA, Collins PW, et al. A review of inherited platelet disorders with guidelines for their management on behalf of the UKHCDO. Br J Haematol 2006;135(5):603–33.
77. Nurden AT, Freson K, Seligsohn U. Inherited platelet disorders. Haemophilia 2012;18(Suppl 4):154–60.
78. Drachman JG. Inherited thrombocytopenia: when a low platelet count does not mean ITP. Blood 2004;103(2):390–8.
79. Balduini CL, Cattaneo M, Fabris F, et al. Inherited thrombocytopenias: a proposed diagnostic algorithm from the Italian Gruppo di Studio delle Piastrine. Haematologica 2003;88(5):582–92.
80. Seligsohn U. Treatment of inherited platelet disorders. Haemophilia 2012;18(Suppl 4):161–5.

Platelet Transfusion Therapy

Perumal Thiagarajan, MD[a],*, Vahid Afshar-Kharghan, MD[b]

KEYWORDS

- Platelet transfusion • Alloimmunization • Transfusion triggers • Pathogen reduction

KEY POINTS

- In the United States, platelets are collected in citrate anticoagulants from single units or by apheresis procedure.
- To prevent bleeding in thrombocytopenic patients, it is a common practice to transfuse platelets when platelet counts reach a trigger threshold (prophylactic transfusion).
- The transfusion of all blood products including platelets can cause viral infection, such as hepatitis B, C, West Nile virus, and HIV, although the modern nucleic acid–based testing has reduced the risk to a very low level.
- Platelet transfusions are considered risky in patients with thrombotic thrombocytopenic purpura because it can exacerbate the microvascular thrombosis.
- Because treatment of alloimmune refractory thrombocytopenia is difficult, costly, and often ineffective, it is critical to prevent alloimmunization.

HISTORICAL PERSPECTIVE

Duke reported the earliest platelet transfusion in a landmark article at the beginning of the last century in 3 patients with idiopathic thrombocytopenic purpura.[1] He achieved temporary cessation of bleeding and an increase in platelet count in 2 patients by transfusing directly the unmodified whole blood. These earlier attempts were limited by lack of platelet concentrates and in vitro activation of platelets. The modern era of platelet transfusion started with demonstration by Gaydos and colleagues[2] that prophylactic transfusions of platelets in patients receiving chemotherapy dramatically reduced the incidence of fatal bleeding complications and allowed completion of chemotherapy. They also pioneered apheresis techniques in harvesting of platelets for transfusion.[3] The introduction of storage at room temperature, the use of

Supported by a grant from the Veterans Affairs Research Service (P. Thiagarajan).

[a] Departments of Pathology and Medicine, Michael E. DeBakey Veterans Affairs Medical Center, Baylor College of Medicine, 2002 Holcombe Boulevard, Houston, TX 77030, USA;
[b] Section of Benign Hematology, M.D. Anderson Cancer Center, 1515 Holcombe Boulevard, Houston, TX 77030, USA
* Corresponding author. Michael E. DeBakey Veterans Affairs Medical Center, Mail Stop # 113, 2002 Holcombe Boulevard, Houston, TX 77030.
E-mail address: perumalt@bcm.edu

Hematol Oncol Clin N Am 27 (2013) 629–643
http://dx.doi.org/10.1016/j.hoc.2013.03.004
0889-8588/13/$ – see front matter Published by Elsevier Inc.

gas-permeable containers, agitation during storage, and the use of acid citrate as the anticoagulant led to better platelet preservation and increased storage time, allowing widespread availability.[4–6] Platelets have become the second commonest blood components transfused.

PLATELET LIFE SPAN

Circulating platelets have a life span of 10 days and about 10% of platelets are removed every day mainly via the spleen and the liver.[7] What determines the end of platelet life span in the circulation is not known and there are several hypotheses. Phosphatidylserine, a well-known macrophage recognition signal for clearance of apoptotic cells, could play a role.[8–10] In resting platelets, phosphatidylserine is located on the inner leaflet of the membrane bilayer and following platelet activation there is trans-bilayer movement from the inner to the outer leaflet.[11,12] Both an activation-dependent and a senescence-induced pathway leading to a trans-bilayer movement of phosphatidylserine have been described.[13] According to "the multiple-hit model," the life span of platelets is determined by the damages to (or activations of) platelets in the blood circulation. Platelet clearance by macrophages depends on the number of "hits" accumulated during platelet life span in the circulation. Logistic regression analysis of the disappearance curves of labeled transfused platelets by best fitting models suggests a complicated clearance process involving linear (due to senescence) and random (due to activation) components.[14] In recent years, an alternate model, based on forward genetic studies with N-ethyl-N-nitrosourea–induced mutagenesis in mice, suggests platelets are formed with an "internal clock" and their survival is determined by intrinsic mechanisms rather than external hits.[15] Platelets express the Bcl-2 family of proteins Bax and Bak in the mitochondria.[16–18] These proteins govern mitochondrial outer membrane integrity and can be either pro-apoptotic (Bax, BAD, and Bak among others) or anti-apoptotic (Bcl-x). Knock-out of antiapoptotic Bcl-x(L) reduces platelet half-life and causes thrombocytopenia.[18] Deletion of proapoptotic Bak corrects these defects, and platelets from Bak-deficient mice circulate for a longer time than normal platelets. Apoptotic stimuli are thought to activate BH3-domain–containing members of this protein family to initiate Bax/Bak-dependent apoptosis. ABT737, a synthetic BH3 mimetic reagent, induces the mitochondrial pathway of apoptosis by binding to Bcl-2 and Bcl-XL and blocking their inhibitory effect on the proapoptotic Bax and Bak. ABT737 has been used to mimic in vivo senescence and phosphatidylserine exposure in platelets.[19]

There is evidence for a fixed daily requirement of platelets.[7] A large number of studies have shown that platelets support the function of the vascular endothelium, and in animals thrombocytopenia has been shown to increase protein permeability across the endothelium of the lung, ear, thyroid, and heart, which can be reversed by infusion of platelet-rich plasma.[20–23] These data are also consistent with clinical observations that recovery of transfused platelets is decreased in thrombocytopenia and may account for the spontaneous unprovoked bleeding seen in severe thrombocytopenia. Daily obligatory requirement is estimated to be about 7100/μL, about 18% of daily turnover.

The life span of platelets stored at room temperature is remarkably similar to the life span of platelets in the circulation. Platelet recovery after transfusion decreases by 10% for each day of storage outside of the body, which is very close to what is expected from the in vivo life span of platelets. The changes in stored platelets are collectively known as platelet storage lesions.[24–26] These changes result not only in reduced response to agonists but also in an accelerated clearance from the circulation following transfusion.[27] Increased phosphatidylserine expression and caspase-3 activity in stored platelets has been observed[28,29] and phosphatidylserine-expressing platelets are rapidly cleared from the circulation.[8]

Platelets that are stored at $4°C$ rapidly undergo shape change and lose responsiveness to agonists, and the in vivo recovery of cold-stored platelets is poor.[5] The mechanism for the rapid clearance of cold-stored platelets is not known and it was postulated that clustering of the GPIb/V/IX complex on the surface of platelets results in platelet clearance by $\alpha_M\beta_2$ integrin on hepatic macrophages that recognizes the β-N-acetylglucosamine (βGlcNAc)–terminating immature glycans. Masking the penultimate βGlcNAc by galactosylation by uridine diphosphate galactose-galactose prevented phagocytosis of cold-stored murine platelets.[30] However, in a human phase I study, galactosylation with uridine diphosphate galactose-galactose did not prevent the rapid clearance of cold-stored platelets and the clinical relevance of these findings in transfusion medicine is not clear.[31]

PLATELET COLLECTION AND PROCESSING
Single Donor Platelets

In the United States, platelets are collected in citrate anticoagulants from single units or by apheresis procedure. Single-donor blood is collected in citrate anticoagulant containing adenine in a pH of 5.3 to 5.9. The platelet-rich plasma is obtained by centrifugation at room temperature at 2100 g for 2.7 minutes (soft spin). The platelet-rich plasma is again centrifuged at a higher speed (hard spin); the supernatant is transferred in a closed system to another container leaving approximately 40 to 70 mL of plasma with the platelet suspension, and it is stored at room temperature with constant agitation. The typical yield is 5.0×10^{10} platelets per unit.

Apheresis Units

Increasingly, platelets are harvested by the apheresis method. Apheresis platelets are especially useful in collecting from family members, HLA-compatible donors, or individuals with rare phenotype. Apheresis has the advantage of collecting from a single donor that limits donor exposure and provides platelets with consistent quality. The apheresis donor unit contains at least 3×10^{11} platelets per unit. More than 60% of platelets infused in the United States are from apheresis donors. Donors can donate twice a week. The newer automated apheresis instruments are capable of collecting single, double, and even triple apheresis units from a donor and they can be programed to yield optimal amount based on donor hematocrit, height, and weight.

Buffy Coat Platelets

Platelets can also be obtained using the buffy coat method, by centrifuging the whole blood (hard spin), and removing the supernatant platelet-poor plasma and bottom red blood cells, leaving behind the buffy coat, which contains mostly platelets and white blood cells.[32] The buffy coat is further centrifuged to remove white blood cells and red blood cells. Platelets prepared by the buffy coat method are less activated, and in addition to a slightly higher platelet yield, it is easier to institute leukocyte reduction and pathogen reduction technologies in this method. In some blood centers, excess plasma is replaced with a synthetic additive solution, which can prolong the storage time and reduce the amount of plasma transfused to patients. As a result, there is a reduction in the frequency of allergic reaction and possibly in transfusion-related acute lung injury. The buffy coat method and additive solutions are used in many blood centers in Canada and Europe.

Frozen Platelets

A considerable amount of work has been performed on freezing frozen platelets for clinical use.[33] Frozen platelets can be stored for years and platelets with rare phenotypes can be saved for alloimmune thrombocytopenic patients. Typically, platelets are frozen in dimethyl sulfoxide as the cryopreservative and, after thawing, they are concentrated by centrifugation and the cryopreservative is removed and replaced with autologous plasma. Despite the demonstration of hemostatic effectiveness in vivo, the process is expensive and cumbersome with many logistical challenges.[34]

PATHOGEN REDUCTION TECHNIQUES

Platelets are stored at room temperature and sepsis associated with bacterial proliferation is the major cause of morbidity and mortality associated with blood transfusion.[35] The incidence of contamination has been reported between 1 in 1000 and 3000, whereas the risk of a clinically significant septic transfusion reaction was between 1 in 13,000 and 70,000 for single-donor platelets and platelets from whole blood, respectively. Because of this concern, the Food and Drug Administration allows storage of platelets at room temperature for only 5 days, and the American Association of Blood Banks requires a method to limit bacterial contamination. Platelet concentrates are tested for bacterial contamination using a growth-based system 24 hour after collection. This strategy detects only up to 40% of bacterial contamination.[36,37] Consequently, several additional approaches have been under investigation to reduce the incidence of sepsis associated with platelet transfusions. Testing on the day of transfusion adds a measure of safety by detecting highly contaminated units. Platelet concentrates or apheresis units are now tested within 4 hours before transfusion. A currently available test based on the detection of lipoteichoic acid and lipopolysaccharide has a detection limit of 10^4 to 10^5 colony forming units per milliliter.

Another approach that is being actively tested is pathogen inactivation during storage, which is already implemented by certain countries.[38] Psoralens and riboflavin along with ultraviolet (UV) radiation are being evaluated. Psoralens are compounds that intercalate into the helical regions of DNA and RNA. Upon UV radiation, adducts are formed between psoralen and the nucleic acids, rendering it incapable of replication. Amotosalen, a novel psoralen, has been shown to inactivate a variety of bacteria and viruses in platelet concentrates.[39] UV radiation reduces amotosalen concentration to very low levels. In addition to Psoralens, other photosensitizers have been tried for pathogen inactivation.[40] Methylene blue and riboflavin have been investigated for pathogen inactivation. Methylene blue plus visible light is known to induce DNA damage primarily at guanine bases. Riboflavin interacts with nucleic acids and enhances UV damage that results in direct electron transfer, production of singlet oxygen, generation of hydrogen peroxide, opening of purine ring, and DNA strand breakage. The advantage of riboflavin over methylene blue and psoralens is that riboflavin is an endogenous physiologic compound (vitamin B2). Recently, a novel procedure that uses short-wave UV light, without addition of any photoactive agent, has been developed.[41]

In addition to inactivating bacteria and virus, pathogen inactivation offers several other advantages for platelet transfusion. The pathogen inactivation process will be effective in the prevention of cytomegalovirus infection, allowing more flexibility by omitting irradiation and testing for cytomegalovirus antibodies. This technology will also be effective against other transfusion-associated infection, such as malaria, and may allow the relaxation of donor deferral because of travel to endemic areas. Because infection is the major limitation for platelet storage, pathogen inactivation may allow extension of platelet storage beyond the current period of 5 days. Pathogen inactivation may also eliminate the current practice of bacterial detection before platelet transfusion. Inactivation of contaminating white blood cells will reduce the graft-versus-host disease and possibly alloimmunization. The disadvantages of the pathogen reduction process include added cost and the concerns about the long-term safety of potentially mutagenic agents used in this process.

PROPHYLACTIC AND THERAPEUTIC TRANSFUSIONS

To prevent bleeding in thrombocytopenic patients, it is a common practice to trans-fuse platelets when platelet counts reach a trigger threshold (prophylactic transfusion) (**Fig. 1**). Because most platelet transfusions are administrated to patients with hema-tologic malignancies, it is not a surprise that most of the studies on platelet transfusion are conducted in these patients. The risk of spontaneous bleeding in a patient with leu-kemia increases when platelet counts are less than 20,000/µL, and this number was considered to be the threshold for platelet transfusion in the 1960s.[2] At that time, the antiplatelet effect of aspirin was not appreciated and aspirin was commonly pre-scribed to these patients for fever. Subsequent studies, when aspirin was no longer prescribed, revealed that a threshold of 10,000/µL could safely replace 20,000/µL in afebrile patients with no significant coagulopathy.[42] The American Society of Hematol-ogy,[43] the American Society Clinical Oncology,[44] and the British Committee for Stan-dards in Haematology (BCSH)[45] have recommended a platelet count of 10,000/µL as a transfusion threshold. The same threshold is applicable to patients after hematopoi-etic stem cell transplantation or patients with solid tumors who developed thrombocy-topenia during the course of chemotherapy, with the possible exception of patients with bladder tumors or necrotic tumors, who should probably receive prophylactic

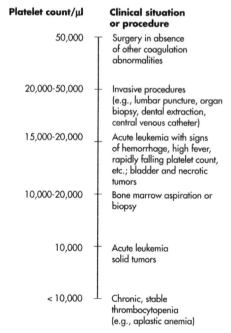

Platelet count/µl	Clinical situation or procedure
50,000	Surgery in absence of other coagulation abnormalities
20,000-50,000	Invasive procedures (e.g., lumbar puncture, organ biopsy, dental extraction, central venous catheter)
15,000-20,000	Acute leukemia with signs of hemorrhage, high fever, rapidly falling platelet count, etc.; bladder and necrotic tumors
10,000-20,000	Bone marrow aspiration or biopsy
10,000	Acute leukemia solid tumors
< 10,000	Chronic, stable thrombocytopenia (e.g., aplastic anemia)

Fig. 1. Threshold for platelet transfusions. (*From* Goodnough LT. Transfusion medicine. In: Goldman L, Schafer AI, eds. Goldman's Cecil medicine, 24th ed. Philadelphia: Elsevier Saunders; 2012; with permission.)

platelet transfusion with platelet counts less than 20,000/µL.[44] Some studies have used successfully an even more restrictive threshold of 5000/µL in patients with acute leukemia in the absence of fever.[46] In patients with acute promyelocytic leukemia the risk of bleeding is very high and the threshold of 20,000/µL is appropriate.[47] In patients with chronic, severe, and stable thrombocytopenia, such as those with aplastic anemia or myelodysplastic syndrome, the recommendations for platelet transfusion are less clear. Most hematologists will not transfuse prophylactically in these patients, unless there is evidence of bleeding. Prophylactic platelet transfusion is indicated in preparation for invasive procedures in thrombocytopenic patients. Most invasive procedures (placement of central venous catheter, transbronchial biopsy, gastrointestinal endoscopy, and biopsy) can be performed with platelet counts greater than 40,000 to 50,000/µL.[45,48] A platelet count of 20,000/µL is adequate for lumbar puncture and bone marrow biopsy,[44] although BCSH recommended platelet counts higher than 50,000/µL for lumbar puncture and no platelet transfusion for bone marrow biopsy regardless of the severity of thrombocytopenia, providing adequate surface pressure is applied to the biopsy site.[45] Circulating red blood also influences platelet function by scavenging endothelial cell nitric oxide, a vasodilating agent that inhibits platelet function.[49,50] The venous blood hematocrit has been shown to correlate inversely with the bleeding time. Furthermore, anemia increases the shear stress and nitric oxide production by endothelial cells at sites of injury. Correcting the anemia in thrombocytopenic patients has been proposed to improve platelet function.[49]

There are several studies on determining the optimal dose of prophylactic platelets. A randomized controlled trial comparing standard-dose (3–6 × 10^{11}) and low-dose (1.5–3 × 10^{11}) platelet transfusion to patients that expected to have platelet counts less than 10,000/mL for 10 days (strategies for transfusion of platelets [SToP] trial) did not support any benefit from low-dose strategy, which required more frequent transfusion episodes and was associated with a higher rate of severe bleeding,[51] although the higher rate of bleeding did not reach statistical significance because of an early termination of the trial due to safety concerns. In another prospective randomized study assessing the efficiency of transfusing 2 doses (0.5 × 10^{11}/10 kg vs 1 × 10^{11}/10 kg), it was found that the higher dose resulted in a longer transfusion interval and decreased the number of transfusion episodes.[52] Although this practice may improve quality of life by decreasing the frequency of transfusions, there was no clinically significant impact on bleeding complications. Furthermore, administering more platelets may diminish endogenous thrombopoiesis as platelets bind to thrombopoietin.[53] In the Platelet Dose Study (PLADO trial) low, medium, and high doses of platelets were compared (1.1 × 10^{11}, 2.2 × 10^{11}, and 4.4 × 10^{11} per square meter of body surface, respectively).[54] Low-dose strategy was associated a decreased number of platelets transfused but an increased number of transfusion episodes per patient. There was no difference regarding bleeding incidences between low-platelet and high-platelet dose groups, in contrast to the concern raised by the SToP trial. Another important result of the PLADO trial was that the characteristics of transfused platelets, such as source (apheresis or random donors), ABO compatibility, and duration of storage before transfusion, had an impact on the posttransfusion increment in platelet counts but no significant effect on the prevention of bleeding.[54] A higher increment in platelet counts after transfusion of apheresis or ABO-matched platelets was shown by several other studies even before completion of the PLADO trial.[55,56]

Despite the common practice of prophylactic platelet transfusion, it has not been proven that this approach is superior to the therapeutic-only strategy, which limits transfusion of platelets only to bleeding in thrombocytopenic patients. A retrospective study on 3000 thrombocytopenic patients did not find any relationship between the morning platelet count or the lowest platelet count and the risk of bleeding on that day.[57] An ongoing prospective randomized study on thrombocytopenic patients with hematologic malignancies will compare the safety of therapeutic-only approach to prophylactic strategy (TOPPs trial).[58] Bleeding patients with thrombocytopenia should receive platelet transfusion with the goal of achieving a platelet count greater than 50,000/μL, except in patients who underwent cardiopulmonary bypass. Platelet functions are abnormal in these patients[59] and they should receive platelets even when their platelet counts are greater than 50,000/μL. In uremic patients with bleeding or an anticipated invasive procedure, correction of uremia by dialysis and administration of 1-deamino-8-D-arginine vasopressin or cryoprecipitate are recommended. Platelet transfusion can be considered in these patients if the other interventions are ineffective.

COMPLICATIONS OF PLATELET TRANSFUSIONS

Transfusion of all blood products including platelets can cause viral infection, such as hepatitis B, C, West Nile virus, and HIV, although the modern nucleic acid–based testing has reduced the risk to a very low level.[60] Bacterial infection has been discussed previously in this article. The noninfectious complications such as volume overload, febrile nonhemolytic transfusion reactions (FNHTR), transfusion-related acute lung injury, and alloimmunization are the most common after platelet transfusion.

Allergic reactions are often seen with platelet transfusion and manifest as itching and urticaria in the absence of fever.[61] Allergic reactions are caused by soluble substances present in donor plasma and mediated by the Immunoglobulin E response and histamine release in recipients. Administration of antihistamine reagents such as 25 to 50 mg diphenhydramine before platelet transfusion can reduce the frequency of allergic reactions. Temporary discontinuation of platelet transfusion and administration of diphenhydramine is adequate in the treatment of mild allergic reactions. In the absence of fever or unstable vital signs, transfusion of the same platelet unit can be resumed. If the allergic reaction reoccurs, a new unit of platelet should be transfused. In the presence of recurrent allergic reactions to different units of platelet products and after an anaphylactic reaction, removal of plasma and washing of platelet should be considered. Severe anaphylaxis after transfusion is rare and can occur in recipients who are deficient in Immunoglobulin A, C4, or haptoglobin.[62–64] Treatment of an anaphylactic reaction after platelet transfusion requires administration of epinephrine, corticosteroid, and vasopressors and airway support.

Another common complication associated with platelet transfusion is FNHTR. Since the introduction prestorage leukocyte reduction, the incidence of FNTHR has decreased.[65–67] FNHTR can manifest as fever, chills, nausea, vomiting, and dyspnea during transfusion, but can also occur minutes or hours after completion of transfusion. Most FNHTR are due to cytokines released from contaminated neutrophils in stored platelet products that accumulate during storage.[68] Fresh platelet units (less than 2 days old) and removal of plasma decrease the frequency of FNHTR.[67,69] In a minority of cases (6%), the recipient's antileukocyte antibodies reacting to donor neutrophils cause FNHTR.[67] In the presence of fever, it is difficult to differentiate between FNHTR, acute hemolytic reaction, and sepsis. As a result, transfusion of platelets coinciding with fever should be discontinued and not restarted with the same unit. Administration of meperidine is very effective in reducing chills,[70] but antihistamine reagents are ineffective in FNHTR and corticosteroid only acts after a few hours. In the absence of the resolution of fever, the possibility of bacterial infection should be investigated.

PROTHROMBOTIC EFFECT OF PLATELET TRANSFUSIONS

Platelet transfusions are considered risky in patients with thrombotic thrombocyto-penic purpura because it can exacerbate the microvascular thrombosis. There have been several case reports and small series describing dramatic thrombotic episodes temporally related to platelet transfusion.[71–73] In contrast with these earlier reports, these complications are not observed in recent years.[74,75] Early institution of aggressive plasma exchange therapy possibly prevents these complications. Based on this analysis, it is prudent not to withhold platelets in bleeding thrombocytopenic patients with thrombotic thrombocytopenic purpura who are on plasma exchange. Platelet transfusions are also thought to be contraindicated in heparin-induced thrombocyto-penia/thrombosis syndrome based on a few case reports. A recent retrospective review of 37 patients with this syndrome who have received platelet transfusions found no evidence of thrombotic events.[76]

ALLOIMMUNIZATION

A lack of adequate increment in platelet counts after transfusion, due to alloantibodies, is a major clinical problem, particularly in patients with chronic thrombocytopenia who require frequent transfusion of blood products. The posttransfusion platelet count is important in evaluating the response to platelet transfusion. Following transfusion, platelet recovery is about two-thirds of the transfused platelets, and approximately 30% to 35% of the transfused platelets are normally pooled in the spleen. Platelet recovery is almost 90% following splenectomy. To assess recovery, it is essential to measure platelet counts at 1 hour and at 18 to 24 hours after transfusion. Corrected count increment (CCI) is used as an objective measure of assessing the efficacy of transfusion. The CCI equals (posttransfusion count − pretransfusion count × body surface area [M^2] divided by the number of platelets).[77] If after 2 separate transfusions, the increment is less than 4500 to 5000/μL at 1 hour and less than 2500 at 18 to 24 hours, then that patient has refractoriness to platelet transfusion.[78] In clinical practice, it is not always possible to calculate CCI, as most treating physicians do not have the number of platelets transfused. Empirically, platelets refractoriness is suspected after transfusion if the absolute increase is less than 2000/μL per random donor platelet concentrate or less than 10,000/μL for apheresis unit.[79] It is also not always practical to get 1-hour posttransfusion platelet counts and some clinicians use 10-minute posttransfusion counts to assess platelet recovery. In most of the platelet-refractory patients, nonimmune factors, such as fever, sepsis, disseminated intravascular coagulation, medications (amphotericin, antibiotics, heparin), and splenomegaly, contribute to refractoriness.[80] ABO mismatch between donor platelets and recipient, and platelets storage for more than 48 hours, reduces posttransfusion platelet recovery.[81]

The immune factor responsible for platelet refractoriness is the presence of anti-bodies against human leukocyte antigens (HLA), especially HLA-A and HLA-B, expressed on platelets, and only rarely of antibodies against platelet-specific anti-gens, such as HPA-2 and HPA-5.[78] HLA-C antigens are expressed at very low levels on platelets and platelets do not express HLA class II antigens; they are not considered to play a role in immunologic platelet refractoriness.[82] Patients develop HLA antibodies after exposure to HLA alloantigens present on fetal white blood cells (previous pregnancies) or contaminating white blood cells (previous transfusion of blood products). Transfusion of ABO-mismatched platelets also increases the risk of alloimmunization to HLA antigens.[83] The presence of HLA antibodies can be confirmed by various immunologic assays.[84] Not all patients with HLA antibodies are refractory to platelet transfusion. In a study on leukemic patients during induction chemotherapy, 45% of patients receiving pooled random donor platelets developed alloantibodies, 16% developed refractoriness, and 13% developed alloantibodies and refractoriness.[85,86]

Because treatment of alloimmune refractory thrombocytopenia is difficult, costly, and often ineffective, it is critical to prevent alloimmunization. Leukoreduction is an effective way of preventing alloimmunization to HLA antigens.[85] In the TRAP trial (To Reduce Alloimmunization to Platelet Study), reduction of leukocytes by filtration of platelets decreased the frequency of alloimmunization from 45% to 18%, and refractoriness from 16% to 7%[85]; these results were confirmed by subsequent studies.[87] The type of platelet products (random donor vs apheresis) did not affect the frequency of alloimmunization.[85] γ-Irradiation and nucleic acid–based pathogen reduction techniques render the white blood cells incapable of stimulating or binding to allogeneic cells and prevent alloimmunization as effectively as leukoreduction.[88,89] Even though γ-irradiation (5000 rad) does not affect platelet functions in vitro,[90] the in vivo recovery is decreased after γ-irradiation.[81]

Transfusion of refractory thrombocytopenic patients due to alloantibodies with HLA compatible platelets results in an increase in platelet counts.[91] HLA-compatible platelets can be identified by selecting donors with the best-matched HLA profile.[92] Platelets need to be matched at A and B loci only because they do not express HLA-C or HLA-D antigens.[82] A large pool of apheresis donors and active cooperation between clinician and transfusion center are necessary for an adequate supply of compatible donors. HLA-compatible donors can often be obtained from siblings and other family members. Transfusion-associated graft-versus-host disease is a potential complication and all HLA-matched blood products should be irradiated to avoid this complication.[93]

Even with the traditional HLA-A and HLA-B loci matching, HLA-compatible transfusion increases the platelet counts in only half of the patients.[91] Conversely, successful transfusion of HLA antigen-mismatched platelets to alloimmunized patients has been reported.[91] A more refined HLA matching using a molecularly defined algorithm (HLA Matchmaker), initially used in renal transplants, has been used in platelet matching.[94] It is based on the fact that a set of triplet amino acids in the exposed part of class I major histocompatibility complex antigens is responsible for the immunoreactivity of the alloantibodies. The program computes the total number of triplet mismatches between the donor and recipient HLA repertoire. Certain HLA types, despite being classified as mismatch by conventional compatibility assessment, will have a compatible sequence and therefore are suitable. This approach has the potential to expand donor selection for alloimmunized thrombocytopenic patients.[95]

Pretransfusion platelet cross-matching has been used by some centers to provide compatible platelets for patients with alloantibodies.[79,96–98] Random platelets are tested against patient's serum using solid-phase assays or by flow cytometry. It is more cost-effective than HLA matching, avoids unnecessary platelet transfusions, and takes less time in identifying suitable donors. In one report, more compatible units were identified among HLA-typed donors by cross-matching method than by HLA antigen matching.[99] Although platelet-specific antigens are rarely the cause of platelet refractoriness, these assays have the advantage of detecting them. Despite the availability of several such tests, their clinical use in predicting platelet recovery is not clear.[100] Other therapeutic approaches to platelet refractoriness, such as infusion of intravenous immunoglobulin, transfusion of vinblastine-loaded platelets, and immunoadsorption of plasma using staphylococcal protein–A column, are controversial and are not accepted as effective treatments.[78]

FUTURE DIRECTIONS

Since the introduction of clinical platelet transfusions half a century ago, there has been a remarkable progress in the safety and efficacy of this process. However, several questions still need to be answered, including the appropriate platelet count trigger for platelet transfusion, especially in the pediatric population. Because the supply of platelets is always limited, there is continuing effort to develop guidelines for the optimal use. A multidisciplinary "think-tank" conference identified the need for randomized clinical trials for optimal clinical use of platelets and the impact of newer pathogen reduction technologies.[101] Furthermore, effort has been made in developing platelets substitutes.[102] Human embryonic stem cells represent an alternate source for platelets.[103] Mature megakaryocytes have been induced from these cells to form platelet-like particles. These in vitro generated platelets display integrin $\alpha IIb\beta 3$ activation and spreading in response to ADP or thrombin. Further refinement of this technology may allow another source of platelets in future.

REFERENCES

1. Duke WW. The relation of blood platelets to hemorrhagic disease. JAMA 1983; 250:1201–9.
2. Gaydos LA, Freireich EJ, Mantel N. The quantitative relation between platelet count and hemorrhage in patients with acute leukemia. N Engl J Med 1962; 266:905–9.
3. Freireich EJ. Origins of platelet transfusion therapy. Transfus Med Rev 2011;25: 252–6.
4. Murphy S, Gardner FH. Platelet storage at 22 degrees C: role of gas transport across plastic containers in maintenance of viability. Blood 1975;46:209–18.
5. Filip DJ, Aster RH. Relative hemostatic effectiveness of human platelets stored at 4 degrees and 22 degrees C. J Lab Clin Med 1978;91:618–24.
6. Slichter SJ. Preservation of platelet viability and function during storage of concentrates. Prog Clin Biol Res 1978;28:83–100.
7. Hanson SR, Slichter SJ. Platelet kinetics in patients with bone marrow hypoplasia: evidence for a fixed platelet requirement. Blood 1985;66:1105–9.
8. Rand ML, Wang H, Bang KW, et al. Procoagulant surface exposure and apoptosis in rabbit platelets: association with shortened survival and steady-state senescence. J Thromb Haemost 2004;2:651–9.
9. Pereira J, Palomo I, Ocqueteau M, et al. Platelet aging in vivo is associated with loss of membrane phospholipid asymmetry. Thromb Haemost 1999;82: 1318–21.
10. Schlegel RA, Callahan MK, Williamson P. The central role of phosphatidylserine in the phagocytosis of apoptotic thymocytes. Ann N Y Acad Sci 2000;926: 217–25.
11. Zwaal RF, Schroit AJ. Pathophysiologic implications of membrane phospholipid asymmetry in blood cells. Blood 1997;89:1121–32.
12. Thiagarajan P, Tait JF. Binding of annexin V/placental anticoagulant protein I to platelets. Evidence for phosphatidylserine exposure in the procoagulant response of activated platelets. J Biol Chem 1990;265:17420–3.
13. Schoenwaelder SM, Yuan Y, Josefsson EC, et al. Two distinct pathways regulate platelet phosphatidylserine exposure and procoagulant function. Blood 2009; 114:663–6.
14. Lotter MG, Heyns AD, Badenhorst PN, et al. Evaluation of mathematic models to assess platelet kinetics. J Nucl Med 1986;27:1192–201.

15. Dowling MR, Josefsson EC, Henley KJ, et al. Platelet senescence is regulated by an internal timer, not damage inflicted by hits. Blood 2010;116:1776–8.
16. Zhang H, Nimmer PM, Tahir SK, et al. Bcl-2 family proteins are essential for platelet survival. Cell Death Differ 2007;14:943–51.
17. Bertino AM, Qi XQ, Li J, et al. Apoptotic markers are increased in platelets stored at 37 degrees C. Transfusion 2003;43:857–66.
18. Mason KD, Carpinelli MR, Fletcher JI, et al. Programmed anuclear cell death delimits platelet life span. Cell 2007;128:1173–86.
19. Dasgupta SK, Argaiz ER, Mercado JE, et al. Platelet senescence and phosphatidylserine exposure. Transfusion 2010;50:2167–75.
20. Lo SK, Burhop KE, Kaplan JE, et al. Role of platelets in maintenance of pulmonary vascular permeability to protein. Am J Physiol 1988;254:H763–71.
21. Aursnes I. Increased permeability of capillaries to protein during thrombocytopenia. An experimental study in the rabbit. Microvasc Res 1974;7:283–95.
22. Gimbrone MA Jr, Aster RH, Cotran RS, et al. Preservation of vascular integrity in organs perfused in vitro with a platelet-rich medium. Nature 1969;222:33–6.
23. McDonagh PF. Platelets reduce coronary microvascular permeability to macromolecules. Am J Physiol 1986;251:H581–7.
24. Cauwenberghs S, van Pampus E, Curvers J, et al. Hemostatic and signaling functions of transfused platelets. Transfus Med Rev 2007;21:287–94.
25. Rao AK, Murphy S. Secretion defect in platelets stored at 4 degrees C. Thromb Haemost 1982;47:221–5.
26. Rao AK, Niewiarowski S, Murphy S. Acquired granular pool defect in stored platelets. Blood 1981;57:203–8.
27. Murphy S. Radiolabeling of PLTs to assess viability: a proposal for a standard. Transfusion 2004;44:131–3.
28. Shapira S, Friedman Z, Shapiro H, et al. The effect of storage on the expression of platelet membrane phosphatidylserine and the subsequent impacton the coagulant function of stored platelets. Transfusion 2000;40:1257–63.
29. Perrotta PL, Perrotta CL, Snyder EL. Apoptotic activity in stored human platelets. Transfusion 2003;43:526–35.
30. Hoffmeister KM, Josefsson EC, Isaac NA, et al. Glycosylation restores survival of chilled blood platelets. Science 2003;301:1531–4.
31. Wandall HH, Hoffmeister KM, Sorensen AL, et al. Galactosylation does not prevent the rapid clearance of long-term, 4 degrees C-stored platelets. Blood 2008;111:3249–56.
32. Murphy S. Platelets from pooled buffy coats: an update. Transfusion 2005;45:634–9.
33. Schiffer CA, Aisner J, Dutcher JP, et al. A clinical program of platelet cryopreservation. Prog Clin Biol Res 1982;88:165–80.
34. Johnson LN, Winter KM, Reid S, et al. Cryopreservation of buffy-coat-derived platelet concentrates in dimethyl sulfoxide and platelet additive solution. Cryobiology 2011;62:100–6.
35. Palavecino EL, Yomtovian RA, Jacobs MR. Bacterial contamination of platelets. Transfus Apher Sci 2010;42:71–82.
36. Dumont LJ, Kleinman S, Murphy JR, et al. Screening of single-donor apheresis platelets for bacterial contamination: the PASSPORT study results. Transfusion 2010;50:589–99.
37. Blajchman MA, Beckers EA, Dickmeiss E, et al. Bacterial detection of platelets: current problems and possible resolutions. Transfus Med Rev 2005;19:259–72.

38. Reesink HW, Panzer S, McQuilten ZK, et al. Pathogen inactivation of platelet concentrates. Vox Sang 2010;99:85–95.
39. Lozano M, Knutson F, Tardivel R, et al. A multi-centre study of therapeutic efficacy and safety of platelet components treated with amotosalen and ultraviolet A pathogen inactivation stored for 6 or 7 d prior to transfusion. Br J Haematol 2011;153:393–401.
40. Seghatchian J, de Sousa G. Pathogen-reduction systems for blood components: the current position and future trends. Transfus Apher Sci 2006;35: 189–96.
41. Seghatchian J, Tolksdorf F. Characteristics of the THERAFLEX UV-Platelets pathogen inactivation system - an update. Transfus Apher Sci 2012;46:221–9.
42. Rebulla P, Finazzi G, Marangoni F, et al. The threshold for prophylactic platelet transfusions in adults with acute myeloid leukemia. Gruppo Italiano Malattie Ematologiche Maligne dell'Adulto. N Engl J Med 1997;337:1870–5.
43. Slichter SJ. Evidence-based platelet transfusion guidelines. Hematology Am Soc Hematol Educ Program 2007;172–8.
44. Schiffer CA, Anderson KC, Bennett CL, et al. Platelet transfusion for patients with cancer: clinical practice guidelines of the American Society of Clinical Oncology. J Clin Oncol 2001;19:1519–38.
45. Guidelines for the use of platelet transfusions. Br J Haematol 2003;122:10–23.
46. Gmur J, Burger J, Schanz U, et al. Safety of stringent prophylactic platelet transfusion policy for patients with acute leukaemia. Lancet 1991;338:1223–6.
47. Falanga A, Rickles FR. Pathogenesis and management of the bleeding diathesis in acute promyelocytic leukaemia. Best Pract Res Clin Haematol 2003;16: 463–82.
48. McCullough J. Overview of platelet transfusion. Semin Hematol 2010;47:235–42.
49. Valeri CR, Khuri S, Ragno G. Nonsurgical bleeding diathesis in anemic thrombocytopenic patients: role of temperature, red blood cells, platelets, and plasma-clotting proteins. Transfusion 2007;47:206S–48S.
50. Valeri CR, Cassidy G, Pivacek LE, et al. Anemia-induced increase in the bleeding time: implications for treatment of nonsurgical blood loss. Transfusion 2001;41:977–83.
51. Heddle NM, Cook RJ, Tinmouth A, et al. A randomized controlled trial comparing standard- and low-dose strategies for transfusion of platelets (SToP) to patients with thrombocytopenia. Blood 2009;113:1564–73.
52. Sensebe L, Giraudeau B, Bardiaux L, et al. The efficiency of transfusing high doses of platelets in hematologic patients with thrombocytopenia: results of a prospective, randomized, open, blinded end point (PROBE) study. Blood 2005;105:862–4.
53. Stefanich E, Senn T, Widmer R, et al. Metabolism of thrombopoietin (TPO) in vivo: determination of the binding dynamics for TPO in mice. Blood 1997; 89:4063–70.
54. Slichter SJ, Kaufman RM, Assmann SF, et al. Dose of prophylactic platelet transfusions and prevention of hemorrhage. N Engl J Med 2010;362:600–13.
55. Triulzi DJ, Assmann SF, Strauss RG, et al. The impact of platelet transfusion characteristics on posttransfusion platelet increments and clinical bleeding in patients with hypoproliferative thrombocytopenia. Blood 2012;119:5553–62.
56. Shehata N, Tinmouth A, Naglie G, et al. ABO-identical versus nonidentical platelet transfusion: a systematic review. Transfusion 2009;49:2442–53.
57. Friedmann AM, Sengul H, Lehmann H, et al. Do basic laboratory tests or clinical observations predict bleeding in thrombocytopenic oncology patients? A

reevaluation of prophylactic platelet transfusions. Transfus Med Rev 2002;16: 34–45.

58. Stanworth SJ, Dyer C, Choo L, et al. Do all patients with hematologic malignancies and severe thrombocytopenia need prophylactic platelet transfusions? Background, rationale, and design of a clinical trial (trial of platelet prophylaxis) to assess the effectiveness of prophylactic platelet transfusions. Transfus Med Rev 2010;24:163–71.

59. Woodman RC, Harker LA. Bleeding complications associated with cardiopulmonary bypass. Blood 1990;76:1680–97.

60. Stramer SL, Wend U, Candotti D, et al. Nucleic acid testing to detect HBV infection in blood donors. N Engl J Med 2011;364:236–47.

61. Perrotta PL, Snyder EL. Non-infectious complications of transfusion therapy. Blood Rev 2001;15:69–83.

62. Vassallo RR. Review: IgA anaphylactic transfusion reactions. Part I. Laboratory diagnosis, incidence, and supply of IgA-deficient products. Immunohematology 2004;20:226–33.

63. Shimada E, Tadokoro K, Watanabe Y, et al. Anaphylactic transfusion reactions in haptoglobin-deficient patients with IgE and IgG haptoglobin antibodies. Transfusion 2002;42:766–73.

64. Lambin P, Le Pennec PY, Hauptmann G, et al. Adverse transfusion reactions associated with a precipitating anti-C4 antibody of anti-Rodgers specificity. Vox Sang 1984;47:242–9.

65. Yazer MH, Podlosky L, Clarke G, et al. The effect of prestorage WBC reduction on the rates of febrile nonhemolytic transfusion reactions to platelet concentrates and RBC. Transfusion 2004;44:10–5.

66. Hillyer CD, Josephson CD, Blajchman MA, et al. Bacterial contamination of blood components: risks, strategies, and regulation: joint ASH and AABB educational session in transfusion medicine. Hematology Am Soc Hematol Educ Program 2003;575–89.

67. Heddle NM. Pathophysiology of febrile nonhemolytic transfusion reactions. Curr Opin Hematol 1999;6:420–6.

68. Heddle NM, Klama L, Singer J, et al. The role of the plasma from platelet concentrates in transfusion reactions. N Engl J Med 1994;331:625–8.

69. Riccardi D, Raspollini E, Rebulla P, et al. Relationship of the time of storage and transfusion reactions to platelet concentrates from buffy coats. Transfusion 1997;37:528–30.

70. Winqvist I. Meperidine (pethidine) to control shaking chills and fever associated with non-hemolytic transfusion reactions. Eur J Haematol 1991;47:154–5.

71. McCarthy LJ, Danielson CF, Miraglia C, et al. Platelet transfusion and thrombotic thrombocytopenic purpura. Transfusion 2003;43:829 [author reply: 829–30].

72. Harkness DR, Byrnes JJ, Lian EC, et al. Hazard of platelet transfusion in thrombotic thrombocytopenic purpura. JAMA 1981;246:1931–3.

73. Gordon LI, Kwaan HC, Rossi EC. Deleterious effects of platelet transfusions and recovery thrombocytosis in patients with thrombotic microangiopathy. Semin Hematol 1987;24:194–201.

74. de la Rubia J, Plume G, Arriaga F, et al. Platelet transfusion and thrombotic thrombocytopenic purpura. Transfusion 2002;42:1384–5.

75. Swisher KK, Terrell DR, Vesely SK, et al. Clinical outcomes after platelet transfusions in patients with thrombotic thrombocytopenic purpura. Transfusion 2009; 49:873–87.

76. Refaai MA, Chuang C, Menegus M, et al. Outcomes after platelet transfusion in patients with heparin-induced thrombocytopenia. J Thromb Haemost 2010;8: 1419–21.

77. Daly PA, Schiffer CA, Aisner J, et al. Platelet transfusion therapy. One-hour post-transfusion increments are valuable in predicting the need for HLA-matched preparations. JAMA 1980;243:435–8.

78. Rebulla P. A mini-review on platelet refractoriness. Haematologica 2005;90: 247–53.

79. Hod E, Schwartz J. Platelet transfusion refractoriness. Br J Haematol 2008;142: 348–60.

80. Doughty HA, Murphy MF, Metcalfe P, et al. Relative importance of immune and non-immune causes of platelet refractoriness. Vox Sang 1994;66:200–5.

81. Slichter SJ, Davis K, Enright H, et al. Factors affecting posttransfusion platelet increments, platelet refractoriness, and platelet transfusion intervals in thrombocytopenic patients. Blood 2005;105:4106–14.

82. Datema G, Stein S, Eijsink C, et al. HLA-C expression on platelets: studies with an HLA-Cw1-specific human monoclonal antibody. Vox Sang 2000;79:108–11.

83. Carr R, Hutton JL, Jenkins JA, et al. Transfusion of ABO-mismatched platelets leads to early platelet refractoriness. Br J Haematol 1990;75:408–13.

84. Detection of platelet-reactive antibodies in patients who are refractory to platelet transfusions, and the selection of compatible donors. Vox Sang 2003; 84:73–88.

85. Leukocyte reduction and ultraviolet B irradiation of platelets to prevent alloimmunization and refractoriness to platelet transfusions. The Trial to Reduce Alloimmunization to Platelets Study Group. N Engl J Med 1997;337:1861–9.

86. Pavenski K, Freedman J, Semple JW. HLA alloimmunization against platelet transfusions: pathophysiology, significance, prevention and management. Tissue Antigens 2012;79:237–45.

87. Seftel MD, Growe GH, Petraszko T, et al. Universal prestorage leukoreduction in Canada decreases platelet alloimmunization and refractoriness. Blood 2004; 103:333–9.

88. Asano H, Lee CY, Fox-Talbot K, et al. Treatment with riboflavin and ultraviolet light prevents alloimmunization to platelet transfusions and cardiac transplants. Transplantation 2007;84:1174–82.

89. Jackman RP, Heitman JW, Marschner S, et al. Understanding loss of donor white blood cell immunogenicity after pathogen reduction: mechanisms of action in ultraviolet illumination and riboflavin treatment. Transfusion 2009;49:2686–99.

90. Moroff G, George VM, Siegl AM, et al. The influence of irradiation on stored platelets. Transfusion 1986;26:453–6.

91. Duquesnoy RJ, Filip DJ, Rodey GE, et al. Successful transfusion of platelets "mismatched" for HLA antigens to alloimmunized thrombocytopenic patients. Am J Hematol 1977;2:219–26.

92. Bolgiano DC, Larson EB, Slichter SJ. A model to determine required pool size for HLA-typed community donor apheresis programs. Transfusion 1989;29: 306–10.

93. Grishaber JE, Birney SM, Strauss RG. Potential for transfusion-associated graft-versus-host disease due to apheresis platelets matched for HLA class I antigens. Transfusion 1993;33:910–4.

94. Duquesnoy RJ. HLAMatchmaker: a molecularly based algorithm for histocompatibility determination. I. Description of the algorithm. Hum Immunol 2002;63: 339–52.

95. Nambiar A, Duquesnoy RJ, Adams S, et al. HLAMatchmaker-driven analysis of responses to HLA-typed platelet transfusions in alloimmunized thrombocytopenic patients. Blood 2006;107:1680-7.
96. Kickler TS, Braine H, Ness PM. The predictive value of crossmatching platelet transfusion for alloimmunized patients. Transfusion 1985;25:385-9.
97. Sintnicolaas K, Lowenberg B. A flow cytometric platelet immunofluorescence crossmatch for predicting successful HLA matched platelet transfusions. Br J Haematol 1996;92:1005-10.
98. Gelb AB, Leavitt AD. Crossmatch-compatible platelets improve corrected count increments in patients who are refractory to randomly selected platelets. Transfusion 1997;37:624-30.
99. Petz LD, Garratty G, Calhoun L, et al. Selecting donors of platelets for refractory patients on the basis of HLA antibody specificity. Transfusion 2000;40:1446-56.
100. Levin MD, van der Holt B, de Veld JC, et al. The value of crossmatch tests and panel tests as a screening tool to predict the outcome of platelet transfusion in a non-selected haematological population of patients. Vox Sang 2004;87:291-8.
101. Josephson CD, Glynn SA, Kleinman SH, et al. A multidisciplinary "think tank": the top 10 clinical trial opportunities in transfusion medicine from the National Heart, Lung, and Blood Institute-sponsored 2009 state-of-the-science symposium. Transfusion 2011;51:828-41.
102. Blajchman MA. Substitutes and alternatives to platelet transfusions in thrombocytopenic patients. J Thromb Haemost 2003;1:1637-41.
103. Takayama N, Nishikii H, Usui J, et al. Generation of functional platelets from human embryonic stem cells in vitro via ES-sacs, VEGF-promoted structures that concentrate hematopoietic progenitors. Blood 2008;111:5298-306.

Index

Note: Page numbers of article titles are in **boldface** type.

Hematol Oncol Clin N Am 27 (2013) 645–655
http://dx.doi.org/10.1016/S0889-8588(13)00049-X
0889-8588/13/$ – see front matter © 2013 Elsevier Inc. All rights reserved.

hemonc.theclinics.com

O

Optical aggregometry, 419–420

P

Paris-Trousseau (Jacobsen) syndrome, 470–472
PF4/H complexes, and immune response in heparin-induced thrombocytopenia, 542
Phosphoinositide hydrolysis, role in platelet activation, 392
Platelet count ratio, 424
Platelet disorders, 381–643
    congenital thrombocytopenia, **465–494**
    drug-induced thrombocytopenia, **521–540**
    genetic dissection of platelet function in, **443–463**
    heparin-induced thrombocytopenia, **541–563**
    immune thrombocytopenia, **495–520**
    inherited membrane glycoprotein disorders, **613–627**
    inherited platelet function disorders, **585–611**
    platelet transfusion therapy, **629–643**
    thrombotic thrombocytopenic purpura and atypical hemolytic uremia syndrome,
        565–584
Platelet function, genetics of, in health and disease, **443–463**
    clinical analyses, 450–453
        nonplatelet microRNA studies of thrombotic risk, 451–452
        platelet microRNA studies in human diseases, 451
        platelet proteomics and cancer, 453
        platelet transcriptomics in essential thrombocythemia, 450
        proteomic applications in thrombosis, 452–453
    clinical features, 444–445
        genetic risk factors for cerebrovascular/cardiovascular diseases, 445
        genetics of functional platelet responses, 445–445
    etiology and pathogenesis, 445
        platelet molecular machinery, 445
    laboratory features of, 445–450
        platelet microRNA transcriptomic studies, 447–448
        platelet proteomic studies, 448–450
        transcriptomic analyses focusing on platelet mRNAs, 447
    relevance of, 443–444
    therapeutics and prognosis, 453–457
        biomarkers identification and phenotypic prediction, 453–455
        microRNAs as biomarkers, 455
        protein target identification using integrated platforms, 455–457
    inherited disorders of, **585–611**
    associated with transcription factor deficiencies, 600–601
    diagnosis of, 602–603
    disorders of platelet granules, 589–593
    disorders of platelet procoagulant activity, 599–600
    disorders of secretion caused by defects in platelet signaling, 593–599
    miscellaneous associated disorders, 601
    others, 600
    overview, 587–589

Moving?

Make sure your subscription moves with you!

To notify us of your new address, find your **Clinics Account Number** (located on your mailing label above your name), and contact customer service at:

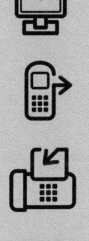

Email: journalscustomerservice-usa@elsevier.com

800-654-2452 (subscribers in the U.S. & Canada)
314-447-8871 (subscribers outside of the U.S. & Canada)

Fax number: 314-447-8029

Elsevier Health Sciences Division
Subscription Customer Service
3251 Riverport Lane
Maryland Heights, MO 63043

*To ensure uninterrupted delivery of your subscription, please notify us at least 4 weeks in advance of move.

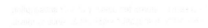

Printed and bound by CPI Group (UK) Ltd, Croydon, CR0 4YY

03/10/2024

01040440-0012